Doctor to Doctor

Classic Teachings of William A. Ellis, D.O. Pioneer Health Physician

Robert H. Strickland, MS, Editor

Doctor to Doctor

The Classic Teachings of

William A. Ellis, D.O.

Pioneer Health Physician

Compiled and Edited by

Robert H. Strickland, M.S.

Illustrated by: Robert H. Strickland and W. Sue Strickland

Published by:

Robert H Strickland Associates LLC
P. O. Box 1388
Everett, Washington 98206-1388 USA
Phone/Fax: 425-258-6796

Library of Congress Control Number: 2016908975

Strickland, Robert H. 1944

Doctor to Doctor / by Robert H. Strickland

p. 438 cm.

Includes index.

ISBN 978-0-9635919-6-8

Disclaimers

The concepts, techniques, and opinions expressed in this book are strictly those of the late William A. Ellis, D.O. **The Editor is not a licensed health professional and offers no advice whatsoever regarding the treatment of any disease condition. This book is a historical document containing accurately transcripted material from Dr. Ellis' lectures, unaugmented personal notes, and recollections of conversations with Dr. Ellis during the period 1977-1985.** Nothing in the Editor's narrative is to be construed as an endorsement by the Editor of Dr. Ellis' opinions.

The Editor's notes dispersed throughout this book serve only to introduce Dr. Ellis, orient the reader regarding his career, and point to modern resources that may relate to Dr. Ellis' opinions. **The notes are not to be taken as an endorsement of any resource referred to by the Editor.** Many of these resources are accessible through internet links. However, because of the volatility of the internet and its service providers, there is no assurance that any link will remain operational.

This book is intended for licensed health practitioners only, who are required by law to use their own experience and judgement while serving individuals under their care. Use of this book by unlicensed persons for self-management of health problems or for providing service to other individuals is not authorized, and any attempt to do so is strongly disapproved and cautioned against.

For suspected medical problems, one should seek licensed professional care, heed sound medical advice, and participate in recommended treatment. In addition, anyone beginning a fitness or nutrition program should first consult a reputable, licensed health care provider for clearance and probable supervision.

Therefore, the estate of William A. Ellis, D.O., the Editor, the publisher, and the listed vendors, along with their associates, relatives, and heirs disclaim any responsibility and liability in connection with any actions taken or not taken based on the content of this book.

Contents

Dedications

William A. Ellis, D.O.

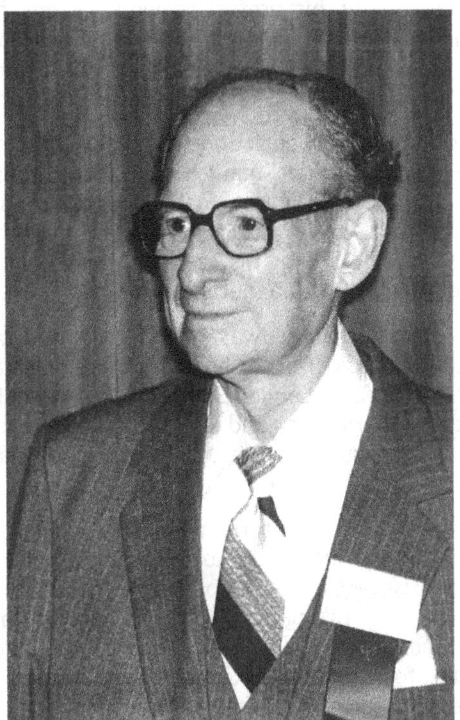

Editor: Naturally, 30 years after his passing, Dr. Ellis is not among us to provide a dedication for this book. Therefore, I provide one for him, below, from memories of our many personal conversations and first-hand knowledge of events. A few thanks are sprinkled throughout.

Dr. Ellis expressed great affection and admiration for the many people that passed through and significantly affected his life, and he was quick to praise others. Many of these are described below, and their mention constitutes a dedication. Omission from this dedication in no way minimizes anyone's contribution to Dr. Ellis' life and career.

Very influential in his life was his father, engineer/inventor Humphrey A. Ellis, a stern parent who demanded that his son display a high degree of discipline. He encouraged his son's natural curiosity and analytical mind. It was his father that inspired Dr. Ellis to start thinking about the human body as a system of levers and pulleys and the role that alignment plays in efficiency of movement.

Although he held his wife and five children in high esteem, Dr. Ellis was also a stern head of the household. Often, patients would come to his home to be treated after hours, a duty that he would accept without question, even though it was an imposition on the family. Dr. Ellis believed that he was a doctor 24 hours a day, seven days a week; and this left no time for nurturing a family. Eventually, his profession won out and he went out on his own. Although seemingly satisfied with this choice, he often mentioned that he regretted his family having to endure more than they should have. He did express that he was fortunate to have their continued love and support, which he never doubted.

Dr. Ellis enjoyed working for the Musebeck Shoe Company after his osteopathic residency, because the job made it possible for him to travel the country, treat thousands of customers, meet other professionals with which he could share information, and build knowledge and confidence for the long career to come. He particularly admired Ransom Dinges, D.O. (pronounced "din-jess") for his teaching ability and for his collaboration in identifying blood tests relating to protein metabolism.

Also, Dr. Ellis said many times that he was thankful for the personal and professional friendships he made with hundreds of other health professionals around the world. Among these were Virginia Livingston, M.D., Lendon Smith, M.D., Linda Clark; Robert Atkins, M.D., Dale Alexander, Beatrice Trum Hunter; and countless others, as well as the 300 or so practitioners worldwide that enlisted Dr. Ellis to help with their patients in the last years of his career.

Additionally, Dr. Ellis enjoyed the long-term friendship of Dolly Ware, of Ware Funeral Homes, who was responsible for bringing him to the Dallas-Fort Worth area to work, and Dr. Lois Allen, a research scientist at the Texas College of Osteopathic Medicine. These ladies rendered assistance one evening, taking Dr. Ellis to the hospital following a serious medical emergency. Also, he was indebted to Josephine Karbach, R.N. and wife of Armin Karbach, D.O., of Arlington, Texas, for providing excellent care for Dr. Ellis during the rigorous radiation treatment schedule that characterized his valiant fight with lymphatic cancer.

In that regard, it must be said that Dr. Ellis' son, Brad, took up the challenge of taking care of his father, accompanying him on trips to clinics and hospitals as far away as Mexico, acquiring medication on a regular basis. During these trips, they were able to resolve misunderstandings and build the type of relationship that they had both wanted and needed. Dr. Ellis said that he had always been very proud of Brad, and that Brad's impressive role in the last part of his father's life and the tender, loving care rendered by Brad's wife, Owanna, was greatly appreciated. She loved Dr. Ellis deeply, providing daily attention and healthy meals during his last days at their home in California.

Robert H. "Bob" Strickland, M.S.

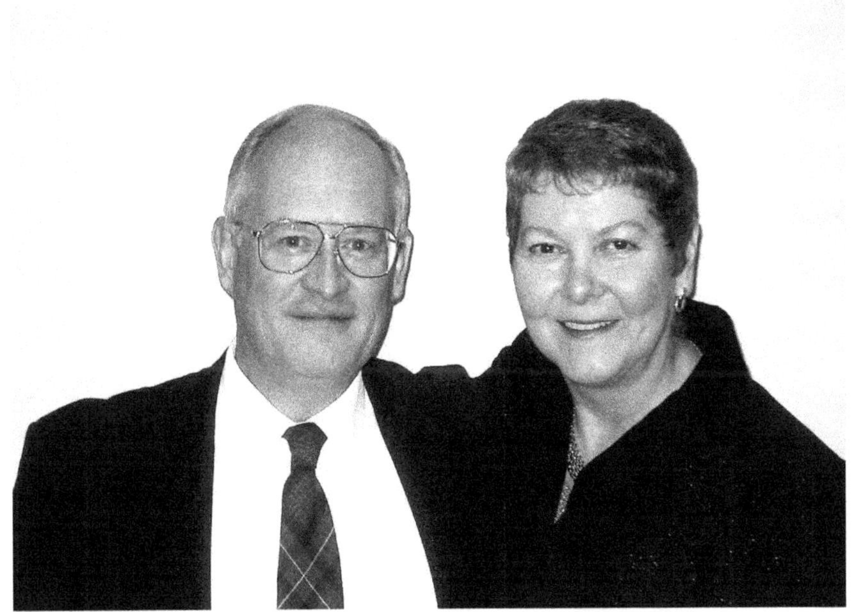

I dedicate this book to the following:

My wife, Sue, who loved Dr. Ellis as much as I did, but who let me finish his book in my own time. Dr. Ellis and I began collaborating on the book in 1984; this was right before he began a struggle with a fatal illness. When he passed away, the wind went out of my sails, so to speak, and the project languished for an unbelievable 30 years. Sue never admonished me for putting off the project, and I have always had her love and support, regardless of the delay.

Pioneers of the health and physical culture movement, such as Dr. John Harvey Kellogg (1852-1943), Bernarr Macfadden (1868-1955), Gayelord Hauser (1895-1984), and Paul Bragg (1895-1976), who, even though holding some mistaken beliefs and misguiding a few followers, weathered criticism to put health issues before the people, who have every right to evaluate them. My favorite among these pioneers is Jack LaLanne (1914-2011), who made me, a 10-year old, aware of the benefits of proper diet and exercise through his television program of the early 1950's. Over the years, Jack got it right!

The great number of health physicians and other health care professionals – M.D., D.O., D.C., D.D.S., R.N., N.D., D.V.M., nutritionists, trainers, etc. – that I have known over the years. I respect these people greatly for their choices of professions and for risking their careers to benefit the people under their care. May they be able to overcome any unjustifiable restrictions placed on them to achieve what is necessary for their patients.

Acknowledgements

Robert H. "Bob" Strickland

I acknowledge the support, sensitive proofreading, and suggestions of my wife, Sue – the former W. Sue Gentry from Albany, Missouri. She has the sharpness of eye, the broadbased knowledge of many disciplines, the consistency, and the desire necessary to do an amazing job. Any author or publisher would do well to have this level of excellence available.

I had known Dr. Ellis for about four years before I met Sue, and Dr. Ellis was the only objective person I trusted to see if she would meet my exacting requirements for a life partner. He gave her a strong endorsement after their first meeting – a two-hour private conversation. That was good enough for me, and, as of the publication date of this book, Sue and I will have been married for over 30 years. Sue has a marvelous perspective on the man and has reminisced with me about our times with him. Without each other, this project would never have been completed.

Those That Helped Me Along the Way

Thanks to the following people who helped me gain an appreciation of the disciplines described in this book.

To Brad Ellis, for his patience and for allowing me to retain a mountain of Dr. Ellis' personal correspondence and reference materials. Without my access to this collection, it would be difficult to impossible for Dr. Ellis' work to be made available to new generations of health professionals.

To Joe Oneal and the late Stan Bynum of Nutri-Dyn (now Progressive) for hiring me as an inside technical representative in 1978. It was a huge challenge to gear up to a different way of thinking about maintaining one's health. It was there I met Dr. Ellis, beginning a 10-year friendship that I might never have had the privilege of enjoying without having answered a small Nutri-Dyn ad in the Dallas Morning News.

To the late Frank DeLuca of Biotics Research Corporation, who hired me in the same capacity for his company. It was a close business relationship with Dr. Ellis that allowed me almost daily contact with him on a professional basis. This constant interaction provided me a completely new way of understanding the body and the techniques of maintaining it, and it bestowed upon me the responsibility of sharing what I have learned whenever and wherever necessary.

To my dear friend and co-worker during the Nutri-Dyn and Biotics years, Iola Murray, for attending to the dozens of administrative and clerical duties while I was developing materials for Biotics, learning from Dr. Ellis, helping the outside sales force, and fielding the many calls that occurred throughout the day. Her talent and dedication puts her among the very best.

To Lew Hulvey, D.C. of Judsonia, Arkansas, for 37 years of friendship, support, and advice from his personal standpoint; it is remarkable how congruent his beliefs about health are with those of Dr. Ellis.

To Denis DeLuca, Bill Sparks, and the rest of the folks at Biotics Research Corporation for an ongoing personal and professional friendship spanning more than 35 years. Their products are thoughtfully formulated, manufactured under highly sanitary conditions, and of consistently high quality. Their products make sense from a scientific standpoint and continue to be at the core of my and my wife's supplement regimen, which we both hope to enjoy into a very productive old age.

Those Who Provided Direction and Materials

Thanks to the following who made their own significant contributions to the book.

Alan Cantwell, M.D.
Aries Rising Press
PO Box 29532
Los Angeles, CA 90029
(www.ariesrisingpress.com)
Email: alancantwell@sbcglobal.net.

Lynn Donches, Chief Librarian
Rodale Library
400 South Tenth Street
Emmaus, PA 18098-0099
Phone: 610-967-8729

Owanna Ellis for providing a picture of William A. Ellis, D.O. ("Bampi" to his family)
Picture courtesy of the Consumer Health Organization of Canada, taken on Friday, March 30, 1985 at the Total Health '85 Convention in Toronto, the last convention that Dr. Ellis attended.

Helen Faria, Admin
Former Managing Editor, *Medical Sentinel*
http://www.haciendapub.com/medicalsentinel
The official, peer-review journal of the Association of American Physicians and Surgeons (AAPS). The *Medical Sentinel* is committed to publishing scholarly articles in defense of the practice of private medicine, the tenets and principles set forth in the Oath of Hippocrates, individually-based medical ethics, and the sanctity of the patient-doctor relationship.

David Forgie, D.C., and Grant Bjornson, D.C. for providing a very important transcript of Dr. Ellis' lecture and demonstration for the Alpha Chi Beta group at Canadian Memorial Chiropractic College, Toronto, Ontario, Canada, December 2-4, 1977.

Dr. Forgie: http://www.rothesaychiropractic.ca
Dr.Bjornson: http://www.canpages.ca/website/business/210701?website=http%3A%2F%2Fbobcaygeonchiropractic.ca%2F

David H. Freedman
c/o Atlantic Media Company
600 New Hampshire Ave., NW
Washington, DC 20037

Oneta Hansen for providing a picture and history of her father, Ransom Dinges, D.O.

Debra Loguda-Summers, Curator/Special Projects
Museum of Osteopathic Medicine, SM
and International Center for Osteopathic History
800 West Jefferson
Kirksville, MO 63501
Toll Free: 1 866 626 ATSU Ext. 2359

Wes Miller
Foot-So-Port Shoe Company (formerly Musebeck and Health Spot companies)
Oconomowoc Business Center
405 E. Forest Street
Oconomowoc, WI 53066

Robyn Oro, Cataloging Assistant
D'Angelo Library
Kansas City University of Medicine and Biosciences
1750 Independence, MO 64106-1453
Phone: 816-654-7267

Steve Zoltai, Collections Librarian & Archivist
CMCC Health Sciences Library
Canadian Memorial Chiropractic College
6100 Leslie Street
Toronto, ON M2H 3J1
(416) 482-2340 x206

Pixabay
Braxmeier & Steinberger GbR (VAT Reg.No.: DE297456622),
Hans Braxmeier, Donaustraße 13, 89231 Neu-Ulm, Germany
Phone: +49 (0)731 / 800 1660
info(at)pixabay.com (https://pixabay.com/)

Foreword

As the years pass, fewer people that knew William A. "Dr. Bill" Ellis, D.O. (February 25, 1906-September 16, 1986) remain among us. The patients, colleagues, and lay persons that are alive have probably not forgotten him, and most of them, I assume, have fond memories.

Editor: Except for the chapters containing information solely for the use of licensed health professionals, there is a companion book for prospective and current patients; it is titled *Doctor to Patient*. Its purpose is to educate readers so that they are better informed about what a health practitioner using *Doctor to Doctor* is attempting to achieve. It also serves as a standalone resource for other health advocates. Copies of both books are available from the same sources.

Dr. Ellis was born in New Jersey, the son of an inventor, Humphrey Ellis. He graduated from Philadelphia Osteopathic College in 1931 and spent the next 50-odd years making people more healthy. He was a large man – 6'2" tall, with a personality bigger than life – an extrovert in a bow tie, with a beaming smile and warm (size 16) handshake. The intelligent understood his opinionated manner; catching on right away that Dr. Ellis was dedicated to health, deeply studied, widely traveled, and intensely interested in helping others. The ignorant might have branded him as arrogant, but nothing could have been further from the truth. What he had was confidence, and rightly so. Dr. Ellis excelled at many endeavors. He was skilled in many sports, and one may have branded him a jock in college.

WILLIAM A. ELLIS

Phi Sigma Gamma; Basketball, 1, 2, 3, 4; Baseball, 1, 2, 3, 4; Golf, 2, 3, 4; Bowling, 2, 3, 4; Tennis, 2; Interclass Swimming, 1, 2; Athletic Editor, *Synapsis*, 3; Athletic Editor, *Axone*, 2; Business Manager, *Axone*, 3, 4; Neo Honorary Society.

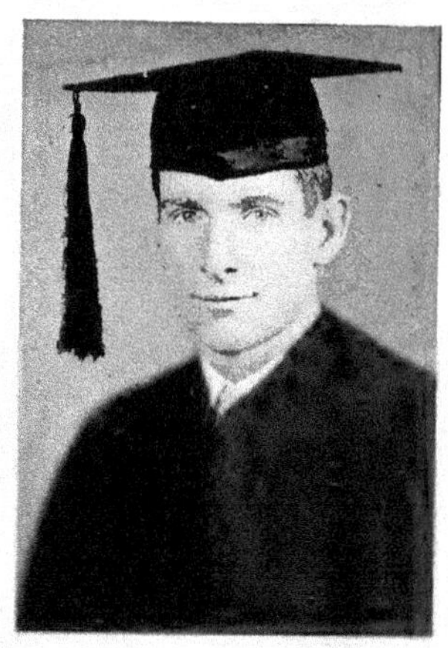

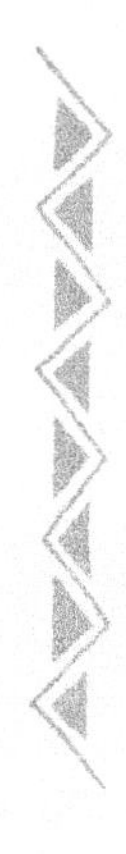

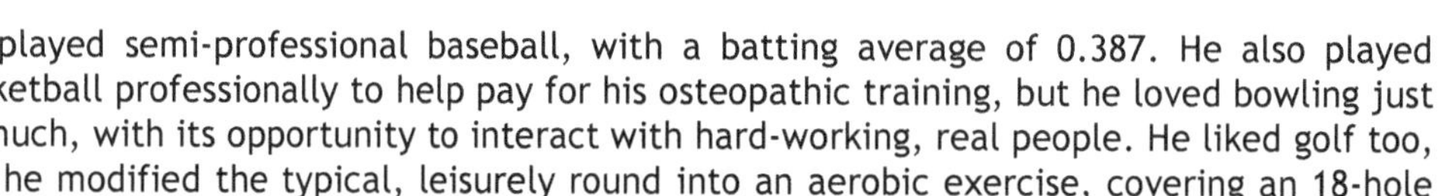

He played semi-professional baseball, with a batting average of 0.387. He also played basketball professionally to help pay for his osteopathic training, but he loved bowling just as much, with its opportunity to interact with hard-working, real people. He liked golf too, but he modified the typical, leisurely round into an aerobic exercise, covering an 18-hole course in roughly 2/3 of the usual time!

Dr. Ellis had pretty rigid social and religious beliefs, shaped by a stern upbringing, but he would listen to, reflect upon, and even incorporate others' ideas, if they were plausible. He had no use for phonies, shysters, or even closed-minded people – especially when it concerned health issues or nutritional products. In his personal notes, Dr. Ellis wrote that he had studied the makeup of the National Science Board, the policy-making body for the National Science Foundation, for the period from 1957 to 1973. He found that, of the 78 scientists officially listed as "academic", 62 were on the payroll of large corporations.

Dr. Ellis was just as outspoken and critical about individuals and companies misrepresenting their products and treatments. I remember one instance when Dr. Ellis warned the president of a nutritional supplement company that he would throw him out of his hotel room. This was in response to the individual attempting to tell Dr. Ellis what to say during his upcoming lecture sponsored by the very same company! At 72 years old, Dr. Ellis was robust enough to accomplish it, and he lectured without restrictions.

What was Dr. Ellis About?

Dr. Ellis was a family practitioner and surgeon; he delivered hundreds of newborns, and he was an expert in foot and postural disorders. His favorite activity, however, was working with patients to restore good health. In pursuit of this goal, he read scholarly journals, studied anecdotal information, attended all types of medical and health-related conferences and trade shows, and tested various modalities in his own practice. To determine what disease condition was present, like any skilled physician or other health practitioner, Dr. Ellis would begin with a clinical diagnosis, assessing a patient's symptoms. This assessment, along with a review of the patient's medical history, a physical examination, and various tests, would enable him to make a medical diagnosis.

His goal was always to eliminate pathology and restore a patient's anatomy and physiology to homeostasis. He constantly refined his concept of normal, and he used various modalities to normalize patients' test results. His treatments involved osteopathic manipulations, adjustment of the diet, internal cleansing procedures, and nutrient supplementation. He considered a proper diet to be the most important consideration, with careful attention being paid to the individual's ability to digest and assimilate dietary protein. In shaping his beliefs, four individuals figure prominently in Dr. Ellis' professional life, and they are discussed below.

Weston A. Price, D.D.S.

Dr. Ellis suffered a physical breakdown himself in 1936 and began a serious study of nutrition, if for no other reason than to find solutions to his own problem. Soon thereafter, he became a proponent of the beliefs of Dr. Weston A. Price, D.D.S. (1870-1948). After 1930, Dr. Price devoted most of his study to nutrition, studying carefully the diets of various cultures around the world. In 1939, he published *Nutrition and Physical Degeneration*, in which he concluded that the Western diet, including flour, sugar, and processed vegetable fats were the major cause of of nutritional deficiencies, leading to dental disease. This book was valuable to Dr. Ellis.

Francis M. Pottenger, Jr., M.D.

Francis M. Pottenger, Jr., M.D. (1901-1967) was also a proponent of Dr. Price, and he operated the Pottenger Sanatorium, which his father had founded for treatment of tuberculosis in Monrovia, California. Dr. Pottenger provided liver, butter, cream, and eggs to convalescing patients, and he gave adrenal cortex supplements to treat exhaustion. His meat and milk studies with cats are often quoted.

Pottenger's meat study resolved that the animals fed an all-raw diet of 2/3 meat, 1/3 raw milk, and cod liver oil remained healthy, while those on a diet of 2/3 cooked meat, 1/3 milk, and cod liver oil developed health problems which were passed on to subsequent generations of progeny. Problems with parasites, skin diseases, and allergies increased from 5% to 90% in the third generation of deficient cats. Their bones became soft, as well. Later, it was shown that supplementing the deficient diets with the essential amino acid taurine could offset the detrimental effects, presumably through augmentation of protein synthesis.

Pottenger's milk study cats were fed 1/3 raw meat and 2/3 milk. What was varied was the way the milk was processed. Cats given raw milk were healthier than those given pasteurized, evaporated, sweetened condensed, or raw metabolized vitamin D milk.

Melvin Page, D.D.S.

Melvin E. Page, D.D.S. (1894-1983) was also a proponent of the teachings of Weston A. Price, D.D.S. He was the son of a physician. After one year in college, Dr. Page quit school to teach school in rural Montana. After two years, he decided to return to the University of Michigan where he obtained a Doctorate of Dental Surgery degree. In 1919, He began a successful dental practice in Muskegon, Michigan, inventing dentures based on sound engineering principles that minimized bone loss.

His research into bone loss led him to Dr. Weston Price's work with primitive people, and he started his investigations at Mercy Hospital and Hackley Hospital in Muskegon. He ran more than two thousand blood chemistries and discovered that no absorption of bone (and no cavities) occurred when the calcium to phosphorus ratio were in a proportion of 10 to 4 in the blood (2.5:1). The Department of Dental Research of the United States Air Force confirmed his findings of the calcium/phosphorus ratio to be correct 42 years later. Dr. Page also found, according to test readings, that the blood sugar level should be at 85, plus or minus 5 (Sclavo test).

In 1940, Dr. Page resettled in St. Petersburg, Florida, remaining there until his death. At the age of 84, he still walked a mile to and from his office almost daily. He believed that body chemistry, when properly balanced by proper nutrition and other factors, will not only prevent dental problems but will naturally affect the rest of the body as well. His treatment philosophy was simple and logical, as follows.

- The harmful effects of the use of white sugar and refined carbohydrates can't be ignored.
- The harmful effects of using chemical additives and other food preservatives for the sake of shelf life upsets body chemistry.
- Using whole food vitamin concentrates, minerals and digestive enzymes to supplement daily food intake might be necessary.
- Milk is not the perfect food for everyone.

Dr. Page used small doses of endocrine extracts to balance the body chemistry. When patients were in his facility, he was able to check and recheck the blood chemistry, especially the calcium/phosphorus (Ca/P) ratio, every three to four days. His Page Food Plan was developed during this time because he noticed that certain foods upset body chemistry more than others. Dr. Ellis worked and studied with Dr. Page during breaks from his practice.

In the early 1960s Dr. Page found himself and his method of practice under scrutiny from the federal government when he was indicted for practicing outside his scope of practice. After a lengthy trial in which Dr. Page introduced over 3,600 case studies and was able to substantiate his findings with over 40,000 blood tests as well as 35 years of research, a federal judge found him not guilty. The judge went on to reprimand the American Medical

Association (AMA) and the Food and Drug Administration (FDA) for not trying to figure out what he was doing rather than harassing him.

In 1972, Dr. Page was invited to present his work at the World Congress of the Federacion Dentaire International in Mexico City. For over 40 years, his work has been a source internationally for many scientists, dentists, physicians and writers interested in the field of nutrition and health. At the University of Pennsylvania School of Dental Medicine Centennial celebration, a department wing was named the "Melvin E. Page, D.D.S. Oral Medicine Diagnostic Laboratory," recognition by his peers for his nutritional work.

Note: See the article about Dr.Page at http://ifnh.org/product-category/educational-materials/pioneers-of-nutrition/dr-melvin-e-page/.

Royal Lee, D.D.S.

Royal Lee, D.D.S. (1895-1967) had an interest in nutrition from youth. In his senior year of dental school, he presented The Systemic Causes of Dental Caries, written when he was 16 years old and explaining the relationship among tooth decay, vitamin deficiency, and the endocrine glands. Although a practicing dentist, he was an inventor with several patents in his name, including a speed governor for electric motors.

In 1929, Dr. Lee introduced a natural food-based supplement in the "most potent and bioavailable form", which he named Catalyn. It was derived from defatted wheat germ, carrots, nutritional yeast, bovine adrenal, liver, spleen, and kidney, dried pea (vine) juice, dried alfalfa juice, mushroom, oat flour, soy bean lecithin, and rice bran extract. The demand was great enough to necessitate creation of a new company, the Vitamin Products Company, later called Standard Process. Dr. Ellis used Standard Process products extensively in his own practice.

In time, Dr. Lee introduced other nutritional tools for practitioners to use in treating their patients, such as Phosfood Liquid in 1931, for support of calcium metabolism and sympathetic nervous system function. By 1934 the demand by physicians convinced Dr. Lee to separate the various vitamin complexes into separate products (vitamins A through G) for more precise clinical application. From 1935 through 1939 he introduced five new products: Drenamin (adrenal support), organic minerals (parasympathetic support), soy bean lecithin, lactic acid yeast (proper pH for healthy functioning of the gastrointestinal system), and wheat germ oil perles (one of the richest sources of natural vitamin E complex).

The 1940s saw a wide variety of specific nutritional products added to the Vitamin Products Company line. In the 1950s, Dr. Lee developed a type of glandular product, that he termed protomorphogen extracts, produced by a process he patented. These were not simply desiccated glandulars but "uniquely-derived nucleoprotein-mineral extracts."

In 1941, Dr. Lee organized the Lee Foundation for Nutritional Research to engage in research and coordinate and communicate nutritional breakthroughs from laboratories around the world. The Foundation was the world's largest clearinghouse for nutritional information for doctors, agriculturists, and homemakers. During its existence the Lee

Foundation disseminated millions of pieces of literature and hundreds of thousands of books on health and nutrition. In 1947 he coauthored a book with William Hanson entitled *Protomorphology, Study of Cell Autoregulation*, a study of biological growth factors and a survey of the problems of aging. The Standard Process company continues to offer these products to health care professionals.

Note: See the article about Dr. Lee written by David L. Morris, B.S., D.C. at http://www.westonaprice.org/health-topics/royal-lee-dds-father-of-natural-vitamins/.

Clinical Research Groups

Dr. Ellis often used the phrases "our research" and "our opinion" in his lectures. What he meant by these references is that he was part of one or more large groups that included physicians, nurses, dentists, nutritionists, academic researchers, physicists, chemical engineers, chemists, public health officials, and allied health professionals. He was a member of the Jarvis Group, established and maintained in the 1930s and 1940s by D. C. Jarvis, M.D. Membership included many other licensed practitioners.

Members of such groups routinely shared information with each other via letter and telephone, as well as during conventions, trade shows, workshops, and seminars. Many were authors of books. The constant ebb and flow of information was scrutinized by numbers of people with critical minds who had a common purpose: to elevate the state of health of all individuals. Therefore, the information was freely exchanged; there was no secrecy. Being a member and president (1955) of the American College of Osteopathy, Dr. Ellis was aware of the value of all types of research in the furtherance of his chosen profession and looked forward to new developments with great enthusiasm.

How did a patient fare on a new treatment? Were there any unexpected results? Did the patient die? What would you suggest for treating a particular disease? Certainly, some far out ideas were expressed within these study groups, but their lack of success usually became apparent, or the ideas were not taken favorably by the group. The point is that well-educated health professionals were evaluating burgeoning notions all of the time. Was it scientific research? No; much of it did not adhere to the tenants of experimental design. Were the conclusions useful in clinical practice? Yes, especially In the absence of "reliable evidence-based results" from the study of specific nutrition-based methodologies.

Naturally, this visibility made all participants vulnerable to the Gestapo tactics of the Food and Drug Administration and state medical boards. Were some disreputable persons within these groups for their own gain? Probably; and these individuals should have been and often were stopped in their tracks by their peers. However, the harassment of honest, well-meaning practitioners continued for a very long time, with many practitioners losing their licenses. Some relief came in the form of legislation introduced in Congress by Senator William Proxmire in the 1970s.

As we shall see in the following sections, there are medical researchers and science journalists that doubt the reliability of much evidence-based research results, as published in many scholarly journals. Their reasons will be apparent from the excerpts that have been selected, and the reader may find the entire articles at the links or in the journals indicated.

The Later Years

When Dr. Ellis retired in 1972, he sold his practice in Tarentum, Pennsylvania and moved to the Dallas/Fort Worth area to begin consulting on laboratory tests to licensed health practitioners. During this period, he was a personal consultant to over 300 physicians worldwide, and he lectured extensively at various health conferences, trade shows, and smaller, regional events, in the United States, Canada, and some foreign countries. He did not apply for a license in Texas or any other state, confining his work with patients to only those of other, licensed professionals.

Neutralization of Health Doctors (Dr. Ellis)

Over the years, there have many cases in which authorities have pursued and ruined the careers of health doctors, many of which were honest, caring, and capable. I have known many of them personally. The court says, "Wait another 60 days." Then, after that time period, the court says, "We're not ready, wait another 60 days." Every time they do that, it costs you another $1,000 in lawyer's fees, and finally you run out of money! So then you sign their edict, and it stops you from using the modality in question any longer.

Some doctors are not going that way; they are paying their lawyers one set fee regardless of how long it takes. This is the way to do it, and you can do this until the matter is resolved, then you have something to go to court with and do some fighting. This is the only way it can be done. They've proven their innocence very conclusively, like the last trial out in San Diego on B17, or Amygdalin or Laetrile, what ever you want to call it; the authorities took these people into court for smuggling because they were advocating its use. But no one had ever been picked up at the border for smuggling. But the authorities went in and raided them, tore their offices apart, and arrested them for using it.

Two California M.D.s – John Richardson and James Privitera – had their licenses taken away from them; the other three accused were lay people; one was an attorney, Richard K. Stacer, who represents the Cancer Federation Inc. When this came into court, the three appellate judges who, acting as the jury, realized what a hot issue this was, brought in all of the judges of the Appellate courts. They threw out all of the charges and then reprimanded the state prosecutors for starting it, because they didn't have any evidence to prove what they were talking about even as far as B17 was concerned. The court also reprimanded the California Health Association for the illegal laws on their books and for the lack of making necessary changes in them.

Editor: The case is described in the *Cancer Defeated Newsletter #151*, at http://www.cancerdefeated.com/newsletters/Laetrile-How-Much-Proof-Do-They-Need.html.

In 1979, the state of California appealed the reversal and reinstated the conviction in a five to two vote, with the Chief Justice and one other Justice voting in the minority. They tried to stop people like Dr. Alan Nittler, M.D., who used very few drugs and medicines but specialized in vitamins and minerals and lost his license. It's still under appeal (as of 1982), yet he cannot practice while it's under appeal in the state of California, according to the way their courts are set up out there. Here's a great guy, but the only objection I have is that he uses 400-800 pills/day for his patients and I can't believe anyone can digest and assimilate than many pills.

There is also Don Kelly, a dentist in Grapevine, Texas who lost his license because he didn't examine people's mouths. He just told patients what was wrong and went ahead and treated them. Now he's a nutritionist in Whittier, Washington, with a practice four times bigger than the one in Texas. All you have to be is a nutritionist; you don't need a license if you want to do something about it.

Evidence-based Research

In their article in the *British Medical Journal* entitled, *Evidence-based medicine: what it is and what it isn't* (BMJ 1996;312:71), doctors David L Sackett, William M C Rosenberg, J A Muir Gray, R Brian Haynes, and W Scott Richardson attempt to clarify the role of evidence-based research (external clinical evidence) in a clinicians practice. Some direct quotes from that article are given below. You may find the entire article on the Internet at http://dx.doi.org/10.1136/bmj.312.7023.71.

"It's about integrating individual clinical expertise and the best external evidence....

Evidence-based medicine is the conscientious, explicit, and judicious use of current best evidence in making decisions about the care of individual patients. **The practice of evidence-based medicine means integrating individual clinical expertise with the best available external clinical evidence from systematic research.** By individual clinical expertise we mean the proficiency and judgment that individual clinicians acquire through clinical experience and clinical practice....

Good doctors use both individual clinical expertise and the best available external evidence, and neither alone is enough. Without clinical expertise, practice risks becoming tyrannized by evidence, for even excellent external evidence may be inapplicable to or inappropriate for an individual patient. Without current best evidence, practice risks becoming rapidly out of date, to the detriment of patients....

Evidence-based medicine is not cookbook medicine. Because it requires a bottom up approach that integrates the best external evidence with individual clinical expertise and patients' choice, it cannot result in slavish, cookbook approaches to individual patient care. External clinical evidence can inform, but can never replace, individual clinical expertise, and it is this expertise that decides whether the external evidence applies to the individual patient at all and, if so, how it should be integrated into a clinical decision. Similarly, any external guideline must be integrated with individual clinical expertise in deciding whether and how it matches the patient's clinical state, predicament, and preferences, and thus whether it should be applied."

David H. Freedman has been an *Atlantic Magazine* contributor since 1998. In his October 4, 2010 article, published in the November 2010 issue, *Lies, Damned Lies, and Medical Science*, he states, "Much of what medical researchers conclude in their studies

is misleading, exaggerated, or flat-out wrong. Though the results of drug studies often make newspaper headlines, you have to wonder whether they prove anything at all. Indeed, given the breadth of the potential problems raised at [a meeting I attended at the University of Ioannina, Greece medical school's teaching hospital], can any medical-research studies be trusted? So why are doctors — to a striking extent — still drawing upon misinformation in their everyday practice?" **Here are some more quotations from that article.**

"Dr. John Ioannidis, who has spent his career challenging his peers by exposing their bad science....[is] what's known as a meta-researcher, and he's become one of the world's foremost experts on the credibility of medical research. He and his team have shown, again and again, and in many different ways, that much of what biomedical researchers conclude in published studies — conclusions that doctors keep in mind when they prescribe antibiotics or blood-pressure medication, or when they advise us to consume more fiber or less meat, or when they recommend surgery for heart disease or back pain — is misleading, exaggerated, and often flat-out wrong.

He charges that as much as 90% of the published medical information that doctors rely on is flawed. His work has been widely accepted by the medical community; it has been published in the field's top journals, where it is heavily cited; and he is a big draw at conferences. Given this exposure, and the fact that his work broadly targets everyone else's work in medicine, as well as everything that physicians do and all the health advice we get, Ioannidis may be one of the most influential scientists alive. Yet for all his influence, he worries that the field of medical research is so pervasively flawed, and so riddled with conflicts of interest, that it might be chronically resistant to change — or even to publicly admitting that there's a problem....And sure enough, he goes on to suggest that an obsession with winning funding has gone a long way toward weakening the reliability of medical research.

He first stumbled on the sorts of problems plaguing the field, he explains, as a young physician-researcher in the early 1990s at Harvard....A new "evidence-based medicine" movement was just starting to gather force, and Ioannidis decided to throw himself into it, working first with prominent researchers at Tufts University and then taking positions at Johns Hopkins University and the National Institutes of Health. He was unusually well armed: he had been a math prodigy of near-celebrity status in high school in Greece, and had followed his parents, who were both physician-researchers, into medicine. Now he'd have a chance to combine math and medicine by applying rigorous statistical analysis to what seemed a surprisingly sloppy field. "I assumed that everything we physicians did was basically right, but now I was going to help verify it," he says. "All we'd have to do was systematically review the evidence, trust what it told us, and then everything would be perfect."

It didn't turn out that way. In poring over medical journals, he was struck by how many findings of all types were refuted by later findings. Of course, medical-science "never minds" are hardly secret. And they sometimes make headlines, as when in recent years large studies or growing consensuses of researchers concluded that mammograms, colonoscopies, and PSA tests are far less useful cancer-detection tools than we had been told; or when widely prescribed antidepressants such as Prozac, Zoloft, and Paxil were revealed to be no more effective than a placebo for most cases of depression; or when we learned that staying out of the sun entirely can actually increase cancer risks; or when we were told that the advice to drink lots of water during intense exercise was potentially fatal; or when, last April, we were informed that taking fish oil, exercising, and doing puzzles doesn't really help fend off Alzheimer's disease, as long claimed. Peer-reviewed studies have come to opposite conclusions on whether using cell phones can cause brain cancer, whether sleeping more than eight hours a night is healthful or dangerous, whether taking aspirin every day is more likely to save your life or cut it short, and whether routine angioplasty works better than pills to unclog heart arteries.

But beyond the headlines, Ioannidis was shocked at the range and reach of the reversals he was seeing in everyday medical research. "Randomized controlled trials," which compare how one group responds to a treatment against how an identical group fares without the treatment, had long been considered nearly unshakable evidence, but they, too, ended up being wrong some of the time. "I realized even our gold-standard research had a lot of problems," he says. Baffled, he started looking for the specific ways in which studies were going wrong. And before long he discovered that the range of errors being committed was astonishing: from what questions researchers posed, to how they set up the studies, to which patients they recruited for the studies, to which measurements they took, to how they analyzed the data, to how they presented their results, to how particular studies came to be published in medical journals.

This array suggested a bigger, underlying dysfunction, and Ioannidis thought he knew what it was. **"The studies were biased," he says. "Sometimes they were overtly biased. Sometimes it was difficult to see the bias, but it was there." Researchers headed into their studies wanting certain results — and, lo and behold, they were getting them.**

We think of the scientific process as being objective, rigorous, and even ruthless in separating out what is true from what we merely wish to be true, but in fact it's easy to manipulate results, even unintentionally or unconsciously. "At every step in the process, there is room to distort results, a way to make a stronger claim or to select what is going to be concluded," says Ioannidis. "There is an intellectual conflict of interest that pressures researchers to find whatever it is that is most likely to get them funded."

He chose to publish one paper, fittingly, in the online journal PLoS Medicine, which is committed to running any methodologically sound article without regard to how "interesting" the results may be. In the paper, Ioannidis laid out a detailed mathematical proof that, assuming modest levels of researcher bias, typically imperfect research techniques, and the well-known tendency to focus on exciting rather than highly plausible theories, researchers will come up with wrong findings most of the time. His model predicted, in different fields of medical research, rates of wrongness roughly corresponding to the observed rates at which findings were later convincingly refuted: 80% of non-randomized studies (by far the most common type) turn out to be wrong, as do 25% of supposedly gold-standard randomized trials, and as much as 10% of the platinum-standard large randomized trials. The article spelled out his belief that researchers were frequently manipulating data analyses, chasing career-advancing findings rather than good science, and even using the peer-review process — in which journals ask researchers to help decide which studies to publish — to suppress opposing views.

The other paper...zoomed in on 49 of the most highly regarded research findings in medicine over the previous 13 years, as judged by the science community's two standard measures: the papers had appeared in the journals most widely cited in research articles, and the 49 articles themselves were the most widely cited articles in these journals.....Ioannidis was putting his contentions to the test not against run-of-the-mill research, or even merely well-accepted research, but against the absolute tip of the research pyramid. **Of the 49 articles, 45 claimed to have uncovered effective interventions. Thirty-four of these claims had been retested, and 14 of these, or 41%, had been convincingly shown to be wrong or significantly exaggerated.** If between a third and a half of the most acclaimed research in medicine was proving untrustworthy, the scope and impact of the problem were undeniable. That article was published in the *Journal of the American Medical Association.*

On the relatively rare occasions when a study does go on long enough to track mortality, the findings frequently upend those of the shorter studies. (For example, though the vast majority of studies of overweight individuals link excess weight to ill health, the longest of them haven't convincingly shown that overweight people are likely to die sooner, and a few of them have seemingly demonstrated that moderately overweight people are likely to live longer.)

And so it goes for all medical studies, he says. Indeed, nutritional studies aren't the worst. Drug studies have the added corruptive force of financial conflict of interest. The exciting links between genes and various diseases and traits that are relentlessly hyped in the press for heralding miraculous around-the-corner treatments for everything from colon cancer to schizophrenia have in the past proved so vulnerable to error and distortion, Ioannidis has found, that in some cases you'd have done about as well by throwing darts at a chart of the genome. (These studies seem to have improved somewhat in recent years, but whether they will hold up or be useful in treatment are still open questions.) Vioxx, Zelnorm, and Baycol were among the widely prescribed drugs found to be safe and effective in large randomized controlled trials before the drugs were yanked from the market as unsafe or not so effective, or both.

"Often the claims made by studies are so extravagant that you can immediately cross them out without needing to know much about the specific problems with the studies," Ioannidis says...."**Even when the evidence shows that a particular research idea is wrong, if you have thousands of scientists who have invested their careers in it, they'll continue to publish papers on it. It's like an epidemic, in the sense that they're infected with these wrong ideas, and they're spreading it to other researchers through journals.**"

Though scientists and science journalists are constantly talking up the value of the peer-review process, researchers admit among themselves that biased, erroneous, and even blatantly fraudulent studies easily slip through it. *Nature*, the grande dame of science journals, stated in a 2006 Editorial, "Scientists understand that peer review per se provides only a minimal assurance of quality, and that the public conception of peer-review as a stamp of authentication is far from the truth." **What's more, the peer-review process often pressures researchers to shy away from striking out in genuinely new directions, and instead to build on the findings of their colleagues** (that is, their potential reviewers) in ways that only seem like breakthroughs – as with the exciting-sounding gene linkages (autism genes identified!) and nutritional findings (olive oil lowers blood pressure!) that are really just dubious and conflicting variations on a theme.

Most journal Editors don't even claim to protect against the problems that plague these studies. University and government research overseers rarely step in to directly enforce research quality, and when they do, the science community goes ballistic over the outside interference. The ultimate protection against research error and bias is supposed to come from the way scientists constantly retest each other's results – except they don't....Of those 45 super-cited studies that Ioannidis focused on, 11 had never been retested. **Perhaps worse, Ioannidis found that even when a research error is outed, it typically persists for years or even decades.** He looked at three prominent health studies from the 1980s and 1990s that were each later soundly refuted, and discovered that researchers continued to cite the original results as correct more often than as flawed – in one case for at least 12 years after the results were discredited.

Doctors may notice that their patients don't seem to fare as well with certain treatments as the literature would lead them to expect, but the field is appropriately conditioned to subjugate such anecdotal evidence to study findings. Yet much, perhaps even most, of what doctors do has never been formally put to the test in credible studies, given that the need to do so became obvious to the field only in the 1990s, leaving it playing catch-up with a century or more of non-evidence-based medicine, and contributing to Ioannidis's shockingly high estimate of the degree to which medical knowledge is flawed. That we're not routinely made seriously ill by this shortfall, he argues, is due largely to the fact that most medical interventions and advice don't address life-and-death situations, but rather aim to leave us marginally healthier or less unhealthy, so we usually neither gain nor risk all that much.

But we expect more of scientists, and especially of medical scientists, given that we believe we are staking our lives on their results. The public hardly recognizes how bad a bet this is. The medical community itself might still be largely oblivious to the scope of the problem, if Ioannidis hadn't forced a confrontation when he published his studies in 2005.

But his bigger worry, he says, is that while his fellow researchers seem to be getting the message, he hasn't necessarily forced anyone to do a better job. He fears he won't in the end have done much to improve anyone's health. "There may not be fierce objections to what I'm saying," he explains. "But it's difficult to change the way that everyday doctors, patients, and healthy people think and behave."....It's not that he envisions doctors making all their decisions based solely on solid evidence – there's simply too much complexity in patient treatment to pin down every situation with a great study. **"Doctors need to rely on instinct and judgment to make choices," he says. "But these choices should be as informed as possible by the evidence. And if the evidence isn't good, doctors should know that, too. And so should patients....**If we don't tell the public about these problems, then we're no better than nonscientists who falsely claim they can heal," he says. "If the drugs don't work and we're not sure how to treat something, why should we claim differently?

We could solve much of the wrongness problem, Ioannidis says, if the world simply stopped expecting scientists to be right. That's because being wrong in science is fine, and even necessary – as long as scientists recognize that they blew it, report their mistake openly instead of disguising it as a success, and then move on to the next thing, until they come up with the very occasional genuine breakthrough. **But as long as careers remain contingent on producing a stream of research that's dressed up to seem more right than it is, scientists will keep delivering exactly that.**

"Science is a noble endeavor, but it's also a low-yield endeavor," he says. "I'm not sure that more than a very small percentage of medical research is ever likely to lead to major improvements in clinical outcomes and quality of life. We should be very comfortable with that fact."

David H. Freedman is also the author of the book *Wrong: Why Experts Keep Failing Us – And How to Know When Not to Trust Them.* Here are some quotations from that book, as they appeared in the June 10, 2010 issue of *Atlantic Magazine.*

"A good doctor, it is presumed, scans the journals for the results of these studies to see what works and what doesn't on which patients, and how well and with what risks, modifying her practices accordingly. Does it make sense to prescribe an antibiotic to a child with an ear infection? Should middle-aged men with no signs of heart disease be told to take a small, daily dose of aspirin? Do the potential benefits of a particular surgical intervention outweigh the risks? Studies presumably provide the answers. In examining hundreds of these studies, **Dr. Ioannidis did indeed spot a pattern – a disturbing one. When a study was published, often it was only a matter of months, and at most a few years, before other studies came out to either fully refute the findings or declare that the results were "exaggerated"** in the sense that later papers revealed significantly lesser benefits to the treatment under study. Results that held up were outweighed two-to-one by results destined to be labeled "never mind."

What was going on here? The whole point of carrying out a study was to rigorously examine a question using tools and techniques that would yield solid data, allowing a careful and conclusive analysis that would replace the conjecture, assumptions, and sloppy assessments that had preceded it. The data were supposed to be the path to truth. And yet these studies, and most types of studies Ioannidis looked at, were far more often than not driving to wrong answers. They exhibited the sort of wrongness rate you would associate more with fad-diet tips, celebrity gossip, or political punditry than with state-of-the-art medical research.

The two-out-of-three wrongness rate Ioannidis found is worse than it sounds. He had been examining only the less than one-tenth of one percent of published medical research that makes it to the most prestigious medical journals. In other words, in determining that two-thirds of published medical research is wrong, Ioannidis is offering what can easily be seen as an extremely optimistic assessment. Throw in the presumably less careful work from lesser journals, and take into account the way the results end up being spun and misinterpreted by university and industrial PR departments and by journalists, and it's clear that whatever it was about expert wrongness that Ioannidis had stumbled on in these journals, the wrongness rate would only worsen from there.

Ioannidis felt he was confronting a mystery that spoke to the very foundation of medical wisdom. How can the research community claim to know what it's doing, and to be making significant progress, if it can't bring out studies in its top journals that correctly prove anything, or lead to better patient care?...**Nor did the problems appear to be unique to medicine: looking at other branches of science, including chemistry, physics, and**

psychology, he found much the same. "The facts suggest that for many, if not the majority, of fields, the majority of published studies are likely to be wrong," he says. Probably, he adds, "the vast majority."

Putting trust in experts who are probably wrong is only part of the problem....So what if experts are usually wrong? That's the nature of expert knowledge – it progresses slowly as it feels its way through difficult questions. Well, sure, we live in a complex world without easy answers, so we might well expect to see our experts make plenty of missteps as they steadily chip away at the truth. I'm not saying that experts don't make any progress, or that they ought to have figured it all out long ago. I'm suggesting three things:

- We ought to be fully aware of how large a percentage of expert advice is flawed; we should find out if there are perhaps much more disconcerting reasons why experts so frequently get off track other than "that's just the nature of the beast"
- We ought to take the trouble to see if we can come up with clues that will help distinguish better expert advice from fishier stuff.
- And, by the way, if experts are so comfortable with the notion that their efforts ought to be expected to spit out mostly wrong answers, why don't they work a little harder to get this useful piece of information across to us when they're interviewed on morning news shows or in newspaper articles, and not just when they're confronted with their errors?

What About the Media?

In his January 2, 2013 *Atlantic Magazine* article, *Survival of the wrongest*, David H. Freedman discusses how personal-health journalism ignores the fundamental pitfalls baked into all scientific research and serves up a daily diet of unreliable information. Here are some direct quotes from that article.

"In all areas of personal health, we see prominent media reports that directly oppose well-established knowledge in the field, or that make it sound as if scientifically unresolved questions have been resolved. The media, for instance, have variously supported and shot down the notion that vitamin D supplements can protect against cancer, and that taking daily and low doses of aspirin extends life by protecting against heart attacks. Some reports have argued that frequent consumption of even modest amounts of alcohol leads to serious health risks, while others have reported that daily moderate alcohol consumption can be a healthy substitute for exercise. Articles sang the praises of new drugs like Avastin and Avandia before other articles deemed them dangerous, ineffective, or both.

What's going on? The problem is not, as many would reflexively assume, the sloppiness of poorly trained science writers looking for sensational headlines, and ignoring scientific evidence in the process. Many of these articles were written by celebrated health-science journalists and published in respected magazines and newspapers; their arguments were backed up with what appears to be solid, balanced reporting and the careful citing of published scientific findings.

But personal-health journalists have fallen into a trap. Even while following what are considered the guidelines of good science reporting, they still manage to write articles that grossly mislead the public, often in ways that can lead to poor health decisions

with catastrophic consequences. Blame a combination of the special nature of health advice, serious challenges in medical research, and the failure of science journalism to scrutinize the research it covers.

...Gary Schwitzer, a former University of Minnesota journalism researcher and now publisher of health care-journalism watchdog HealthNewsReview.org,...conducted a study in 2008 of 500 health-related stories published over a 22-month period in large newspapers. The results suggested that not only has personal-health coverage become invasively and inappropriately ubiquitous, it is of generally questionable quality, with about two-thirds of the articles found to have major flaws. **The errors included exaggerating the prevalence and ravages of a disorder, ignoring potential side effects and other downsides to treatments, and failing to discuss alternative treatment options.** In the survey, 44% of the 256 staff journalists who responded said that their organizations at times base stories almost entirely on press releases.

When science journalism goes astray, the usual suspect is a failure to report accurately and thoroughly on research published in peer-reviewed journals....the findings of published studies are beset by a number of problems that tend to make them untrustworthy, or at least render them exaggerated or oversimplified....Biostatisticians have studied the question of just how frequently published studies come up with wrong answers. **A highly regarded researcher in this subfield of medical wrongness is John Ioannidis, who heads the Stanford Prevention Research Center,....[he] has determined that the overall wrongness rate in medicine's top journals is about two thirds, and that estimate has been well-accepted in the medical field.**

Another frequent claim, especially within science journalism, is that the wrongness problems go away when reporters stick with randomized control trials (RCTs)....**Ioannidis and others have found that RCTs, too (even large ones), are plagued with inaccurate findings, if to a lesser extent. Remember that virtually every drug that gets pulled off the market when dangerous side effects emerge was proven safe in a large RCT.**

Why do studies end up with wrong findings?...To cite just a few of these problems:

- **Mismeasurement - To test the safety and efficacy of a drug,...**scientists must rely on animal studies, <u>which tend to translate poorly to humans</u>, and on various short-cuts and indirect measurements in human studies that they hope give them a good indication of what a new drug is doing. The difficulty of setting up good human studies, and of making relevant, accurate measurements on people, plagues virtually all medical research.
- **Confounders - Study subjects may lose weight on a certain diet, but was it because of the diet, or because of the support they got from doctors and others running the study?**
- **Publication bias - Research journals, like newsstand magazines, want exciting stories that will have impact on readers.** That means they prefer studies that deliver the most interesting and important findings....since scientists' careers depend on being published in prominent journals, and because there is intense competition to be published, scientists much prefer to come up with the exciting, important findings journals are looking for — even if its a wrong finding....A reporter who accurately reports findings is probably transmitting wrong findings.

It's not nearly enough to include in news reports the few mild qualifications attached to any study (the study wasn't large, the effect was modest, some subjects withdrew from the study partway through it). **Readers ought to be alerted, as a matter of course, to the fact that wrongness is embedded in the entire research system, and that few medical research findings ought to be considered completely reliable, regardless of the type of study, who conducted it, where it was published, or who says its a good study.**

When a reporter, for whatever reasons, wants to demonstrate that a particular type of diet works better than others or that diets never work, there is a wealth of studies that will back him or her up, never mind all those other studies that have found exactly the opposite (or the studies can be mentioned, then explained away as flawed)....**Questioning most health-related findings isn't denying good science; its demanding it.**

Yet in health journalism (and in science journalism in general), scientists are treated as trustworthy heroes, and journalists proudly brag on their websites about the awards and recognition they've received from science associations, as if our goal should be to win the admiration of the scientists we're covering, and to make it clear we're eager to return the favor....given what we know about the problems with scientific studies, anyone who wants to assert that science is being carried out by an army of Abraham Lincolns has a lot of explaining to do. Scientists themselves don't make such a claim, so why would we do it on their behalf? We owe readers more than that. Their lives may depend on it."

1 Your Health is Your Responsibility

My main objective is to make you think. Don't just look at the propaganda; don't just look at the salespeople or the advertising; 95% of what I see on television today is unbelievable. It is there to sell the product and has nothing to do with the quality of the product. This is especially true in the food field. Stay away from it.

Life to me is like a three-legged stool. As long as the three legs are in balance, the top of your stool is perfectly horizontal; therefore, you don't have any problems. But if one leg gets a little bit shorter than the other two, the top of your stool is going to turn off to the side. That becomes your problem of life because you constantly keep sliding off the stool.

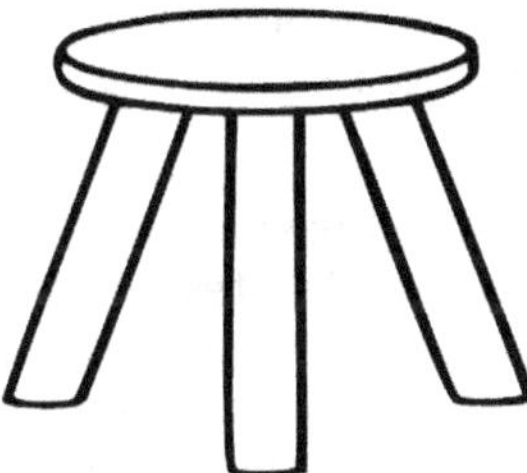

What do these three legs stand for? They stand for the intellectual, the spiritual and the physical. So you see, you have to fortify each a little every day to make sure you can solve your problems and stay on a horizontal plane. Remember that at all times.

My father taught me as a youth that, if I had not learned one new thing each day, that day was wasted and would never come back. The other thing he said to me was, "Son, no matter how stupid an individual is, he knows one thing that you do not know, and it pays you to listen to it." As I have gone around and picked up the gems from so many of these doctors, friends, and lay people whom I have helped, they'll say, "Doctor, I want to tell you about something I've learned from somebody way back who was a herbologist....", or something like that. I listen to them, even though I might not have any respect for them; I still listen. If I can take 10 gems from 10 people, I may extract something that works out very well for people. Another thing that my father used to say was, "When you're green, you grow; when you're ripe, you rot!" Think about that one.

Editor: At the time Dr. Ellis made these statements to his audience (1985), he had just appeared on Ed Busch's syndicated America Overnight radio show. He received over 370 letters and 111 telephone calls as a result of his appearance. This response was astounding, as the show was only two hours long, beginning at midnight.

Socialized medicine does not work. And I know one thing, I would never practice under it myself. I saw this coming years ago. One of my good friends was down in Washington, He said, "You know, we're developing a book. It's a blue book in which we're going to put down the name of all diseases, and then we're going to put under that how you're to treat them. It's going to be up to you as a doctor to make the diagnosis; then if you don't treat it in accordance with what we have put into that blue book, you will lose your license." Linda Clark, probably the best research nutritionist that writes books, once said to me, "When you write, make sure you don't have a reference to one thing. When you make a statement, state that it's strictly your opinion. Otherwise you too can be arrested." See? We've lost our freedom of speech. That's the same thing that I do.

When you go against the consensus of medical opinion (nobody can describe the consensus of medical opinion), they believe that their opinions are worth more than yours, because you're different from them. **One of the things I think that has kept me out of trouble more than anything else in my years of practice is that I have gotten results. You've got to have good results! I stick my chin out further than anybody I know because I just happen to be one of those dogmatic people who believes that God taught me these things, and that's what I'm going to teach. As long as I know what I know, I'm going to teach it to anybody.**

I lecture over the whole world. So far, I have represented the United States in 37 foreign countries and have lectured in 41 of the 50 states. I have a lot of friends, many of whom are doctors. We start asking, "Do you have a wholistic center in your area?" They say, "Oh yes!" and then explain. I reply, "But they are not wholistic." I have not yet found one that is a total wholistic health center in the United States. The reasons why are that doctors are trying to commercialize on this image. If they can go out and do a better job than what I'm doing, shame on me. That's just the way I feel. I'll teach anybody anything and everything I know if they want to sit down and listen. If I can't stay ahead of them with all of the things that I have picked up over this world, then it's my fault, it's not theirs. Let them go out and do it. The more of us that think in terms of health, the better we're going to come out in the end.

Take Charge of Your Health

It is vitally important for each thinking adult to inform himself with respect to how he should live, what habits he should retain, and which ones he shall discard. Many of the simplest habits, such as smoking and drinking alcohol, are just as harmful as the vicious or immoral ones! Eating sweet rolls and drinking tea can get you into trouble just as certainly as alcohol and tobacco.

What has nature designed for you as a plan for healthy living? Do you have any idea? Well, carry on reading! Poor health is primarily a result of poor eating (nutritional) habits. **You, and only you, have the power of decision regarding what foods you eat; therefore, the choice is up to you! As my father used to say, "Regardless how bad any situation is, if you want to be truly honest with yourself, you can always find out where you were at fault!" Such is a wonderful revelation, because it is the first step in taking charge.**

If you are seriously interested in making the desired corrections, they are within your capabilities, because a wealth of information is now available concerning diet and nutrition. **However, a doctor is only as good as the cooperation he receives from his patient; so, when you start a program, stick with it long enough to get results.** Do not allow yourself to get discouraged! Often, when the body starts to change from the diseased state to the healthy state, reactions will take place that may make you feel like the cure is worse than the disease. These reaction periods last for about 10 days, so simply prepare yourself for it, and be determined that you will keep working toward the worthwhile reward ahead! Consider these issues:

- Surgery can remove an organ or part after it is too badly diseased to function; but surgery cannot heal or replace the organ or part.
- Drugs may alleviate or remove the symptoms of a disease, but they cannot remove the cause of the disease.
- Manipulations will aid structural or body balance and restore a certain amount of circulation and nerve flow to the affected organ or part, but they cannot change the quality of the blood or nerve fluids that are flowing to that organ or part.
- The mind can alter one's attitude about life, but it cannot completely deal with the physical causes of disease. You must learn as much as you can about the natural laws before you can understand why only one or two techniques is not sufficient.

Holistic health takes a complete commitment, intelligent eating habits, proper sleep, proper attitude, and proper physical care. It is nothing less, and you cannot cheat the system by omitting any one of the above. You can only cheat yourself directly and your loved ones indirectly! You must be disciplined. If you're not willing to follow all of the rules and regulations set down by your health doctor, you're not going to get anywhere.

Can we now move forward, determined that we are going to learn as much as we can and apply it with dedication? Good, I'm glad that you have decided to accept the responsibility for your own health! After all, when you get sick, it is you who have allowed your body to deteriorate by not keeping it free of toxins and neglecting to give it the vitamins, minerals, enzymes, coenzymes, hormones, proteins, fats, and carbohydrates that it needs and deserves. Incidentally, have you been breathing clean air and drinking pure water?

When you maintain good habits, you act as a good example for the non-believer. If you desire to work as part of a group, you can join organizations such as the Natural Food Associates or the Organic Food Group; their philosophy is to bring wholesome and nutritious foods back into the general marketplace.

Public Image of the Body

How does industry and, consequently, the general public envision the human body? They do so in terms of information that is part of commercial, so-called nutritional campaigns that give rise to food fads. Over the years, the calorie theory has had its rise to fame and its decline to oblivion. The vitamin principle, the chemical characterization of foods in an attempt to fit the food to the body by a detailed analysis of the assumed need at the time, has not worked either. Neither of the methods nor the assumptions upon which they were based successfully dealt with the problems of health; the people who were so analyzed were looking for a crutch. **None of the techniques restored health to the degree desired. Why? Because none of the theories took into account the fact the body is more than a crude chemical laboratory or furnace that simply burns up food for the human engine.** The human body is much more complex than their systems analyses could handle.

If you really want to appreciate the extent of the health problem, consider the following figures (as of 1985). The U.S. Public Health Service published the facts that there are only three million healthy persons in the United States today. With a population of 186 million, this means that only one in 62 are healthy! Additionally 76,000 persons are being admitted into our hospitals every day – 49,000 of these for the first time; and the figures are rising. Fifty percent of all hospital beds are being filled with mentally deficient patients, and this figure is also rising. Many patients are the unwitting victims of the American, commercially influenced and directed way of life; clever propaganda and advertising mislead people into buying and using unfit foods that cannot even support the life of bacteria and mold, much less support the life of a human being.

Just because one may eat a product without dropping dead or immediately falling ill is no proof that the product is even a marginally suitable item for consumption. Most deficiencies do not appear for weeks, months, or, perhaps, years later – when the cause of the problem is long forgotten and ignored!

As you can see, our most difficult task is to fight the constant bombardment of the people with this ill-conceived media attack on the viewing and listening public. The sole interest of companies who advertise in this way is to sell products and maximize profits. As P. T. Barnum once said, "If you tell a lie big enough and often enough, the greatest majority of people will believe it."

The Pharmaceutical Industry

Drug trusts are stopping us from getting the truth. You know, all colleges today are subsidized by industry. If they get subsidized high enough, believe you me, they are going to teach what is in accordance to get that money from that industrial grant. I see this in my own colleges. I have been kicked out of a couple of osteopathic colleges because I tell them that all they are doing is turning out a bunch of pseudoosteopaths and a bunch of half-assed medics. I got kicked out of my own college (Philadelphia Osteopathic College) for telling them, "You better realize that you're in a rut, and until you get out of that rut you had better look out. It's going to get deeper, the sides are going to fall in, and that's going to be the funeral of the osteopathic profession."

That funeral almost happened, because a month later, after I made that statement to the executive director in Chicago, California's osteopathic group seceded from the American Osteopathic Association, and osteopaths were given the opportunity to receive a small M.D. license for $65. Now they've reversed the law, with the courts determining that it was illegal, and 2,000 of these California osteopaths that had received their small M.D. licenses reapplied for their D.O. licenses. They found out that they did not want to be M.D.s. I would not want to degrade myself that low.

General Health Tips

To get started, below are listed tips for a healthier life. Some activities need to be developed without delay, while others can be incorporated over time, but only with sincere application on your part. Most of these are repeated and expanded upon in later portions of this book. For now, read them over and resolve to be open-minded. You may copy this list and share it with others.

1. Be aware of your health needs. Be aware of your disease possibilities like cavities in your teeth, sinusitis, infections, constipation, sores and cuts that do not heal rapidly, and being overweight.
2. Rest and relax according to your individual need. For some people, eight hours of sleep is sufficient; others need six. Some others need ten.
3. Form a regular bowel habit. Drink a full glass of water upon arising to aid peristalsis. If you are reducing in weight and working toward your normal weight, you should have two or three movements daily. Report irregularities such as constipation or excessively loose movements to a physician.
4. Breathe fresh air and get some sunlight, but not too much!
5. Enjoy life. We live today, on yesterday's experiences to make a better tomorrow.
6. See a health doctor who's interested in making you healthy; do not see a disease doctor who's only interested in relieving your symptoms. When you're at your doctor's office, look at him; does he look healthy? If he's healthy himself, he'll be able to teach you how to get healthy. But if he looks sick, or is big and fat, how can he tell you to reduce your weight or get your health back? Start to become a healthy doctor.
7. Get a health survey done at least once a year. This consists of your blood, hair, and urine analysis. Have your doctor check your blood chemistry levels of Total Protein, Albumin, and Globulin to see if you have sufficient hydrochloric acid (HCl) in your stomach to digest proteins and fats. There's no such condition as over acidity of he stomach. Today, bottle-fed babies start running out of sufficient HCl in their late teens and early twenties. Most everybody over 50 years old needs HCl supplements.
8. Follow the instructions about which foods and drinks to consume and to avoid, as shown in Specific Food Recommendations. Remember, if you eat junk foods, you will have a junky body. Eat health or natural foods, and you will be naturally healthy.
9. Read the book written by Jane Armstrong, *Pick your Poison*. Study what's in foods that you eat. Avoid all food containing artificial coloring. These dyes are highly cancer-causing.

10. The most important factors in your diet to get in balance are proteins, vitamins, and minerals. Vitamins are the catalysts that make the minerals become the enzymes. Protein is needed in every single function of the body. Vitamins and minerals must be in their proper balance and in ratio to one another, otherwise they will break down and not perform properly. This to me is the basic cause of disease.

11. Do not overcook protein with high temperature. Keep it on the rare side, and cook at an internal temperature of 138° F.

12. Be careful with salt. Have your doctor check your blood levels of sodium and potassium for proper balance. If not balanced, they destroy circulation and make you nervous. You may need to consume salt to maintain the balance; be absolutely sure about the levels in the blood before reducing salt intake.

13. Learn how to blend food so that you can eat it digestibly.

14. Eat foods that can spoil but eat them before they spoil.

15. Include adequate bulk type food such as bran, celery, lettuce, etc.

16. Include food rich in B17 (the seeds of all fruit have it, with the exception of citrus seeds, especially peaches, pears, apples and apricots.)

17. Do not eat food that you know produces gas.

18. Chew your foods thoroughly; they must be near liquid before swallowing.

19. Do not use aluminum cookware or aluminum foil on foods, as it has been found to devitalize food.

20. Drink at least 8-10 eight-ounce glasses of fluid daily. The body needs this amount to carry on all functions. you perspire an amount equal to the amount of urination per day. Avoid hot or excessively cold beverages.

21. Drink distilled water and supplement to your mineral deficiencies. Before drinking spring, well, or even city water, have it analyzed and checked with the health doctor to see if it's good to drink. **Do not drink chlorinated water** or ingest organic chlorides in any form, as they are now found to cause cancer and have also been found to destroy HCl formation in your stomach.

22. Exercise daily; it's a must for health. Walk or swim two miles a day or ride a bicycle 10 miles a day. That comes out of the International College of Fine Nutrition program.

23. Learn how to balance your body. Research has shown that 62% of the population has an anatomical short leg. The standing X-ray of the lumbar spine and pelvis is the method to ascertain which leg and how much. Use both a heel and sole lift for balance; do not build up only the heel.

24. Avoid using synthetic chemicals for your skin and hair, such as cosmetics, colognes, hair tints, and dyes. For ladies, don't wear bras and panty hose made from synthetic materials, but use cotton panties.

25. Do not smoke, keep away from the smoke of others. Second-hand smoke is worse than first-hand smoking, because you mix it with the carbon dioxide coming out of your breath, and it changes the chemistry of the nicotine and sulfuric acid from the paper.

26. Avoid chemicals in your environment, such as in paint and solvents used to clean tools.
27. Avoid all aerosol containers, such as found in insecticide, deodorant, and air fresheners.
28. If you have to wear dark glasses outside, get a full spectrum lens. Do not use fluorescent bulbs; use Spectrolights.
29. Avoid radiation from microwave towers, microwave ovens, and television sets (color is three times worse than black-and-white).

Break the Laws and Pay the Price

Many people make a serious mistake in assuming that their bodies are their own to do with as they desire. Our Creator lends bodies to individuals during their short stays on this earth, so that they may express themselves physically, emotionally, mentally, and spiritually. For this loan, like any other kind of loan, our Creator demands payment; but this payment, unlike any other financial obligation, is very reasonable. The payment consists of diligent care and nourishing of these bodies in full conformity to the terms and conditions as outlined by our Creator in the Holy Scriptures. These laws have been known throughout the ages as Natural Laws.

Man, throughout the ages, has taken great delight in his attempt to break these laws. No man can break the divinely created laws of God. He may violate them, but he cannot break them. Every so often, one reads in the newspaper of someone who tries to break the law of gravity by jumping out of a twenty-story building. None of these individuals break the law of gravity, but they break almost every bone in their bodies when they hit the sidewalk!

No man, no matter how hard he may try, can escape his vital relation to the universe, as it is forever fixed by these laws. These laws are absolutely non-yielding and are constantly and vigorously enforced by powers beyond any man's control. Remember, each time you break these laws, you must pay! There is no escape; there is no chance of not being caught! You will be penalized by worry, disease, fear, confusion, discontent, insecurity, anger, insanity, and a broken life; then you head for the underground bungalow.

You cannot go to a doctor and say, "I've broken all of the laws of God and nature, but I expect to get better because you're going to give me some miracle pills." It just doesn't work that way. Conformity to these laws always brings its own rewards. As proof of this statement, remember Proverbs 3:1-2 that says, "My son, forget not my law; but let thine heart keep my commandments. For length of days and long life and peace, shall they add to thee."

Editor: Dr. Ellis saved the following list from an Ann Landers column in the Saturday, July 23, 1983 edition of the *Dallas Morning News*. It is entitled *Golden rules make life a bit easier.* The rules in bold type relate more closely to the previous words about the Natural Laws, but all of them are worthy of consideration.

If you open it, close it.

If you turn it on, turn it off.

If you unlock it, lock it up.

If you break it, admit it.

If you can't fix it, call in someone who can.

If you borrow it, return it.

If you value it, take care of it.

If you make a mess, clean it up.

If you move it, put it back

If it belongs to someone else, and you want to use it, get permission.

If you don't know how to operate it, leave it alone.

If it's none of your business, don't ask questions.

If it ain't broke, don't fix it.

If it will brighten someone's day, say it.

2 Protein Nutrition

I don't want you to believe anything I tell you just because I say it. But before you condemn it, try it out over a long enough period of time to prove whether I'm right or wrong. That to me, is the key to understanding all of these concepts.

We have statistics on a 160-pound man, so we're going to talk about him. We don't have one on women, so we're going to have to say that they are both the same, or as close as possible. In a 160-pound, man, you have 100 pounds of water, 29 pounds of protein, 25 pounds of fat, five pounds of minerals, one pound of carbohydrates, and one quarter of an ounce of vitamins. That ought to surprise a few of you.

Some of the things you're going to read are going to blow your top, because you've been propagandized by industry so long that you think so many of the things they tell us are truthful, when they are exactly the opposite; they are absolutely wrong. Like health advocate Elizabeth Rodston said, "In my 20 years of lecturing on better health through better food, I have found that few people will listen or make changes in their buying or eating habits, until they are either old enough, sick enough, or smart enough to desire to do so." She continues, "Be one of the smart ones who will learn to prevent disease through supernutrition before getting sick or old."

Just as a building is only as good as the weakest brick in its structure, the human body is only as strong as the weakest cell. You had better take care of every cell, and they are up in the trillions. It is estimated that your brain has 26 billion. So it is important that you think in terms of treating the total body – not Isolated parts. You have to treat everything. You have to get the ingredients in that body and the bloodstream and, if into spinal manipulation, normalize the nerve supply to the organs and other systems.

Physiology and Diet

Today, every school student has the opportunity to learn, in the study of human physiology, that the cells of the body are constantly being rebuilt. Some parts of the body are renewed as often as once a month. Much of the body is renewed every year, but the bones of the skeleton require about seven years for their complete replacement. The bloodstream constantly brings fresh building material to every cell and carries away the waste products of metabolism. **The only way the body is able to rebuild itself is from the material carried to it by the bloodstream.** If any part lacks health and efficient function, it is because the material brought by the blood has been unsuitable for the task of maintaining healthy tissue. The only source from which the blood can derive these rebuilding materials is by absorption through the walls of the intestines of food substances that have been put into the digestive tract – ingested foods. Therefore, the fact that you are unhealthy shows that you have failed to put the proper substances into the digestive tract. **Unless you have been subjected to external injury, the lack of nutritional factors is the cause of your disease.**

Importance of Protein to Metabolism

How important are proteins? Researchers at the University of Illinois Medical School have demonstrated that proteins are the most important substances in our diet. Their report, published in the late 1940s, was of great interest to physicians who wanted to apply the principles stated therein to their patients.

It is the lack of available protein that causes one to get old! Sufficient protein containing all of the amino acids is required for body synthesis and producing protein tissues for repair and maintenance of muscle, hair, fingernails, heart, brain, and all vital organs, in addition to enzymes and hormones secreted by the ductless glands. Indeed, without utilizable protein, there is no life. There is no disease, illness, or abnormality in the body that is not, in some way, related to protein metabolism.

- There are protein molecules in the bloodstream (albumin and globulin are two) that are carriers for other materials such as enzymes, minerals, fats, sugars, vitamins, and hormones.
- Enzymes and many hormones are themselves protein in nature.
- The red blood cells are mainly protein, the oxygen-carrying component, hemoglobin, being a globular protein.
- All of the endocrine glands unite molecules of proteins with molecules of other substances to form hormones. For example, thyroid protein plus iodine equals thyroxine, pancreas protein plus zinc equals insulin.
- Through the action of proteolytic enzymes and vitamin and mineral catalysts, proteins are broken down into amino acids. These are absorbed and assimilated through the intestinal wall and carried through the portal circulation to the liver.

  Two of the 10 essential amino acids, arginine and histidine, are vital to growing youngsters. The body uses 26 amino acids, and 16 of these can be synthesized in the liver, primarily from the 10 essential ones. Methionine, another essential amino acid, is a precursor to the important lipotropic factors, choline and inositol. Interestingly, all of the essential amino acids must be present in the body and in sufficient quantity at the same time. Otherwise, the nutritional effectiveness of the entire group is impaired.

Proteins are not stored in the body in the form in which they are ingested. The assimilated amino acids are transformed into storage proteins, the predominant one being albumin. This albumin is the internal source of amino acids; the diet is the external source. However, the amino acids will not be utilized unless there is a normal complement in the body of gonadal or sex hormones. Adults tend to expend protein excessively. Business and social pressures, insufficient rest, pregnancy, and lactation all cost more protein than most of us can spare. The body that doesn't have a regular dietary supply of protein must steal protein from wherever it can to keep going. Any cell might be robbed. The joints are the first to be looted. As the body uses more proteins and if the stored supply is inadequate, they may be taken from any tissue, even though the tissues involved may not be able to spare any of their own protoplasmic proteins.

At the stage of senility, lack of steroids from the adrenal cortex may be a cause of protein deficiencies. In many arthritics, there is anemia, secondary in nature with all evidences of inflammation – characteristic of usage of proteins at an accelerated rate. A patient with a high fever uses proteins more rapidly and presents a greater hypoproteinemia than one who may not be eating enough proteins. **In arthritis or bursitis, the body will make an effort to maintain serum albumin (storage protein) levels by taking protoplasmic albumin from the joint surfaces themselves. The more taken, the more severe is trauma to the joints.** Cortisone or ACTH, by releasing albumin from the muscle tissues, makes it available to the blood and thus to the joint surfaces, decreasing the irritability and inflammation – the arthritic manifestations in the joints. However, as you notice, this is done at the expense of the muscle tissue! This leads to protein depletion in other tissues even though the arthritic symptoms have been relieved. Remember that, for a gram of protein available in the bloodstream, the healthy joint surface requires 30 times as much.

When protein intake equals protein usage, a balance exists and is expressed in terms of nitrogen balance. If more protein is used than is replaced by ingestion and assimilation, a negative nitrogen balance exists. **An excellent criterion of protein availability to the tissues is the state of the skin, hair, and fingernails. Coarse, brittle hair that falls out easily; dry, hard skin that wrinkles easily or is not elastic; and fingernails that crack, split or do not grow properly are all indications of inavailability of proteins.** This inavailability of sufficient amounts of protein can be caused by inefficient intake in the diet, poor mastication, poor digestion, poor absorption, poor assimilation (aberrant enzyme, vitamin, and mineral metabolism), and improper levels of the sex hormones. Other signs of protein deficiency are fatigue, sensitivity to cold, evident pallor, allergies, most edema, hypertension, and a negative attitude. In fact, children who are highly nervous, irritating, defiant, and mischievous are those children who are eating large amounts of sugars and starches. They eat very little protein-rich foods!

Quoting from the article, *Arthritis Isn't Hopeless to This Doctor, Prevention* magazine, July 1968, interview with Dr. Ellis, "...especially among older people, **proteins go through the system largely undigested. But the human body is such that, at any cost, it will keep the blood supply of protein (albumin) constant and adequate. If the protein does not come from the blood, the body will draw it out of the tissues. If the protein is taken from the bursas, the collagen will break down and bursitis will develop. If from the tendons, tendosynovitis will result. If from the joints, arthritis; if from the muscles, rheumatism.**

The water supply in most of our major cities hasn't helped the situation any. For example, the pH of Pittsburgh's drinking water, which should be around 7, was 8.2 a few years ago. Now it is 8.8. They pour alkalai (calcium and magnesium carbonate (lime), sodium hydroxide, aluminum sulfate (alum), iron chloride) into the reservoir to encourage coagulation and flocculation to reduce dirt and bacteria. But these same alkalies raise the likelihood of painful arthritis."

Dr. Ellis' Own Physical Breakdown

The reason why I learned so much about digestion and assimilation of food was because I had a physical breakdown at age 29. I found out that I had no production of hydrochloric acid in my stomach at all – absolutely none. At that time, I made my own hydrochloric acid. I had to carry it in a glass-stoppered bottle with a glass straw and dropper everywhere I went. I would get an eight-ounce glass of water, pull out the bottle, and put 10 drops into the glass. When I wanted to drink it, I would use the straw and have to curl my tongue and suck it up because if it hit my teeth, it would dissolve them.

Today we have betaine hydrochloride tablets. Also, we are lucky to have protein supplements in the form available today. When I started out trying to get a protein supplement, we didn't have them on the market. We had to drink raw meat drippings.

Protein Intake

First, we must eat a variety of protein sources animal and vegetable. When we tell a patient that he is deficient in proteins, he will usually say, "But doctor, I eat plenty of meat or protein food!" This shows how necessary it is to know the difference between eating sufficient amounts of protein foods and eating sufficient amounts of protein foods that contain the essential amino acids in the proper ratios!

One of my physician professors tells a story about a patient of his who, as a boy, made a vow that, when he was successful, he would eat only T-bone steaks. He worked very hard and finally attained a successful status, so he began eating only T-bone steaks. A short time later, he was doing some extra heavy work, and his back started to ache. He tried, unsuccessfully to rid himself of the pain by the usual methods. Thereupon, he presented himself to my physician professor for help. At first, the physician failed, but in an off-handed conversation, he learned about the exclusive diet that his patient had chosen for himself. The physician remembered having read in one of our reliable textbooks that T-bone steaks do not contain all of the essential amino acids. He placed his patient on a liquid protein/complete essential amino acid supplement, and improvement became evident. The patient had to change his ideas about eating only T-bone steaks and eat all forms of protein or take a liquid protein supplement for the rest of his life! It is true, however, that animal proteins are the best sources of amino acids, although we must not forget that proteins are available in grains, nuts, and fruits.

Are you getting enough protein? One way to determine this is to multiply your weight by two to get the number of protein calories required per day. The best animal proteins are turkey, lamb, beef, fish, fowl, eggs, and gelatin (lacks tryptophan).

Protein Digestion

The first step in halting protein thievery is to have ample protein in the diet. But, it is equally true that the richest protein diet won't prevent a degenerative disease if the protein is poorly assimilated by the system.

Now that we have assured ourselves of what proteins to eat to obtain an adequate amount of the necessary amino acids, what is the next step necessary to ensure that these proteins become available for use by our bodies? Digestion! Here lies a very revealing story for those of you who believe everything you hear and see in advertising propaganda. Let's start at the beginning and work into the needs and problems. First, we must masticate our proteins as we do all food in our mouth to break up the large pieces, mix them with saliva, and thereby prepare them for the other digestive processes to follow.

I was allowed to get into the Stanford Research Institute to talk to a scientist about protein metabolism and the $1,800,000 he got from the government to study it with regard to cancer. He said, "I've been feeding the finest grade of protein to these animals, and they're still all protein deficient." I said, "Are you assuming that because you were giving them protein they were going to have it available?" He said, "Of course." I said, "Well, that is where you are mistaken." I drew out a little chart that I had learned at the University of Illinois Medical School seminar on digestion and assimilation in 1949. He was astounded that he had not been taught this, and when I went back the following year, he was in school trying to learn it. This digestion and assimilation of food is vital.

It is in the stomach that our greatest, and consequently our most serious problem exists. This problem is the widespread lack in our population of gastric digestive power in the form of hydrochloric acid and pepsin. Also essential are inositol, choline, methionine, trypsin, and chymotrypsin. Pepsin, the only digestive enzyme present in the adult stomach, is the stimulator for the production of hydrochloric acid. In fact, peppermint is a stimulator of pepsin production; peppermint tea is beneficial with meals to induce acid production. Acidity is needed to activate the peristaltic wave and open the pyloric valve of the stomach; it also stimulates the emptying of bile from the liver and gallbladder. When the stomach is too alkaline, and fermentation or putrefaction takes place, the gallbladder is falsely triggered, bile is regurgitated back into the stomach, and a burning sensation is experienced (heartburn). People who have an acetone smell on their breath are not digesting their food. The starches and sugars ferment; fats and proteins putrefy. You can tell the difference in that the fermentation gives a breath similar to that of alcoholism. The putrefaction gives a really foul breath. With sufficient stomach acid, the digestion will be complete, and there will be no odors.

There are several methods of determining whether we have an adequate supply of gastric secretions. One may swallow a small collection tube after a test breakfast and directly measure the hydrochloric acid content of the measured volume. A newer test is called Diagnex Blue. This test is conducted by swallowing a couple of these pills and measuring the dye as it is excreted in the urine in a given period of time. **How does a lack of hydrochloric acid manifest itself? Symptoms are a lack of appetite, distaste for meat, burping, a sense of fullness an hour or two after eating, and a burning or itching rectum.**

Scientists have shown that the maximum production of hydrochloric acid is reached in persons of age 25; by the age of 40, it has diminished by 15%. By the age of 65, the production has diminished by 85%. The point is that, the older you get, the less able you are to digest proteins properly.

Remember what I said about advertising on TV, radio, and in magazines? Those companies who propagate such advertising claims would have you believe that everyone is over acidic and that everyone needs antacid tablets! Nothing could be further from the truth! Did you know that the symptoms of an over-acid stomach are exactly the same as those of an alkaline stomach? **With the lack of acid, bile backs up into the stomach, the highly alkaline bile irritates the stomach lining, and a burning develops.**

Why not try a simple test to see if this assumption is correct? The next time you have a full feeling in the stomach, a burning sensation, or if you are burping, take a teaspoon of apple cider vinegar in a small amount of water. You will be surprised how quickly you will feel better! However, if the burning sensation increases, your stomach is truly over-acidic; this is not a common occurrence.

Protein Assimilation

Assimilation is the next important step in protein utilization by the body, and it depends on several factors. We must have adequate vitamins and minerals, especially vitamin C. In this case, vitamin C should include all components of the complex – civatemic acid, ascorbic acid, and bioflavonoids or vitamin P. It is of utmost importance to eat enough raw greens and fresh fruit to get this vitamin C or to take a complete supplement. With the proper balance of vitamins, minerals, and sex hormones, the proteins will be made assimilative. Remember, however, that the sex glands are the only glands that do not continue to function during your entire life. After castration by surgery, after the female menopause, or after the male climacteric, the sex organs cannot contribute to the endocrine balance of the body. If transfer of these duties from the sex glands to the adrenal glands or liver does not take place, a reaction occurs. This is called hot flashes in women and a loss of sex drive and great fatigue in men. Thymus, adrenal, and thyroid tissue are needed.

We must be able to absorb nutrients efficiently. Even when the sex glands are functioning very nicely, we can still inhibit protein assimilation by coating the lining of the stomach and intestinal membranes with mucous. **The most severe, mucous-forming food is milk, and this, I feel is the most notorious cause of malabsorption of nutrients. Suffice to say at this point, even though we eat a high protein diet and have the proper digestive enzyme, vitamins, minerals, and hormonal balance, we can defeat the purpose of protein ingestion by using milk products.** We must have a clean, unclogged bowel wall for the proper absorption and utilization of nutrients. Preservatives, such as potassium nitrate, can have serious effects on the glandular system. I have seen this in my own practice.

Allergic Responses to Protein

Consider now that 29 pounds of protein are found in the average 160-pound man. Proteins come from external sources such as meat, fish, eggs, fowl, and gelatin in one group. Nuts, seeds, and cereals constitute a separate group. A major consideration is the digestibility of them.

From the *Organic Consumer's Report* comes this statement, "Hay fever, asthma, and migraines are related to the body's inability to properly break proteins down completely into amino acids, preparing them to be used as building blocks to repair tissue, etc. This faulty process results in the buildup of uric acid and other toxins. Undigested proteins find their way into the bloodstream, setting up allergic reactions. The usual medical way of treating these allergies is to isolate individual allergens. This method usually involves a restricted diet and often causes the affected person to rely upon drugs to counteract the attacks."

Editor: In *Clin Exp Immunol*. 2008 Sep; 153(Suppl 1): 3-6, titled *Allergy and the Gastrointestinal System*, G Vighi, F Marcucci, L Sensi, G Di Cara, and F Frati listed the clinical manifestations of gastroenteric allergy, including the following quotes. "Gastrointestinal anaphylaxis is a very severe reaction caused by the ingestion of foods such as cow's milk, hen's egg, peanut, fish, and crustaceans.

Allergic eosinophilic oesophagitis is a disease characterized by swelling of the oesophagus caused by massive infiltration of eosinophils. Symptoms can range from severe heartburn to difficulty swallowing, food impaction in the oesophagus, nausea, vomiting and weight loss....A personal or family history of other allergic diseases, such as hay fever, food allergy and asthma, is frequently observed. Various studies have shown that patients with eosinophilic oesophagitis have positive allergy tests to foods, and that avoidance of these foods leads to the resolution of symptoms. Culprit foods include milk, egg, peanut, shellfish, pea, beef, chicken, fish, rye, corn, soy, potatoes, oats, tomatoes and wheat. Of these, the most common food triggers are milk, egg, wheat, rye and beef. Environmental allergens such as pollens, moulds, cat, dog and dust mite allergens may also be involved in the development of eosinophilic oesophagitis.

Food protein enteropathy and food protein enterocolitis/proctitis is an adverse reaction to foods affecting mainly children, mostly aged under 2-3 years. The major causative allergens are milk and soybean. The immunological mechanism is linked to immune complexes and/or cell-mediated reactions, and clinical symptoms include vomiting, diarrhoea, enteropathy with protein loss and malabsorption and failure to thrive.

Oral allergy syndrome (OAS) consists of itching and swelling of the lips, the oral mucosa and the soft palate immediately after eating fruits or vegetables. If the culprit food is ingested despite the local disturbances, gastrointestinal symptoms such as vomiting, abdominal pain and diarrhoea may occur and, more rarely, urticaria and anaphylaxis may also develop. OAS affects approximately 40% of subjects suffering from pollinosis; its pathogenetic mechanism is explained by cross-reacting allergens shared by pollens and vegetable foods."

Acid-Alkaline Balance

There is some misunderstanding about whether a food is acidic or alkaline and what it does to the body's (blood) pH. The blood pH remains very close to 7.4 (alkaline) regardless of what foods are consumed. However, we are concerned with the effect that eating certain foods or drinking certain beverages have on the pH of the urine. **If a food increases the acidity (lowers the pH) of the urine after it is ingested, it is classified as an acid-forming food. If a food increases the alkalinity (raises the pH) of the urine after it has been ingested, it is classified it as an alkaline-forming food.**

The acid-alkaline balance is of utmost importance in protein digestion and synthesis, yet it is often overlooked. **A diet high in protein produces residue that raises urine pH, increasing the chance of forming kidney and bladder stones.** Knowing his or her urine pH helps the individual adjust the diet to lower the pH of the kidneys and bladder. Care must be taken to avoid other alkaline-forming foods such as orange juice, which is highly acidic in the glass, but causes the urine to become alkaline. Others include tomato, and pineapple, with sweet milk running a close second. See Directions for Combining Foods on page 76.

Testing Urine pH

To determine urine pH, you can use a simple do-it-yourself test, using a small piece of chemically-treated testing paper (litmus or nitrozine). **Test the first urine voided upon arising or the first urine voided after breakfast. Both should be acid, pH5.5 or 6 (below 7 is acid, 7.0 is neutral, and above 7 is alkaline). The second test is more important, for it is normal to be most acid about 4:00 AM.**

Restoring Urine Acidity

When the morning urine test indicates over-alkalinity (above pH 7), there are some reliable ways to return the pH of the bladder to acid.

- Follow the advice of Dr. Jarvis' in his book, *Folk Medicine*, which is to take two teaspoons of apple cider vinegar with a little honey in either hot or cold water.
- Another method is to use Digestin, one of the many hydrochloric acid tablet products available in health food stores, at each meal. The Digestin-type of digestive aid is a very good one, made from a combination of betaine HCl from beets, glutamic HCl from grains, plus small amounts of pepsin, bile, and often papain and vitamin B6. Consistent testing will help determine the amount needed by each person, as it is an individual problem.
- Consume bacteria as found in acidophilus or lactic acid fermenting yeast tablets.
- Consume cold processed, unsaturated vegetable oils with a high linoleic acid content. One example of the use of oil is described by Dr. Jarvis. It follows the results from the use of one tablespoon of corn oil at each meal (we don't want

> anybody using corn oil today, as it is sprayed 34 times in its growth process). Sesame and safflower oils are also high in linoleic acid, which when present, insures the synthesis of other valuable fatty acids such as linolenic, and oleic acid.

Walter B. Guy, M.D., prolific researcher in digestion and mineral utilization in the 1930s, attributed over-alkalinity and the resulting infiltration of the salts of urea into the lymph channels to be directly related to arthritis, diseased hearts, kidneys, and swollen joints. Hydrochloric acid is the only acid normally present in human tissue. When deficient, lactic acid, a waste by-product of muscular activity, increases. In the course of elimination, this is broken down to carbon dioxide, to be expelled by respiration, and glycogen, to be retained as tissue food.

3 Food and Diet

"If the doctor of today does not become the dietician of tomorrow, the dietician of today will become the doctor of tomorrow." - Dr. Alexio Carrell, Rockefeller Institute of Medical Research

Benjamin Franklin once wrote, "Would'st thou enjoy a long life, a healthy body, and a vigorous mind, and be acquainted with the wonderful works of God, labor in the first place to bring thy appetite to reason."

What you eat and how you eat it is what you are! You eat for health or you eat for disease; there is no in-between! If you do not buy wholesome food, you are on a disease diet. If you do not prepare it properly, you are on a disease diet. If you do not combine the foods properly, with respect to foods that are eaten at the same time, you are on a disease diet. Furthermore, if you overcook your food, you are on a disease diet. **Are you eating a disease diet?**

Today, as we are living in a chemical world, we have to change our diet to modern standards. We can no longer buy top quality foods (except those that are organically grown); instead, we are forced to accept foods raised for quantity with chemical fertilizers, fungicides, and bactericides. These same foods may be fortified or enriched, while others are processed, medicated, hormonized, pasteurized, degerminated, refined, hydrogenated, hardened, bleached, or what have you!

These processes – additions and subtractions to foods – are used as propaganda to entice the unsuspecting customer to buy and consume these products as being improved upon from the original. Unfortunately, the customer learns too late that this propaganda is not the truth, for, when they have been afflicted with disease, they learn, if they are fortunate enough to be taught, the bitter truth that is the basis of their problems!

The following information is presented so that patients and their physicians can understand the principles of good diet as they relate to their own health. Patients should learn these principles so they can discipline themselves and have an appreciation for what their physician is doing to try to help them. Mutual cooperation is essential.

Physicians should think of what is to follow as valuable personally and professionally. Unless a physician understands the eating habits of patients and makes an effort to modify their undesirable eating habits, he or she cannot successfully treat these patients. Physicians must make it their business to discover these eating indiscretions; one good way to accomplish this is through a 7-Day Diet Journal. When a comprehensive profile is done for a patient, this journal is a necessary part. It is a very simple, but effective, information gathering tool. Just have the patient write down everything he or she eats for a period of seven days.

Editor: At the end of Dr. Ellis' career, he became aware of research involving tests for food, preservative, and coloring intolerances (not allergies) being carried out in San Antonio, Texas and Miami, Florida. He was hopeful that he would be able to incorporate such testing into his comprehensive plan, but the field was not commercialized by the time Dr. Ellis began his struggle with a terminal illness.

Subsequent to Dr. Ellis' passing, researchers developed what is called the ALCAT test and made it available to the public. Current information about this service is found at https://cellsciencesystems.com/patients/alcat-test/. A book about food intolerance and weight control is *Your Hidden Food Allergies Are Making You Fat* by Roger Deutsch and Rudy Rivera M.D., July 23, 2002, available from Amazon.com.

For a list of undesirable food additives, visit the MPH website at http://mphprogramslist.com/50-jawdroppingly-toxic-food-additives-to-avoid/.

Vegetarianism

I don't believe in vegetarianism. I have done over 2,000 blood, hair, and urine analyses on vegetarians. They all have very poor immune systems, and they are always anemic. We see problems as a result of these two factors. So many of these people look like they are a fugitive from a square meal.

In the Bible, there are 233 verses that tell you about eating meat; 83 tell you to eat beef, 61 to eat fish, and six to eat venison; but there's not a single verse that I can find that tells you to be a vegetarian.

Diet vs. Personality

What you eat affects your personality and emotions. Massachusetts Institute of Technology researcher, Dr. Richard Workman, says, "A lack of protein may lead to withdrawal and indifference. Too much sugar makes a person an emotional yo-yo; oversensitive, irrational, and jumpy." When you talk about sugar, the normal yearly consumption of sugar per person is five pounds. In the U.S. last year, the consumption was 140 pounds. The sugar content of most of today's childrens' cereals ranges from five to 55%. Any wonder that there are so many hyperkinetic children today? Not counting the 3,000 additives that Dr. Ben Feingold talks so much about. **The American Diabetic Society years ago made the statement that if the U.S. population continued to eat the amount of processed starches and sugars that they are now doing, everybody in the U.S. will be diabetic within 10 years!** It is very important to eat natural food in its natural state.

When you consider those factors of hypoglycemia, the forerunner of diabetes, figure how many of you with those symptoms and the direction that you're heading if you don't change your diet. Honey is among the best, but take it sparingly. Honey is made up of slow-absorbing sugars, whereas white sugar is a fast-absorbing sugar that overstimulates the pancreas. There's a great push of energy, but then insulin production goes too long and produces hypoglycemia. You get tired and useless again.

Even in the case of diabetes, you can use as much as two tablespoons a day of good blackstrap molasses. The mineral content of the molasses will help to stimulate the activity of developing insulin. You want to remember that insulin is manufactured in the beta cells of the Islets of Langerhans from zinc, chromium, and albumin (that is the part of the protein), and you also have to consider potassium because of what it does to the sugar metabolism within the liver.

Recommended Eating Habits

To ensure the success of this program, a patient must cooperate. Doctors should make sure that the patient keeps in contact with his or her office so that the patient can stay motivated and modifications to the program may be made as necessary.

The following are more instructions.

- **Establish a health diet.** Too often, people decrease their food intake to the point of decreasing metabolism. It is important that you have a normal daily intake of nutritious food. By establishing this habit you will find that you actually eat less and feel better for it! The menus listed below are not to be followed letter by letter, but they are considered to be a pattern of eating by which it is possible for you to achieve a correct balance of carbohydrates, proteins, and fats.
- **Choose your foods wisely.** Taste and hunger should not be the sole reason for food choice, but these foods can be appealing as to appearance and taste. Keep on a high protein, low fat, low calorie diet. This means emphasizing the protein foods such as meat, eggs, fish, fowl, whole grains, and gelatin.

  It is my opinion that it is best for us to eat as many organically raised foods as possible to obtain the highest quality. If prepared properly and eaten slowly with thorough mastication to assure a proper start in digestion, the foods can supply us with the nutrients we need for better health. As Charles F. Kettering said, "We should all be concerned about the future because we will have to spend the rest of our lives there."
- **Avoid the high fat foods** such as oleomargarine, uncooked dressings (mayonnaise, french dressing), heavy pastries, fish packed in oil, the hydrogenated shortenings, and cooked nuts. Use butter sparingly. Use fresh foods preferably. If these are not available, use frozen ones. If at all possible, do not use canned or boxed foods.
- **Eliminate milk and milk products from the diet.** I like the taste of milk, ice cream, and cheese, but I do not eat them! Neither should anyone else!
- **Prepare your food wisely.** Avoid fried food; instead bake, roast, broil, or boil meats. Eat as many raw vegetables as possible each day. When cooking

vegetables, use as little water as possible, and start the vegetables in boiling water so that cooking time will be shorter. Do not overcook!

- **Work toward a good breakfast habit and noon-day meal.** Remember, the foods you eat during the day tend to be burned up during the day. When starchy foods are eaten at night, they are not used by the body for energy, but tend to be stored as fat!
- **Eat foods that can spoil**, but eat them before they spoil!

  By the way, how do you test to find out if bread is any good to eat? Take a slice or two of bread or any bread product. Put it on the top shelf of your kitchen cabinet. Allow it to stay there for 48 hours. Then take a look at it. If mold has developed on it, you can say "Oh, I have good bread!" Naturally, you want to eat it before it gets moldy. Mold only comes on something that is alive. If there is no mold on it, it's dead bread. It's been embalmed already.

  Here is a story about shredded wheat; as told by Dr. Joe Nichols of Henderson, Texas. Dr. Nichols put an open box of shredded wheat in his garage and left it there for six months; no bugs or animals were interested in it. He then brought the open box into his office; it has been there for four years with no bugs; it is just as fresh as five years ago. In another experiment, he ground up the shredded wheat and fed it to a group of rats. He also ground up the box and fed it to another group of rats. In six months, the rats that ate the box were healthier.
- **Eat slowly**, masticate thoroughly, enjoy your food. Never overeat!
- **Eat in quiet.** Do not watch television or listen to talk shows on the radio. Quiet dinner music is fine.

Specific Food Recommendations

The following are specific recommendations in the various categories of foods indicated. The left column lists approved, healthy foods, and the right column lists unhealthy foods to be avoided. See Directions for Combining Foods on page 76 for suggestions on what foods may be eaten together to promote complete digestion.

RECOMMENDED FOODS	FORBIDDEN FOODS
Beverages Chamomile tea, clear tea, mint tea, papaya tea, ginseng tea, misc. herbal teas, Sanka, Pero, Postum Some acceptable ones are Soyalac (a milk substitute made from soybean); Pero, Cafix, Postum (all coffee substitutes), Sun-Gal, Yerba Mate, Mate, and herb and root teas (peppermint, rose hips, etc.).	**Beverages** Alcohol, cocoa, soft drinks, drinks that contain stimulants and depressants. Coffee, decaffeinated coffee, black tea, or any other drink that contains caffeine or acid are diuretics, and they break down kidney function. They also eliminate potassium and the vitamin B complex. **Drink absolutely no milk!**
Bread Rye, soya, whole wheat or bran muffins, whole wheat, sprouted grain	**Bread** All other, white enriched, bleached
Cereals Untoasted buckwheat, corn meal, cracked wheat, millet, steel-cut oatmeal, rice, sesame, fine ground grits, rye, 100% all bran, Vigor Whole grain cereals are superior and should be eaten raw, if possible. However, these may be cooked.	**Cereals** All other refined and bleached flour Corn and wheat should be avoided. Do not eat, under any circumstances, boxed cereals from the grocery store. Avoid processed grain foods such as macaroni, noodles, white rice, and spaghetti.

Cheese None	**Cheese** All forbidden
Dessert Fresh ripe fruit, stewed fruit, gelatin (made from naturally sweetened and colored fruit or fruit juice) Fruit and gelatin salads are acceptable, but not when made with Jello. One should use unsweetened, uncolored, and unflavored gelatin and add fruit and fruit juices.	**Dessert** All pastries, puddings, custards, junket, sauces, Jello (artificially sweetened and colored), ice cream Eat absolutely no pastries, custards, puddings, candy, or ice cream!
Eggs Soft boiled or poached from chickens raised on the ground	**Eggs** In any form from caged chickens
Fats and Oils Butter (unsalted), cold-pressed, unsalted oils such as olive, corn, sesame, sunflower, safflower Only a few of commonly available oils are acceptable for use. The best ones, listed in the order of their acceptability are sesame, flaxseed, sunflower, soy, cottonseed, olive, and corn. The best healthy dressing is one made with cider vinegar and unsaturated oil. Honey may be added as a natural sweetener, and herbs may be used to flavor the mixture.	**Fats and Oils** Oleomargarine Shortening, saturated fats and oils **Avoid all fried foods; they contain dehydrogenated oils.** Mayonnaise and prepared, bottled dressings Canola oil (**Editor:** Dr. Ellis' recommendations were made before canola (rapeseed) oil became popular. Some cautions about ingestion of rapeseed oil are found at http://breathing.com/articles/canola-oil.htm, and http://www.diabetesincontrol.com/component/content/article/64-feature-writer-article/2570&Itemid=8.) Peanut oil (allergenic)
Fish Fresh, white-fleshed, salt-water top feeders	**Fish** All fresh-water, salt-water bottom feeders

Vegetables	**Vegetables**
Raw, frozen, fresh or freshly cooked: artichokes, asparagus, carrots, cauliflower, celery, chives, corn, endive, green leeks, spinach, green peas, green pepper, lentils, lima beans, potatoes, radishes, tomatoes, wax beans, string beans, yams, egg plant, squash, mushrooms, beets, sprouts, mung beans, raw dandelion greens, beet greens, broccoli, Brussels sprouts, raw cabbage, cucumber (unpeeled), lettuce, washed sauerkraut, raw spinach (never cooked), parsley, rutabaga, Swiss chard, onions, turnips, and potatoes (used sparingly, not over once a week) Any vegetables listed under salads Vegetables may be eaten raw or cooked, but cooking should be done with as little water as possible as in wok cookery. Cooking in this sense could be best described as "wilting." Use cayenne pepper and organic garlic, as well as onions. They do not cause digestive problems.	All canned Spices and contents such as black and red peppers or hot peppers. They destroy stomach acidity.

Fruit	**Fruit**
Fresh fruit or water-packed only and preferably between meals, including: apples, pears, apricots, cherries, currants, grapes, guava, mangos, melons, nectarines, papaya, peaches, plums, quince, tangerines, avocados, ripe pineapple, rhubarb, grapefruit and oranges (once a week if the system tolerates), lemons, currants, gooseberries, strawberries, cranberries, blueberries, loganberries, blackberries, raspberries. Fruit is best eaten singly and separately at least three hours after you've had protein. The following dried, unsulfured fruit can be stewed: apples, apricots, dates, figs, prunes, peaches, pears, plums, raisins, dates, apricots. Eaten only very ripe: bananas (use sparingly because they are highly alkalizing) Do not eat acidic and alkaline fruit together.	Canned fruit because they are preserved in sugar. The so-called dietetic fruit are just as bad with their chemical sugar substitute.
Juices	**Juices**
Only fresh juices, consumed within minutes after being made for the best results. These may be selected from lists of permitted fruit and vegetables, including the following green leaves: chicory, endive, escarole, lettuce, Swiss chard, and watercress. Prune and cranberry juices (truly acidic, from malic acid) are better for us as we get older. Vegetable and unsweetened fruit juices are acceptable, but not when packed in metal or plastic. The preferred containers are glass.	All canned juices, and juices with artificial coloring and sweetening Tomato and tomato juice based drinks should be avoided, as should citrus juices.

Meat Lean, grilled, broiled, roasted or baked beef, chicken and turkey (raised on the ground), lamb, and veal. Internal organs: only heart and extra fresh calf liver permitted. Meats should be prepared by broiling at 280° F. They should never be eaten well done; they should be eaten as rare as possible.	**Meat** Bacon, ham, sausage, or pork, most of which are preserved with chemicals, especially nitrates or nitrites. They form the carcinogen classes of nitrosamines, a most potent cancer causer. Cold cuts, luncheon meats, canned meats and hot dogs; as they have the same preservatives, and most of them contain red dye. Smoked or barbecued meats. They are also cancer causers. Beef that has fat in the lining portion of the muscle. This means that the animal was raised on hormones and antibiotics. Do not eat chickens that are raised on wire – the cages.
Milk and Milk Products Butter	**Milk and Milk Products** None except butter
Nuts All types of fresh raw nuts (avoid long term storage to minimize fungus growth; only 10 daily) Seeds and nuts of all kinds (except peanuts) are acceptable, but they should be eaten fresh, never cooked, especially in oil, and in moderation, with no salt, no preservatives, and in moderation.	**Nuts** Roasted and salted Peanuts (allergenic)
Potatoes Baked, boiled and mashed, potato salad, brown rice or corn as a substitute	**Potatoes** French fries, shoestring, pan fried, white rice
Salads The following raw vegetables, shredded or finely chopped, separated or mixed: carrots, cauliflower, celery, chicory, green pepper, lettuce, radishes, Swiss chard, watercress, onions, ripe tomatoes, turnips, Brussels sprouts, broccoli	**Salads** Any salad with fatty or sweetened dressing

Seasoning	Seasoning
Chives, garlic, onion, cayenne pepper, parsley; herbs such as laurel, marjoram, sage, thyme, savory, cumin, oregano; salt substitutes such as Cosalt or other potassium salt	Black pepper, paprika, sodium salt
Soup	**Soup**
Vegetable, barley, brown rice, wild rice, millet	Canned and creamed soup, fat stock, consomme
Sweets	**Sweets**
Unpasteurized honey, unsulfured molasses, raw sugar, or dark brown sugar, carob	Candy, chocolate, white sugar
Any variations in this diet should be done only with a doctor's permission. Avoid all toxic materials including alcohol and tobacco. Keep away from other people that smoke.	

Meat

My favorite meal is nothing but a nice piece of meat and a nice raw vegetable salad, using apple cider vinegar (don't use any other kind of vinegar) with a good oil like sesame oil, sunflower oil, or a good olive oil. I like sesame because it has vitamin T in it to support blood platelets.

One of the big problems with protein in the diet is that so few people know how to cook proteins. We have been teaching what the Pennsylvania Restaurant Association taught us. These professionals did the research on how you should cook meat to get the most good out of it.

Correct Cooking Temperatures

Meat should be cooked at an internal temperature of 138° F. Use a meat thermometer for accuracy. It just takes a little longer. This temperature is in the range of minimum pasteurization temperatures, depending on the length of the cooling time.

Editor: Below is a helpful chart of cooking temperature and time combinations to ensure pasteurization of beef, lamb, and pork from Amazingribs.com. For data on other meats, visit the website.

Table 1: Meat Cooking Temperature vs. Cooking Time

Internal Temperature (^oF)	Cooking Time
130	121 minutes
135	37 minutes
140	12 minutes
145	4 minutes
150	72 seconds
155	23 seconds
158	0 seconds

Most people today and most restaurants, cook meat at an external temperature of 350-400° F, which often carries the internal temperature of the meat too high, robbing it of vital, nutritious juices and making it tougher to digest. Meat juice is the plasma of the cell; it is not blood. When I started in this business many years ago, we didn't have the protein supplements like we can get today at the health food stores. The meat juice remains valuable.

One of the few times that I have ever agreed with the FDA comes from an article in the *Wall Street Journal* of August 1977; it says, "Blood rare beef pre-cooked to fade from the food counters. US to order that the meat be cooked to 145° F."

145° F is pretty close to 138° F, and to have the FDA finally admit this shows that we people in the health field really have something! 145° F does kill the Salmonella, or any other bacteria if it is cooked like that, and you get the temperature on the inside to 138° F and that's when you eat it.

Suggested Cooking Sequence

Here are some stepwise instructions that will help you learn how to cook beef, lamb, and pork properly.

- Depending on the thickness of the meat, select a cooking time that ensures the entire piece will be cooked to completion at the desired internal temperature. You must monitor the internal temperature of the meat with a meat thermometer.
- Rinse the meat and allow it to attain room temperature, but do not let it sit at room temperature very long; otherwise bacteria will multiply, making your job more difficult. Do not salt the meat before cooking!
- Preheat the oven to the desired external temperature. Start with 250° F; put the meat in the oven.
- Allow the meat to warm up as long as necessary for the internal temperature to reach 138° F. To measure the temperature, insert a meat thermometer into the thickest portion of the meat and take a reading for no more than 15 seconds. (Instant-read thermometers are not oven safe and must not be left in the meat while it is cooking.)

- When the internal temperature reaches 138° F, start timing the cooking period. Adjust the external temperature as necessary to maintain the internal temperature.
- At the end of the recommended cooking time, take the meat out of the oven and heat the oven to broiling temperature.
- Put the meat back in the oven and let the broiler sear the surface, creating a crust that will hold in the juices. Let it cook for two to three minutes; the internal temp should remain at 138° F.
- When the crust is formed, pull the meat from the oven. Do not cut it immediately! Let it rest for at least 15 to 30 minutes to allow the juices to finish circulating and settle. The internal temperature of the meat will rise 3-5° F during this time.

Editor: Foodnetwork.com states, "Ground meat is riskier, because a contaminated meat surface is broken into small fragments and spread through the mass. The interior of a raw hamburger usually does contain bacteria, and is safest if cooked well done." Escherichia coli (E. coli) is killed at 155° F, but the USDA minimum safe internal temperature for ground beef is 160° F. Read more at: http://www.foodnetwork.com/recipes/articles/meat-and-poultry-temperature-guide.html?oc = linkback.

Microwave Cooking

What happens to meat in a microwave oven? The protein on the inside is devitalized. The U.S. government did a study of two groups of men for 90 days one group ate microwaved food and the other ate food cooked by conventional means. At the end of 60 days the men that ate the microwaved food were so tired and listless they got rid of the microwave ovens. There is also a radiation factor; read Linda Clark's *Are You Radioactive?* Food cooked in a microwave oven is devitaminized because it cooks at 2,000° F. The food is also demineralized, as indicated by the low values shown in a hair mineral analysis.

The microwave sets up free radicals, better known as peroxides. When eating microwave cooked food, you may just as well reach over and drink a bottle of hydrogen peroxide; it is exactly the same thing. We are seeing such an increase in cancer today that it is astounding. The National Cancer Institute announced that one out of three people living today will have cancer, and one out of six will die. I have not seen the American Cancer Society or the National Cancer Institute advance one single thing in cancer in 45 years; we are no better today. We in the so-called unorthodox field are clearing up 75% of them, if we can get these patients before chemotherapy, radiation, or surgery. Which way do you want to go?

Pressure Cooking

Keep the heat as low as possible.

Barbecue Cooking

Although barbecued meat should be avoided, if one must eat some occasionally, ensure that the heat source is not directly under the food to be cooked. Meat drippings should not be burned and vaporized so that they come in contact with the meat.

Eggs

Eggs are one of the finest protein foods that you can eat. It is a complete protein, but you must know something about them. In the first place, they must be fertile, which means there must have been a rooster around for every 12 hens when those eggs were made, and when you put it in an incubator it could make another chick. They must come from chickens that are raised on the ground and not in cages (on wire). Wire makes it easy for the farmer because all of the droppings go down underneath and are easy to pick up. It's a little more difficult when they're on the ground. But when they are on the ground, they're picking up the gravel which goes into their craws, which is their digestive enzyme system. They pick up the bugs, worms, and all of these things that give them proper nourishment, to make a good egg.

The most important thing to remember is that under the shell of an egg is an enzyme called avidin. If you crack the shell of an egg, avidin destroys the biotin and the pantothenic acid, the two most important parts of the egg. It also neutralizes the lecithin, which is very high in eggs. Place it in boiling water for 30 seconds to deactivate the avidin and kill the bacteria under the shell. If you scramble or fry an egg or put it in an omelet and you're using grease, it's those oils and fats that become polysaturated; you destroy the lecithin and have an unbalanced egg that is harmful.

Editor: in an study published by Durance, T. D. (1991). *Residual Avidin Activity in Cooked Egg White Assayed with Improved Sensitivity. Journal of Food Science*. 56 (3): 707-9. doi:10.1111/j.1365-2621.1991.tb05361.x. A new assay method found residual avidin activity in fried, poached, and boiled (2 minute) egg white to be 33%, 71%, and 40% of the activity in raw egg white. This suggested that cooking times were not sufficient to adequately heat all cold spot areas within the egg white. Complete inactivation of avidin's biotin binding capacity required boiling for over 4 minutes.

Dr. Emmanual Cheraskin at the University of Alabama took a group of dentists whose cholesterols ranged from 600 to well over 1,500 mg%. He wanted them less than two hundred, preferably under 175. On the scale he was using the low normal was 150. He put them on six soft boiled eggs every day. In 90 days, every one of their cholesterols were reduced to less than 200, and most of them were less than 175. You see, proteins burn up cholesterol. Now where does cholesterol come from? Cholesterol is manufactured through the colon and the liver from starches, sugar, and milk products. Less than 15% comes from foods that contain cholesterol, so don't be taken in by the advertising gimmicks they put on television and radio. A few years ago, we knew a man who said "I'll prove something else."

He ate 60 soft boiled eggs daily, for 60 days. This meant in his waking hours he ate a soft boiled egg every three and a half minutes. His cholesterol was 1,600 when he started, it was 145 at the end of 60 days. Surprising, isn't it?

Again, make sure your eggs come from chickens raised on the ground not on wire; 95% are raised on wire. These chickens are loaded with a microorganism called by Dr. Virginia Livingston the Progenitor cryptocides (see Appendix A: Additional Reading); which are found in all people with cancer. To her, it is one of the basic causes of cancer. All people that I know with cancer cannot digest meat properly, so it putrefies and causes cell degeneration. They need HCl, trypsin, and chymotrypsin.

Fats

Unsaturated oils are preferred, and the best is sesame. The linoleic, oleic, and arachidonic acids are highest in sesame oil. The next best is safflower, followed by sunflower oil. In sesame oil is vitamin T; it builds blood platelets required for clotting. You can mix 1/2-1 cup of these oils with butter and keep the mixture in the refrigerator or freezer. At room temperature, It can turn rancid long before you can taste or smell it.

Editor: Dr. Ellis' recommendations were made before canola (rapeseed) oil became popular. Some cautions about ingestion of rapeseed oil are found at http://breathing.com/articles/canola-oil.htm, and http://www.diabetesincontrol.com/component/content/article/64-feature-writer-article/2570&Itemid=8.

Vegetables

There are 65 green, yellow, and red vegetables. Take 10 or 12 of these, and put them through a salad maker. If the particles are very small you won't get into so much trouble because you won't have to chew 40-50 times. It is very rare that I can get anybody to chew more than 5-10 times. It is a case of attacking their food rather than chewing it properly. It is vital to do enough chewing to get the saliva to mix with the food, because it activates the production of hydrochloric acid in your stomach.

Parsley, by the way, is one of the great vegetables that we have, with probably more vitamins and minerals than any other vegetables. Another, if you want to get some potassium, is a raw potato. However, eating from the nightshade family, of which the potato is a member, might increase pain for a person who is arthritic. The part of the potato you want to eat is the skin and the 1/4" under it. That is where the food value is located. The inside is pure starch. If you go to a banquet, where you usually end up with a baked potato and meat, take a spoon, and scoop out the inside of the potato and throw that away. Eat the remainder, and it won't be so harmful to you.

Fruit - Good or Bad?

All fruits are good if they are tree-ripened. There are only four acid residue fruit: prunes, plums, cranberries, and rhubarb. Rhubarb must be eaten raw because it's high in oxalic acid. If cooked, it interferes with calcium metabolism in the body. If it is sour there are insufficient minerals. Rhubarb is sweet and delicious raw.

Acid fruit can be mixed with anything with the exception of alkaline fruit. All other fruit, including tomatoes, leave an alkaline residue. Alkaline fruits are best eaten singly, all by themselves at least three hours after or two hours before eating protein. All fruit is to be eaten between meals and before bedtime if very hungry.

My favorites are grapefruit, oranges, apples, and bananas. Two of those are good, and two are not so good. Citrus is picked green and shipped to you; that's what you buy. It took me six months of fighting with the Florida Citrus Commission to make them agree that there wasn't any vitamin C in oranges. You get vitamin C only from tree-ripened fruit.

The most important thing about bananas is that the skin is real thin. When we were in the Caribbean, I paid a kid fifty cents to go up a tree and get me a banana that was tree ripened. You wouldn't believe the difference in the flavor of that one banana compared to what you have in the stores. All bananas are picked green, then they are shipped to the destination, where they are put into a gas chamber to turn them yellow. Then we think that they are ripe. But, as long as those skins are thick, they are still green. Buy your bananas this week off the stand and eat them next week or the week afterwards. Let the enzymes in the skin work on the banana to ripen it. When they get a lot of black marks all over is when you eat them; then you can use the potassium effectively. Other sources of potassium are avocados and parsley.

Tomatoes - A Fruit to Avoid

Many authors call tomatoes the golden fruit with many vitamins. But I don't believe it. In Ireland, they grow the most beautiful, perfect tomatoes with plants 10 feet high with small tomatoes on them. We went from there to the Soviet Union and Switzerland, and in every country, they would serve you tomatoes and cucumbers for lunch and supper. I eat neither of them, but if you do, remember to eat cucumbers with the green covering on the outside, as that's where the enzyme factors are. If you peel it, you lose all of that and the cucumber is more harmful to you at that particular time.

A cancerous person should not eat tomatoes, it will neutralize the treatment and make the cancer worse. I've done research in cancer since 1936 and help take care of cancer patients as a consultant to doctors. If we can get them before radiation and chemotherapy, we can clear up about 75% of them. I wrote an article, *How to Feed the Cancer Patient.* Gina Larsen was on the reviewing board for the article and refused it because I couldn't explain why Bill Coate had said no tomatoes; she felt they were the finest food you could eat. I couldn't find the documentation on it, because Coate didn't explain it to me.

Cleaning Vegetables and Fruit

Today we are running into a lot of arsenical poisonings because of the sprays being put upon your vegetables. So when I talk about the sprays put on vegetables, let me teach you how to make sure they are fit for you to eat. All of your fruit and vegetables today, practically all of them, have some kinds of pesticides or weedicides, or some other type of spray on them. To remove them, follow these instructions.

- Use plain, unscented household bleach; one tablespoon to a gallon of distilled water.

Editor: Bleach is very caustic; protect your eyes and wash it off of your skin immediately. Watch out for the safety of anyone around you, mop up spills, and do not leave the container open or exposed to children. Do not use spashless bleach; it foams extensively.

- Soak your fruit or vegetables for 15-20 minutes. This will remove most of these pesticides, weedicides, and sprays from the outside.
- Take them out, dry them, and put them into distilled water for another fifteen minutes. This will remove the rest of the residue.

Make the bleach water new each time and throw it out after you finish with it. It works out a whole lot better that way.

A Sample Menu for the Day

Our research has proven that our finest health menus consist of 50% or more protein in our diet; 20% or less of fats, mostly from unsaturated oils, and 30% carbohydrates, mostly from green, red, and yellow vegetables and not heavy starches.

To maintain best health, the largest meal of the day should be breakfast, as that is the energy you work on all of the rest of the day. The second largest meal should be lunch, and the evening meal should be small. This is so that the gastrointestinal tract can have some rest while you sleep. Eat no snacks in the evening. If this order is reversed, I can predict weight gain. Another point to be made is to eat natural foods whenever possible.

Table 2 is a sample menu showing you that it is possible to serve a day's meals that are high in protein, low in fat, and that supply nutrients that add up to better health. There are, of course, many variations; substitutions may be made from the foods listed under Specific Food Recommendations on page 63. There is, however, no substitute for the gelatin.

Table 2: Sample Menu for the Day

Meal or Snack	Components
Breakfast	Select either of the following: • Prune or cranberry juice upon arising, one or two eggs (soft boiled or soft poached), one or two slices of whole grain bread, and a beverage from those listed in the previous chart. (Bread and its products are not usually recommended in combination with a protein food. However, soft boiled or soft poached eggs are digestible when eaten with a moderate portion of whole grain bread, preferably toasted. The same statement cannot be made for meat proteins or eggs that are cooked to a hard consistency.) • Cooked whole grain cereal, honey if desired, cranberry or prune juice, choice of a beverage from those listed in the previous chart.
Mid-Morning	Fruit juice or cold water with one package of gelatin added.
Lunch (sometimes called Dinner)	Broiled ground beef patties (cooked rare to medium rare), raw vegetable salad with dressing, choice of beverage.
Mid Afternoon	Fresh fruit
Dinner (sometimes called Supper)	Vegetable soup with Rye Crisp, choice of meat (prepared as above), vegetables, cole slaw, or salad with dressing; choice of beverage.
Bedtime	For a relaxing sleep, drink cranberry juice, warm bouillon, or cold water to which has been added a package of gelatin.

When I'm on the road I eat mostly soft boiled eggs. There's another thing that you can do with an egg. If you take a raw egg from the icebox, warm it up a little bit under the faucet with warm water then put it into boiling water for 30 seconds to destroy the avidin enzyme. Crack the shell and combine them with cranberry juice in a blender (8 ounces). That is a meal. The acidity of the cranberry juice picks all of the acidity out of the egg so that you would not know it is raw. Cranberry juice, being acid (malic acid that does not break down in the body), helps to digest the protein. You can also add one tablespoon of gelatin. It's an excellent meal. You can also use prune juice, which also contains malic acid. Many times, when I am sitting at home writing my 30-35 letters a day, I don't have much time to take off for lunch, so I'll make this delicious drink, and I'm good for five hours.

When I'm at home I like my organically grown rye, millet, and steel-cut oatmeal. Usually what I do is take a tablespoon of buckwheat, a cup of rye, and a cup of millet. They are the highest in minerals and protein of all cereals. I put it in a double boiler with two cups of distilled water, because no city water that I know of is fit to drink anywhere. While it's cooking, I put it on a low temperature and shave, shower, and dress. That gives me about 25 minutes to finish; I come back to the kitchen and put cranberry juice in the mixture. It's very delicious and lasts me about five to six hours.

You could probably use raw bran, barley, or brown or wild rice as a cereal. Then you don't eat anything else that's all you need at that particular time. Lunches and suppers remain somewhat the same. Of course we have some kind of meat. I would advise at least seven to 21 meals from salt water fish.

Directions for Combining Foods

Proper combining of foods optimizes the digestive processes. **It is possible to eat a variety of foods that interfere with the digestion of certain others. Likewise, it is possible to eat foods that enhance the digestion or, at least, do not interfere with the digestion of the others.** Properly and completely digested carbohydrates yield monosaccharides; improperly and incompletely digested carbohydrates yield the poisonous substances acetic acid and alcohol (fermentation). Completely digested proteins yield amino acids, whereas incompletely digested proteins yield ptomaines and leucomaines (putrefaction), both poisonous substances.

Allergies are a manifestation of improperly digested proteins that enter the bloodstream before they are broken into a sufficiently small fragment; such reactions can be prevented by effecting the eating habits that promote the most efficient digestion all along the alimentary canal. Some suggestions are as follows.

- **Select your proteins wisely.**

  Muscle meat is difficult to digest, even when combined properly with other foods. The best and most digestible source of protein is the egg, and it should be soft boiled or soft poached; never fried, scrambled, or hard boiled.
- **Do not mix proteins with starches (carbohydrates).**

  As proteins move into the stomach, pepsin is secreted, and this triggers the release of hydrochloric acid. Protein digestion requires this acidic environment. However, as the medium becomes more and more acidic, carbohydrate digestion becomes curtailed. Furthermore, the presence of the carbohydrate neutralizes the acid; i.e., the medium that is favorable to the digestion of one is unfavorable to the digestion of the other. Meat and potatoes is, therefore, a poor combination, as is meat and alkaline fruit, starches, and sugars.
- **Do not mix acid (alkaline-forming) fruit with proteins.**

  Alkaline fruit include tomatoes and all fruit except prunes, plums, cranberries, and rhubarb. These should be eaten singly and at least three hours after ingestion of proteins. Acid (acid-forming) fruit, such as prunes, plums, cranberries, and rhubarb, can aid digestion and can be used in the same meal as protein foods. (Rhubarb contains oxalic acid and, on that basis, should be avoided.)
- **Do not mix acid (alkaline-forming) fruit with starches.**

  Citrus fruit or vinegar will inhibit the action of ptyalin, a starch digesting enzyme that originates in salivary secretions. It will not act in even a mildly acidic medium. Proper chewing assures mixing of foods with ptyalin, but the enzyme can become inactivated upon contact with the ingested acids and not be able to work before gastric hydrochloric acid is secreted.

- **Do not mix sugars with starches.**

  Sugars, sweet fruit, and honey ferment if delayed in the stomach. Such a delay can occur if the sweets in the mouth inhibit the formation of ptyalin. This enzyme is necessary for the preparatory stages of starch digestion to trigger the movement on to the intestine where proper digestion of starches takes place. Do not drink sweetened drinks and eat breads at the same time.

- **Eat melons by themselves.**

  Melons are so simple to digest, they move directly to the intestine without inducing the formation of enzymes and hydrochloric acid. If other foods hold the melon in the stomach, it can ferment. It is acceptable to eat berries with melons.

- **Do not drink milk.**

  Man is the only creature that drinks milk beyond the age of weaning. Milk causes mucous in the colon, allergies, and malabsorption of nutrients, and neutralizes the hydrochloric acid in the stomach. Milk should not, consequently, not be taken with any protein. The lesson is don't touch!

Food Combining Charts

The following two charts are for use in choosing foods for combination with each other in the same meal. Those boxes that are connected by lines may be combined. Do not combine foods if their boxes are not connected. For example, whenever you eat protein, meat, fish, fowl, eggs, gelatin, nuts, seeds, or cereal, do not eat bread, potatoes, lima beans, corn, or rice at the same time.

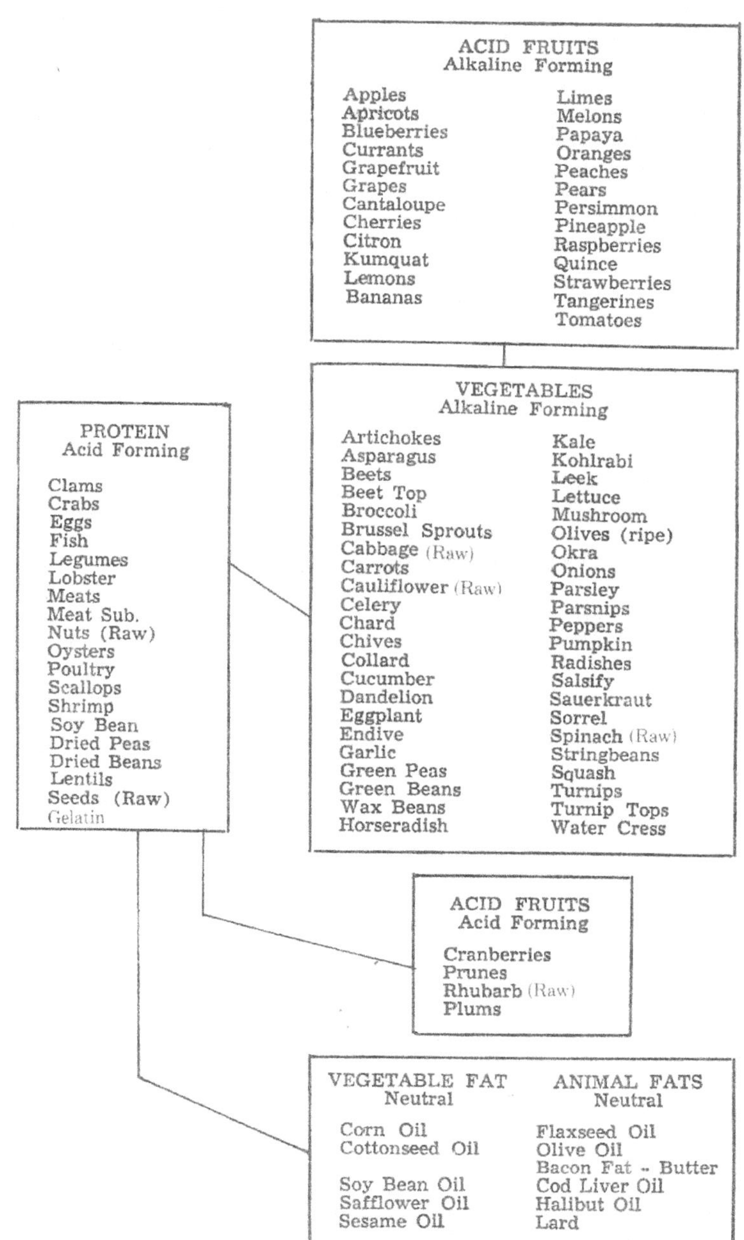

Figure 1: Combining proteins with other foods

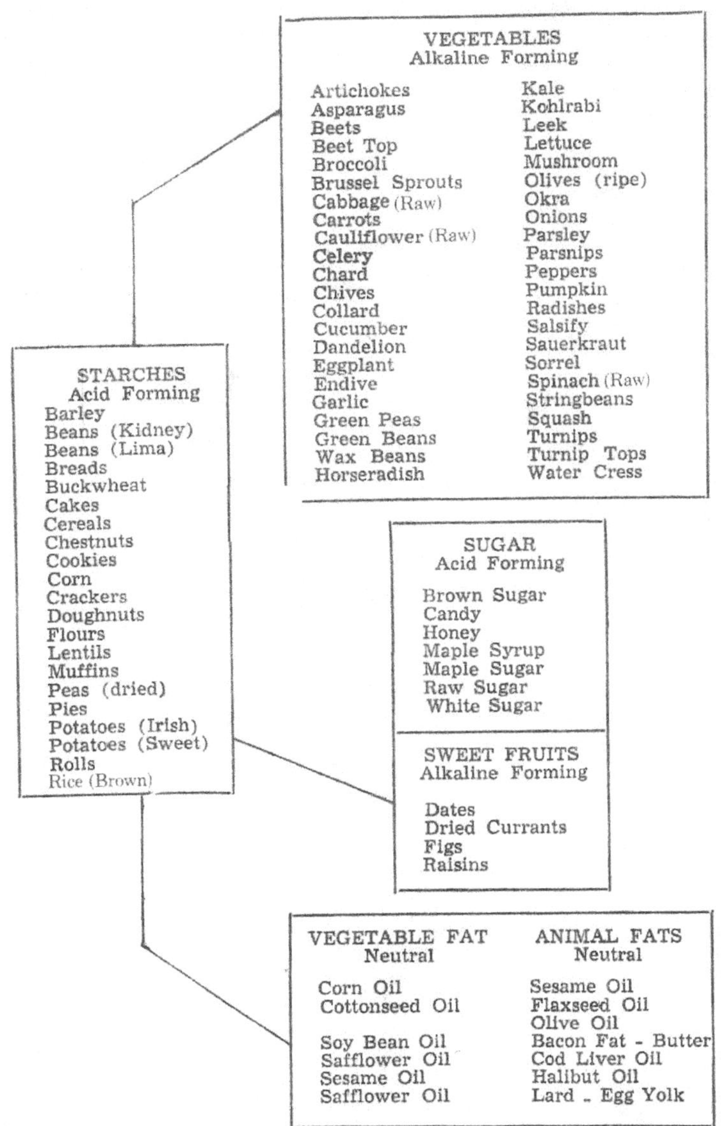

Figure 2: Combining starches with other foods

4 The Water We Drink

I have checked cities in 40 states altogether, and I don't know of a city water supply that's fit for anybody to drink from. Even the Environmental Protection Agency (EPA) has shown that the city water of 89 of the largest cities in the United States has the potential to cause cancer.

What is contaminating the water supplies? Pollution from the air, nitrates and nitrites that farmers put on crops, and pesticides and herbicides that are being used. This amounts to chemical warfare; when the rain comes down where does it pour? Into our lakes and rivers; that's where we are taking the water for drinking. We're going to have to recycle our urine, feces, and everything else to get our water supply, if we don't look out. Because that's where we're going; it's up to each one of us to develop healthy priorities within ourselves and fight to remain healthy.

Making the Headlines

The headline in an article that I saw in a Pittsburgh newspaper says, *Tap water is inferior, the United States reports*. The information in this article was provided by the Department of Health, Education, and Welfare. To the side of the article, it states, "It was not unusual to find undesirable bacteria, arsenic, lead, barium, cadmium and other chemical delicacies in the tap water samples." Believe you me, when you start doing some checking on water, you will find how true it is, because we're doing it all of the time.

There are all kinds of unwanted contaminants in drinking water. For instance, the chemical element cadmium competes with and displaces zinc in the human metabolic processes. Excess cadmium provokes high blood pressure. One place where you pick up cadmium is in your drinking water, the other place is from smoking cigarettes. **Almost everyone in the United States is being poisoned by some type of metal pollutant.**

This is the work of Dr. Henry A. Schroeder, who probably knew more about minerals and their activity within the human body than anyone else that I know of. One of the most important additives to water that we are watching today is chlorine; a cancer link is claimed. When pesticides, weedicides, nitrates, and nitrites are present in the water supply, the added chlorine combines with many of these chemicals and sets up a chloroform type of chemical that is a carcinogen.

Let's look at another headline, *Whatever happened to pure water?* Here's another real good one, *Sewer Seepage, threat to the wells.* The Triple F Foods people in Des Moines, Iowa (covers an area of seven states) have been able to prove that any septic tank or any farmer putting nitrates or nitrites within 10 miles of a spring or well, will cause these contaminants to go into that spring or well. And you see, you're not too safe even with springs or wells today.

Here's the one that came out of the San Francisco Sentinel, *Bad winds blow poison waste, state study warns.* If you ever go out to San Francisco and walk around that bay, you will know what we're talking about, because you can smell it very easily.

Here's the water story on the difference between raw tap water and softened water. **Never use softened water for drinking purposes; the salt or the chemicals that are put in can be most harmful to the human body. The salt gets in there and throws the balance of sodium and potassium right out of line.** It gets you into all kinds of problems, so we tell you very definitely to stay away from it.

Increased concern is found about air and water pollution. This is the Harris survey.

Here comes one out of New Rochelle N.Y. back in 1972, *Clear water isn't necessarily good.*

Editor: For current information on contaminants in water supplies, see the following link. http://water.usgs.gov/nawqa/studies/domestic_wells/.

The Politics of Water

I had a patient that used to come in with vague aches and pains as if he was getting a slight cold, runny nose. I'd get them cleared up and he would be good for maybe two, three, four weeks. Then, he would be back in the office for the same thing all over again. This went on for about six months and I said, "I'd like you to bring me a sample of your water." Now his family lived out in the country, on the side of a hill. He said, "What's the matter? Our water tastes real good. It looks clear you know, nice sandy type of loam out there; everything's fine." I said, "I still want that sample; I'm going to have it analyzed." Which I did.

The analysis came back stating that his water was unfit for human consumption. So we decided to do a little investigating. We found out that six months earlier, on the opposite side of this hill, a new house had been put in, and the septic tank apparently wasn't installed properly, because the overflow started early. It went into the underground water supply that was going through the hill and came up into the opposite side of the hill, where my patient lived.

Of course, from then on we knew what the answer was; they would have to boil it. The only thing that was wrong was the bacteria. So if they use this water for humans or animals, they would have to boil this water, or drill a new well somewhere else, to get away from those bacteria.

In Wisconsin, it took three years to get Dr. Mittelstaedt to realize how important water was in his practice. So, Dr. Oscar Rasmussen, Executive Vice-President of Lorne Pharmical

Company, and I got to talking about water. As research director for Armor and Co., he had a lot of experience with feed lots and farming; he and I lectured many times together.

Finally we got it across to Dr. Mittelstaedt. He still didn't want to believe It, but he went home and drew a circle of 10 miles around Marshfield, Wisconsin. These farmers, were having all of these vague aches and pains; he made every one of them send in a sample of water. Then, the State of Wisconsin did spring water analysis; every one that came back showed that their water was unfit for human consumption. Well, that also meant that their animals were getting the same diseased water, so it wasn't any good for them either. And here you are, right in the middle of the cheese and milk industry, being fed water that wasn't fit for anybody to drink.

What do you think is going to happen to the products coming out of those animals alone? So I said, "Gee that's funny, I guess we'll have to get them on distilled water and mineral supplements." Then Dr. Mittelstaedt drew a circle of 25 miles around Marshfield, Wisconsin and wrote to each town to get a copy of their water analysis. Again he found absolutely not one city's water fit for human consumption.

On the back of one of his own patient's slips that came back from the state, was a note about the number four well in Marshfield. They have five wells that they draw their water out of for the city water supply. The note stated, "This water is very diseased. Don't use it for human consumption." So Dr. Mittelstaedt took it to his attorney and had him notarize it before he turned it in. He then sent it to the water board, saying, "Unfortunately this has come to me and being a health doctor, I am vitally interested to know not only what this well has been doing and what you are going to do with it in the future, but about the other four wells. Have you had them checked? What are you going to do about their future if they also are contaminated? If one is in that area, in all probability, most of them are contaminated." Three years after he issued that challenge, Dr. Mittelstaedt still had not received an answer to his letter, and that number four well was still being used to supply water to the people of that town.

Disaster in the Mouth

If true preventive dentistry were more widely practiced, the American mouth would not be the disaster area that it is. More than 25 million people put their choppers in a glass every night. 95% have cavities – more than one billion cavities and 75% have gum disease. Dental problems are proliferating faster than the nation's dentists can cope with them.

When you get this kind of report, you realize that fluoridated toothpastes aren't stopping cavities, and they don't. They actually do more damage to the gums. If you want to do the best thing, never scrub your teeth. You should never put a toothbrush on them. What you should scrub, is the gums. Get that circulation into that gum, then you won't have that problem with cavitation. Also stay off of sugar.

Rats given fluoride in their drinking water at levels as low as in some cities water systems developed abnormalities that led to miscarriages, still births, and birth defects. One other little thing, fluoride poisoning as a result of ingesting fluoride salts is a serious environmental hazard for both children and adults. Inhalation results in inflammatory changes in the lungs that can progress to pulmonary emphysema. In systemic absorption, the ion binds to circulating calcium causing severe hypocalcemia, tetany, and cardiac arrhythmias. Laundry powders may be one of the main sources of fluoride.

Fluoridation of Public Water Supply

Probably the big one that we talk about most is the work of Dr. Dean Burk, the former head of the cancer division, of the National Cancer Institute in Washington. I don't know much about the use of fluoridation in Canada, but I do know that some of the research done in Toronto and Montreal has shown that if fluoridated water is used for a person on a kidney machine, the patient is always dead within 24 hours. The medical school in Toronto took a look at children between the ages of four and sixteen who were using fluoride toothpaste to stop cavitations in teeth. They found out that these children swallowed between 20% and 26% of the toothpaste.

Dr. Ali H. Mohammed at the University of Missouri, Kansas City, said, "Cities began adding fluoride to their water supply 20-25 years ago and now some 95 million are drinking artificially fluoridated water." This statement appeared in the San Francisco newspapers, but not in Los Angeles. Los Angeles is the only city over a million people in the U.S. that is not fluoridated. The National Health Federation took out ads in a big campaign when this came up on their referendum, and San Francisco voted it down 56 to 44%.

Let's do a little interesting mathematics. Early on, the United States Government, mandated one part per million (ppm) of fluoride in drinking water. They have now reduced it to 0.75 ppm. But for illustration, let's use one ppm; it's easier mathematics. If children swallow a portion of the toothpaste that most everybody is using these days, all users are going to consume additional fluoride. All canned vegetables are packed in fluoridated water, at least they are in the states. Add this to the fluoride that is coming from air pollution, and it is an impossibility for your body to stay at even one ppm; therefore the actual level becomes poisonous. **One thing of great interest to me is that fluoridated water destroys the production of hydrochloric acid in your stomach, an absolute necessity for digesting food, and it antagonizes iodine, needed by a variety of tissues.**

The Fluoride Movement

The fluoride movement was started by a dentist in Deaf Smith County, Texas. He had found that their water was pretty high in calcium fluoride. He wasn't a biochemist, so he didn't realize that calcium fluoride is the natural or organic form. He didn't see that many cavities around there, so he gave credit to it. **The corporations picked this up, because the end product of aluminum manufacturing is the inorganic form of fluoride, sodium silica fluoride.** The only good that it was ever used for was rat poisoning and for etching glass. They had stock piles of it all over the place and didn't know what to do with it to get rid of it. So they hooked onto the idea of this dentist. **They let everybody believe that the inorganic fluorides were the same as the organic fluorides, which is 100% wrong!** Today you're seeing stannous fluorides; these are all in the inorganic form, and that's why they are so harmful to the human body. They make your bones brittle.

You know, when I was practicing over in Grand Rapids and got started on this thing, I went to the dental laboratories that were making false teeth, bridges, and plates. I went to one of them asking, "How much has your dental work increased (having teeth pulled, installing plates, and inserting bridges) since we've been on fluorides?" This was about 10 years after they started it. "Oh," the owner said, "We're doing about 500% more business today than we did before the fluoridation rose, 10 years ago." I should have had him put this in writing. Well I went to every dental lab and got the same answer.

Then I went to all of the suppliers of fracture materials that supplied all our hospitals and the doctors in the area. We found out that the amount of fracture material that they were selling had increased by 800%. So I published this, and it came back to Dr. Protho who was the head of the Health Division, and, of course, we were both on the Kent County Mental Health Board at the time. He brought this up and asked me, "Would you happen to know anything about this? I know you work in this field." I said, "Yes, I'm the one who published it." He said, "Well, you know that's wrong." I said, "No, it isn't doctor. I went around to every one of these dental labs and to every one of the suppliers of fracture material to the hospitals and doctors."

That's when I realized that I should have had it in writing, because that's what he asked me for, "'Where's your proof?" "Well..." I said, "To me, I believe in the honesty of people. If these people are honorable in their business, then I have no reason to doubt them, but if you want to say that they are dishonorable, that's up to you. As far as I am concerned, they are honorable people and I'm going to leave it that way whether you want to believe it or not, it's still true."

Distilled Water

We tell you today, to drink distilled water. Now we hear a lot of people say, "Drinking distilled water demineralizes you." Well, this is not true, there is no research that proves this. The one thing that it doesn't do for you is give you the necessary minerals. As a result of not giving them to you, you can have a depletion occur in the body. That's why we tell you to have a hair analysis to tell you what your minerals are doing in your body. Then, you supplement to your mineral deficiencies. With respect to distillers, I think one of the better ones today, is this New World distiller. It takes little space, and you can hook it right up to your water supply and let it run on a constant basis.

Editor: The New World Distiller Corporation of Gravette, Arkansas is no longer in business. It is suggested that the reader review the selection of distillers on the internet, beginning with http://www.purewaterinc.com/Shop-Water-Distillers.

5 Milk and Milk Products

I believe that milk and milk products are the number one cause of disease! I have found it to be the leading cause of colds, sinus conditions, asthma, bronchitis, and mucous colitis. No moo for you!

Milk is a product made by a human or animal mother to supply adequate food for her offspring. This milk is intended to be the baby's food until its own digestive enzymes begin to be produced in sufficient quantity to digest solid food. When the transfer is appropriate, the mother's breasts dry up and return to their normal size. The cow does the same thing for its calf as a mother does for her baby – if left alone within her natural habitat.

The first recorded incidence of an infant being given cow's milk was in 1793. Since then, many articles have been written, stating that milk is the perfect food for man, supplying all or most of his daily needs. Included among these publications are magazines such as *Life* and *Time*, as well as nutritional periodicals and even literature published by the Department of Agriculture.

I've performed more than 25,000 blood tests for my patients. These tests show conclusively, in my opinion, that adults who use milk products do not absorb nutrients as well as adults who don't. Of course, poor absorption, in turn, means chronic fatigue.

Jefferson Medical College in Philadelphia, in a course on heart attacks and strokes, taught that they have found that milk and milk products to be the greatest single cause of heart attacks in humans. Because of its mucous formation it can be one of the main causes of crib deaths. Milk forms mucous, giving the baby a hard time breathing: they twist and turn getting the bedclothes all over themselves, but they actually suffocate from the mucous in the bronchial tubes. It is published that 30,000 deaths a year are due to milk and milk products.

Dr. Lynn Ferguson of the Ferguson-Droste-Ferguson Rectal Hospital in Grand Rapids, Michigan, stated before a group at the American Medical Association meeting in 1961, that they would have to close the doors of their 200 bed hospital within a year if all people stopped using milk and milk products.

Before a group at the 1962 AMA meeting, a pediatrician from Miami stated that milk is strictly an infant food and should, like toys and rattles, be discarded when the child leaves infancy. *Science News* reported that a growth hormone from the malfunctioning pituitary gland has been isolated from milk. In my opinion, this is one reason why we see large thighs and fannies on our young girls and why boys are growing so tall today. Normally, a cow dries up on the completion of the weaning of its calf; however, today a cow is stimulated first by the continuous milking process, which sends a hormonal stimulus to the pituitary gland to secrete the mammary stimulating hormone. This anterior pituitary hormone is found in the milk that children and adults drink! (*Science Newsletter*, Sept. 24, 1964).

Now as we were discussing the anterior pituitary hormone, these people with the real beautiful type of skins, whitish skins, white texture, beautiful color; this is where you find that anterior pituitary hormone. You can walk up to those people and say, "You're highly allergic to milk." If you take it on a daily basis, you have your body so poisoned, that you don't realize what these symptoms are that are hitting you. But if you stay away from it for 90 days and then try it, you will find out how fast it really hits you.

Milk is the greatest cause of human disease that I know of. I have challenged every milk industry in the world to prove on a scientific basis that cow's milk or goat's milk can be used on human beings without harm. So far, not one of them have accepted my challenge.

In 1978, the *Health View Newsletter* came over, interviewed me, and published *The Truth About Milk* by Dr. William A. Ellis (Letter #14). As a result, the dairy industry immediately challenged me and told me I didn't know what I was talking about. So Sam Biser, the Editor, wrote to them and said "All right, we want you to write a 4,000 word treatise. We'll publish it in opposition. But we want scientific facts."

All we got was propaganda, 4,000 words, so it wasn't published. In December, two and a half years after the first one had been published, came a little excerpt by Robert Kowalski, the head of the American Dairy Council, "If you send me 50¢, we will tell you the truth that was not told by Dr. Ellis in his article *The Truth About Milk*. I sent in my 50¢. I waited the rest of December, all of January, and right up to the last day in February, and I still hadn't received anything. So I sat down and wrote a letter to Mr. Kowalski. "Dear Mr. Kowalski, I noticed this little excerpt in the Health View Newsletter that said that if I sent you 50¢, you would send me the scientific evidence that cow's milk is good for people. I sent you 50¢ back in December." Three months later, I have received nothing and fired back, "Unless you answer this, I am going to turn you over to the Postmaster for using the mails to defraud." Believe it or not, I got the exact same sheets of paper that Sam Biser had received three years before — all propaganda, absolutely nothing truthful about it. No scientific experiments had been done.

Editor: For a recent review on the role of dairy products in the human diet, see *Dairy: Milking It for All It's Worth* by Dr. Loren Cordain, author of *The Paleo Diet* at http://thepaleodiet.com/dairy-milking-worth/. This article reviews the history of how milk became part of the human diet in conjunction with the domestication of animals 10,000 years ago. A short quote from this article reads as follows. "...we are the only species on the planet to consume another animal's milk throughout our adult lives. Humans don't have a nutritional requirement for the milk of another species, nor do any other mammals. An increasing body of scientific evidence supports the evolutionary caution that this dietary practice is not necessarily harmless."

Human vs. Cow's Milk

A calf has four stomachs; a human being, one. We humans simply do not possess the digestive enzymes found in the calf's third and fourth stomachs that allow him to digest milk. So, even if the milk is raw, we cannot digest it properly. Homogenized milk takes three or more hours to be digested and leave the stomach; a human mother's milk leaves the infant's stomach in less than 45 minutes.

The human baby develops his brain first, while the animal develops his bone structure first; therefore, milk for a human, and that for an animal naturally should be different. The calf develops his bone structure first and doubles his weight in the first 30 days. Approximately 90 pounds at birth, it will weigh 1,000 pounds at the end of its weaning period. Growing calves need more protein to enable them to grow quickly in size. Human infants, on the other hand, need less protein and more fat as their energies are expended primarily in the development of the brain, spinal cord, and nerves. In humans, the brain develops rapidly during the first year of life, growing faster than the body and tripling in size by the age of one.

Protein Content

The proteins in milk can be divided into two categories: casein and whey. 100 gm of whole cow's milk (3.3 gm) has more than double the protein of human milk (1.3 gm), and most of this protein is the soluble phosphoprotein, caseinogen. Cow's milk has a ratio of casein to whey proteins of 80:20, while human milk contains these in a ratio of 40:60, respectively. Problematically, in the stomach of human babies, caseinogen is converted by the enzyme rennin (before pepsin formation) to the insoluble casein, a form more difficult for babies to digest.

Probably 50% or more of the protein in cow's milk is wasted. The sole purpose for rennin is milk digestion. As other digestive enzymes and hydrochloric acid appear, rennin disappears. Rennin leaves the human stomach by two years of age, at which time all milk and milk products should be stopped. The protein in human milk is lactalbumin which is soluble and easily digested. It is utilized by the baby easily, with virtually 100% efficiency. A baby raised on mother's milk will have more body flexibility and adaptability.

Fat Content

The total amount of fat in cow's milk is almost equal to that of human milk, but they differ in the type and proportions. Cow's milk contains more saturated fat while human milk contains more unsaturated fat, as shown in Table 3.

Table 3: **Comparison of Fat Content, Bovine vs. Human Milk**

Proportion of Types of Fat in Milk British Food Standards Agency (FSA)	
100 gm of Cow's Milk	**100 gm of Human Milk**
2.5 gm saturated	1.8 gm saturated
1.0 gm monounsaturated	1.6 gm monounsaturated
0.1 gm polyunsaturated	0.5 gm polyunsaturated

The higher level of unsaturated fatty acids in human milk reflects the important role of these fats in brain development. The brain is largely composed of fat, and early brain development and function in humans requires a sufficient supply of polyunsaturated essential fatty acids. The omega-6 fatty acid, arachidonic acid (AA), and the omega-3 fatty acid, docosahexaenoic acid (DHA) are both essential for brain development and functioning. Both are generously supplied in human milk but not in cow's milk.

Other Nutrients

Although human milk contains less calcium than cow's milk, the calcium in human milk is better absorbed into the body than the calcium in cow's milk, again illustrating why human milk is the best source of nutrition during the first year of life. The best source of calcium depends on what you need. If you are going to build the immune system, the best source is calcium lactate. If you want to build the bones, the best source is raw veal bone.

The high protein, sodium, potassium, phosphorus, and chloride content of cow's milk present what is called a high renal solute load; this means that the unabsorbed solutes from the diet must be excreted via the kidneys. This can place a strain on immature kidneys forcing them to draw water from the body, thus increasing the risk of dehydration. Furthermore, cow's milk is low in vitamin C and vitamin D (Department of Health, 1994), and contains less vitamin A than human milk.

Importance of Breast Feeding

Mother's milk transfers immunity to the baby and implants enough intestinal bacteria to be the basis for a lifetime supply needed for resistance to infectious diseases. The most important milk, cow or human, is that milk produced in the first 10 hours after birth. The reasons it is important are threefold:

- Acidophilus bacilli are present for starting the normal intestinal flora for the intestinal tract. They are there only for the first 10 hours.
- An enzyme is present that activates the stomach and the intestinal tract to digest food. It starts all of the digestibility system of the cells. When we have separated calves from their mothers, milked the mothers, and then fed the milk out of the pan to the calves, those calves never develop like the ones that suckle off their mothers' nipples. The reason for it is that the enzyme in the nipple is there to help digest the milk. Air destroys that enzyme.

- A reflex mechanism that takes place during suckling makes the uterus contract, and thus stops the bleeding from the placental attachment area.

Humans are the only ones who do not know how to get from the birth canal to the breast of its mother. As soon as animals are born, they start wiggling and know exactly how to get to the nipples of their mothers. As soon as they get there, they start sucking. This applies to dogs, cats, calves, pigs, or anything else. Of course, that's the way that you are going to stop the mother from bleeding to death. You girls don't have to have that shot in the tail or pituitary extract to stop you from bleeding. All you have to do is put that baby on that breast, but it should be there within a matter of minutes. As soon as that cord stops pulsating, put a clamp on it, cut it, clean the face, and put the baby right up on the breast.

Children should be breast-fed as long as the mother can stand the teeth of the infant. They should get vegetables, etc., only after nine months to one year of age. The digestive enzyme ptyalin does not develop until six or seven months of age. **Some babies are being fed adult food in the first week; the food is not digested in the stomach, but its presence takes away the hunger feeling. They can get some colic and other problems, and this, in our opinion, is a major cause of disease in later life.**

Our research also shows that breast-fed babies do not run out of hydrochloric acid until they are near 50 years of age. Bottle-fed babies are running out in their late teens and twenties, and most are complete achlorhydrics by the time they reach 40 years of age. We know of one child four years of age that has no hydrochloric acid. When I did the analysis on this, I said to the doctor that this was a bottle-fed baby.

It was the first time that the doctor had heard me say that, so he wrote back, "How did you know?" It's very simple when you know this. Seventeen European researchers in 1972 published that the amino acid leucine in milk and milk products stimulated the beta cells of the Islets of Langerhans, causing an increase in insulin production. Thus, there is a basic cause for hypoglyemia. Continued use over a period of time breaks down the beta cells, causing diabetes.

Allergy to Milk

Today, in the United States, 28% of the food consumed is dairy. Up to 50% of whites, 75% of blacks, and 100% of orientals do not have the lactase enzyme in their bodies to handle lactose, the sugar that is in milk. Lactase is produced by the lining of the small intestine and in the majority of humans, this lactase production stops when weaning takes place in infancy. Only in Europe and America does this lactase production continue after weaning. When lactase production does stop, drinking of milk causes flatulence, bloating, and diarrhea. That is why milk is, in every book that I have looked at, number one on the allergy list. The other ones in the top five are chocolate, wheat, corn, and beef. Naturally, lactose-intolerant whites, blacks, and orientals should not touch milk in any form!

Milk is found to be loaded today with the same colon bacillus as found in the bowel. It lines all mucous membranes with excessive mucous, thus making absorption most difficult. Milk stimulates mucous membranes, so basically it is the main cause of colds, sinusitis, asthma, bronchitis, and mucous colitis. Most all degenerative diseases can be found to be more severe in those using milk or milk products. In most cheeses, also in chocolate, is an enzyme called phenylethylamine, and it is one of the main factors in producing migraine headaches.

A Case of Relapse

When I was practicing in Grand Rapids, this young girl, Delores, who looked like she was 25 years old, but actually was 16, came to see me. She was in the high society group of Washington, D.C., where she lived. She had already been through the John Hopkins asthma clinic at Boston University; it is quite well known all over the world. On this trip she had just come through the Mayo Clinic, trying to find out what was wrong – why she had severe asthma.

Well who am I as a little GP, telling these three great institutions that they don't know anything about asthma? So I again started our usual routine on diet and found out that she was drinking, as the propaganda tells you, three glasses of milk a day, eating ice cream, and this type of thing. So I said to her, "Honey, I think you're old enough and intelligent enough to understand what I'm going to talk to you about."

I told her some of these things about milk. I said, "What I want you to do, you're going to be here a week with your aunt." Her aunt was my patient; that's how she got in. "I want you to stay away from all milk products – even foods that contain any milk products – for the next week while you are here; then I'll tell you about the rest of what we want. Now what I want you to do when you go home, and we talked about this last night when we talked about detoxification, is to take the Fleet's Phospho-Soda, and a lemon enema." That night she had a very mild attack. The next six days she had absolutely no attacks of asthma whatsoever.

She came in on her way back to the airport and to Washington. I said to her, "What I want you to do is just stay away completely from all milk or milk products; we'll give you Pneumotrophin (a protomorphogen of the lung tissue) with some vitamin A and C and calcium lactate." Calcium lactate is best used if you are trying to build antibodies to fight infection; it is not a body builder. I asked her mother after the daughter left, "Would you please report to me periodically, so that I know how she is doing."

Well, like so many of these people, you never hear from them. Six months went by, and I finally got a letter from the mother. It said, "Dear Doctor, three months ago, as I was sitting at my desk to write to you a letter to tell you how great Delores has been doing, I got a telephone call from her girlfriend's mother that Delores was having an asthmatic attack. She asked me to come over and bring the bottle of adrenal cortex that a doctor had given her (we always carried it in a little box with a sterile syringe). So I hotfooted it over there; it was only two doors away from where I lived.

Here was Delores, lying on the floor, having the worst attack that she had ever had. I didn't think she was going to make it. I decided to give her a full cc of adrenal cortex. It took her almost 30 minutes to get enough breath back to start talking. I said to her, "I can't understand how, all of a sudden, you have gotten this attack." She said, "Well mother, as you know at these birthday parties they serve this ice cream and cake. I knew I had no business eating the ice cream, so I was nibbling at the cake when my girlfriend's mother came in and said, 'Delores, why aren't you eating your ice cream and cake? Don't you insult my daughter.'"

I told her that we had found a doctor who said that the cause of my asthma was milk products and that I had no business touching them. Her reply was, "What stupid doctor are you going to? Milk's good for everybody, now you eat it!" I still wasn't that sure, but I took a half a teaspoonful of the ice cream, put it in my mouth, and within 20 seconds was on the floor with an asthmatic attack." That almost killed her. So you can be sure that Delores' mother straightened her out so that she would never serve milk products to someone with an allergy again.

Anything involving the lungs – sinus trouble, asthma, bronchitis – these are the things that are really basically allergies. Every allergy book you look at puts milk and milk products as number one on the list. **The only one thing that we want you to use is butter, because it does not have the enzymes or the hormones.**

I was brought before the Dairy Council in Michigan; their vice-president was my patient and was quite quiet, even though he was usually quite vociferous. It was getting to be time to vote on the question of suing me for the statements I was making, because I talk to many clubs, such as Rotary, Kiwanas, Exchange Club, and others.

One of the other members of the council suddenly realized and asked him why he hadn't said anything. He answered, "I just wanted to see how far you are going to go before you hang yourselves. I have had asthma for many years and I heard that this doctor treated differently than others and I have spent thousands of dollars trying to get rid of my asthma. I went to Dr. Ellis, who knew that I owned a dairy and was on the Dairy Council; he challenged me to go off milk products for 90 days and then go back and try one teaspoon of milk or ice cream or cheese. I accepted his challenge and, when I did try the teaspoon of milk, my asthma hit me in a matter of seconds. Then I had to go home and clean myself out again so I could get rid of it. This man knows more about milk than anyone on this Council. If you really want to make him and ruin the milk industry, you go ahead and sue him." They did not.

Pasteurization

Milk was supposedly pasteurized to destroy bacteria; however, for years, the law stated that raw milk could be sold with a bacterial count up to 10,000 bacteria per ml, but grade A pasteurized milk could be sold with a bacterial count up to 100,000 bacteria per ml, and grade B, 200,000. **Pasteurization is not done to destroy bacteria, it is done to destroy the phosphatase enzyme that helps to turn milk sour.** That is why today, with the destruction of the phosphatase enzyme, milk does not turn sour and therefore It does not need refrigeration.

Watch in the middle of the summer when your milk man goes down the street, you won't find any refrigeration on his truck, because he knows darn well that it won't turn sour. In fact, it won't even spoil with the new method. **Also, with the destruction of the phosphatase enzyme was the loss of our ability to assimilate calcium.** In pasteurization, lecithin is lost by the splitting of phosphorus salts. The casein alters its reaction and forms very hard curds. Some, like curds in skim milk take more than five hours to leave the stomach. The sugar of milk becomes caramelized, the citric acid is destroyed, the lime salts become insoluble, and the oxygen content is decreased.

Another of the major purposes of pasteurization of milk is to stabilize flavor. In the process, lysine becomes unavailable due to its incomplete enzymatic digestion and/or actual destruction in some cases. Milk for evaporation purposes is usually grade B, with a permitted bacteria count many times that of grade A milk. Pasteurization kills these bacteria, but it does not remove their dead bodies.

On Pittsburgh television, the Auto Dairy (automated milking system) announced, "We have now a new method of pasteurization and have done an experiment." They brought a group of people in and gave every one of them a glass of milk poured from a gallon jug, saying to them, "This is our old method of pasteurization. Remember what the taste is, the consistency, everything that you can think about it, then we're going to give you another glass of milk treated by the newest pasteurization method."

They all drank the first glass. The facilitator poured each a glass from another gallon jug, which they all drank. The testers all said that they could not tell any difference. Then, the facilitator said, "We want you to know that our newest method is now being done at 2,000° F. You see this jug that I took off the shelf up here, has been sitting there for the past 28 months." For 28 months it was sitting up there without refrigeration! In other words the 2,000° F has destroyed anything that has a chance of spoiling or turning sour, and that's what is being given to people in Pittsburgh, to be classified as milk. Is this the kind of stuff you want in your system? I don't.

What has science shown? Two universities have found that good, strong calves, at about their second or third month, when taken off breast feeding and fed on their own mother's milk that had been pasteurized beforehand, died of heart attacks within eight months.

Some researchers have questioned the possible effects of pasteurization. Does it affect susceptible individuals, especially children, and cause diarrhea, nausea, or vomiting? Another serious question — since wheat and other grains are usually low in lysine and suffer biological change when heated, milk that is heated will not combine to provide a complete protein, as would otherwise result with unheated milk. When pasteurized or homogenized milk is used, this can pose a serious nutritional problem for millions of children.

Other Dairy Products

Ice cream is nothing more than a chemical concoction. It has a small amount of skim milk powder, and 34 chemicals including artificial colors and flavors that have been on the cancer causative list for at least 30 years. Recently the International Association of Cancer Victims and Friends published a list of all of these chemicals and what they do in the body. If you ever read that list you would never put another bit of ice cream in your mouth, believe me. It took the FDA eight years to get red dye #2 out of food, but now some companies have simply mixed it with another to make a new dye that is more poisonous, and still on the market. They are willing to put a chemical on the market and wait until the FDA tells them to stop. No drug should be put on the market until its manufacturer has researched to establish its safety.

Buttermilk today is made from skim milk with streptococcus lactic acid bacteria added. It is then incubated at a carefully controlled temperature until the right acidity is reached. Then, they add yellow butter flecks to some for visual effect. Cottage cheese, in the factory that I visited, is not the old-fashioned Smearcase as we old-timers knew it. Today they add bacteria to skim milk to make it curd. The curds are pulled off and washed with hippuric acid to destroy the bacteria. I don't know how many of you city folks have been around horses after they urinated, but that nice strong odor that you get out of that urine is hippuric acid; I just want to keep you up to date on all of these things! Then they add 13 chemicals, one of which is a drying agent very similar to plaster of paris, and what remains, is sold to you as cottage cheese.

Yoghurt is in the same category. The milk that you get in yoghurt does more harm than the good that you get from the acidophilus bacilli. It's much simpler today to take freeze-dried acidophilus bacilli in a little tablet containing anywhere from six million to 100 million bacteria. You get the beneficial bacteria without milk allergens.

You see, to me anything that is 51% harmful and 49% good you had better stay away from, because it's going to add up and get you. And that's why I quit yoghurt and kefir both. One of my good friends Is the public relations man for a dairy company. He and I fight on this – lots of times on programs – he gets up and tells all of the virtues and good things about milk, and I get up and tell what I'm telling you about milk. So we really confuse the audience. I have found that it takes four days to get over the ill effects of one teaspoon full of any milk product, except butter, so I say to you, "Stay off all milk products for 90 days. Then just try one teaspoonful of milk, or ice cream, or a piece of cheese and watch how fast, within seconds, it clogs up your throat and nose with mucous and gives you a harder time breathing." It really does a job.

Butter is OK

Butter does not contain the enzymes and hormones found in other milk products. Never use axle grease (better known as margarine) anytime. It is too hard to digest. The leucine that stimulates insulin production in the B-cells of the Islets of Langerhans Is not found in butter, but only in milk. **Below is a direct quotation from *Margarine vs. Butter,* published in the *Lancet,* April 6, 1974.**

"The trend throughout the world today is to incorporate an ever-increasing amount of the polyunsaturated fats into human diets. And there is considerable evidence that this practice is not exactly contributing to a glorious old age. Quite the contrary, especially when the source of that polyunsaturated fat (so-called) is margarine, which has taken the place of butter in the butter dishes of more than two-thirds of all Americans.

Recent research points to margarine as a source of a substance which has been termed a far greater health risk than various cholesterol-containing supplements such as beef fat, butter fat, and powdered eggs, which it has supplanted in so many diets. **Dr. Fred Kummerow, a food chemist at the University of Illinois, says that this factor in margarine is causing atherosclerosis – the hardening of the arteries deemed the major triggering cause of coronary heart disease.**

Dr. Kummerow said that while margarine based on soybean oil is high in unsaturated fats in its original form, in actual commercial practice in the United States margarine producers utilize a process that converts a certain percentage of these fats – varying up to 30 per cent – to saturated forms. These converted fats, designed to make the product more stable, are called trans fats. **When Kummerow and his associates fed different types of diets to different groups of swine for eight months and then slaughtered them, they found that the trans fatty acids – margarine base stock – was more atherogenic than various cholesterol-containing substances like beef fat, butter and eggs.**

Even the highly touted polyunsaturated oils can be dangerous to health when they are heated, according to some very important research carried on at the Institute of Nutritional Chemistry at the University of Helsinki. Dr. Rakel Kurkela and his associates raised experimental animals on a standard diet, with a supplement of various fats, either in unheated native form or heated at a frying temperature for 20 hours. These fats were used in two different ways: heated and aerated (in an open dish, exposed to air as in frying) or heated and unaerated in a closed area (like baking). Fresh fats in the native state were also used.

The experiment lasted 10 to 30 days. Weight increases were measured daily. Those of the experimental animals on a diet supplement of butter had approximately the same weight gain whether the butter was heated and aerated or fed in a fresh unheated native state. In contrast, the animals which received unsaturated safflower oil in an unheated native state gained more weight than those raised on the butter. But, those animals receiving safflower oil which was heated and aerated had no weight gain at all. At the end of the 13 days of the experiment, all of the animals of this group were in poor condition. This shows, says Dr. Kurkela, that poisonous substances had formed during the aerating and heating of the oil. When these experiments were continued, all of the animals died.

How do you get the essential fats into your diet without lowering the boom on your chances for a healthy old age? Put the butter back in the butter dish. Natural butter, in moderation, is rich in vitamins A, D and E, which protect it from oxidation. To increase the butter's content of essential fatty acids, try this recipe for a modified butter: mix a half pound of softened butter with a half cup of a good pressed oil. Mold it in your butter dish and keep refrigerated. It tastes delicious. But for cooking, use the plain butter or olive oil. Raw seeds and nuts, freshly cracked, whole wheat and wheat germ are good sources of essential fatty acids. Make sure, though, that the wheat germ is fresh and not rancid.

If you have trouble digesting fats, you can get your essential fatty acids without eating them. Rub them into your skin. Dr. Martin Press and associates at the Royal Postgraduate Medical School at the Unilever Research Laboratory in Sharnbrook, Bedford, England, report that daily skin applications of sunflower seed oil rapidly corrected EFA deficiencies brought about by massive small bowel resections in three patients. In two of the patients, fatty acid patterns virtually returned to normal within 12 weeks. What's more, it took only two to three mg of linoleic acid per Kg to do the job. This, the researchers note, is at least 10 times less than any previous estimates of' the amount required. When rubbed into the skin, they explain, linoleic acid is incorporated directly into circulating lipoproteins, bypassing the liver, where a great deal of it may be oxidized."

Editor: In the years since Dr. Ellis' passing in 1986, there have been many studies on the effects of dairy products in the diet. An extensive review article entitled *White Lies* that supports many of Dr. Ellis' opinions about milk and milk products is posted on the Viva! Health website at http://www.vegetarian.org.uk/campaigns/whitelies/wlreport02.shtml#vvf.

6 Detoxification

When you go to a doctor and are given a drug, a shot, or a prescription will it go into a cell that is filled with toxic material? You are just wasting your money. Get these toxins out of your system so your doctor has a chance to make an accurate diagnosis! Also, following detoxification, an individual's diagnosis will, in all probability, be entirely different from the admitting one!

Everything you eat and the way in that your body handles it depends on how toxic you are; i.e., whether your system needs to be detoxified. "Being toxic" means that the body is reabsorbing toxic materials from the digestive tract. Such materials include not only dyes and other chemicals but, more commonly, the products of inefficient digestive processes.

Digestion

There is a temporal order to the digestion of food, beginning in the mouth. The food must be chewed sufficiently. Most people attack their food and gulp the large particles rather than chew them properly. If the chewing action is complete, the bolus of food contains sufficient amounts of salivary enzymes and is alkaline so that it can trigger the stomach to produce hydrochloric acid.

The churning action of the stomach admixes hydrochloric acid into the food; the bolus now becomes acidic. This acidity triggers the flow of bile, which is highly alkaline. Bile neutralizes the hydrochloric acid as the bolus enters the small intestine, where the pancreatic secretions are favored by an alkaline environment. As the digested materials enter the large intestine, there is again encountered a more acidic environment where bacterial flora further break down the foods and aid in the absorption of whatever products are formed at that stage.

Each successive step depends on the efficiency of the previous one. For the sake of illustration, let's assume that we eat only perfect quality foods in the proper combinations. Eating such good quality foods, how can one become toxic? Generally, by the time a person reaches his late teens or early twenties, he does not produce enough hydrochloric acid or pepsin in the stomach, especially if he has been bottle-fed.

The most important thing in your life is the colostrum in the first two hours after birth. These secretions help establish the way the digestive system will work all of the rest of your life. If you do not get these enzymes and bacteria, improper digestion will be a lifelong problem. In addition, we are in the habit of inadequately chewing our foods. The particles are too large by the time we swallow them, and this does not expose enough surface area for subsequent digestion. An insufficient amount of hydrochloric acid cannot provide enough acidity to induce bile secretion. Therefore, insufficient alkalinity for the optimum environment for pancreatic enzymes to work, etc. This leaves a herculean task for the acidophilus and bifidus bacilli to complete the digestive process. They simply cannot do as much as is required by inadequate digestion above the large intestine. Therefore, they produce undesirable breakdown products that are absorbed back into our bodies and that ruin the environment for the beneficial organisms. It becomes too toxic to support their growth. Inefficient breakdown of protein is termed putrefaction; inefficient breakdown of fats is called rancidification; inefficient breakdown of carbohydrates is termed fermentation. These are generally anaerobic processes that eventually produce an alkaline condition in the intestine with subsequent constipation and gas.

Resorption (reabsorption) of putrefied, rancidified, and fermented substances from the now sluggish bowel manifests itself in bad breath, body odor, and, as mentioned before, constipation. Other indications are a coated tongue, pasty skin, excessive bowel gas, too much oil on the skin, metallic or soapy taste, headaches behind the eyes, fatigue, and irritability. All of these symptoms are quite unnecessary, and the toxic condition should be avoided. Before one is able to sensibly attack any problem concerning health, he must ensure that he is detoxified! It is vitally important to remove the poisonous materials that develop from poor digestion and assimilation and correct your eating habits so that the food becomes available and usable after passing through the proper areas of the digestive system.

Four Avenues of Detoxification

One thing that we have learned is that most people don't know how to detoxify themselves. **You must detoxify the body before you do anything else, because if it's filled with a lot of poisons and toxins, I don't care how many vitamins, minerals, enzymes or hormones, drugs or medicines you ingest; they can't get in. It's already full.** If they do try to get in, they can then push themselves out, and then we start seeing tumor formations. So that's something you definitely don't want to get into. So where do we start as far as detoxification is concerned?

We must understand the four avenues of detoxification — the lungs, the skin, the kidneys, and the bowel. Also, to some extent, the hair removes toxic minerals from the body. This post extension process is slow, however, and is a better indication of the presence of toxic metals than it is a way of eliminating such substances.

Lungs

The one that most people do not think about are the lungs. If you have a bad breath, it means you are constipated, because you're not getting the poisons out of your body any other way, so it's coming up through the lungs and out through the mouth. You can have infections as far as the teeth and the gums are concerned, but we find most bad body odors are caused by one thing — putrefied proteins. If you have a bad odor, but if it's not too bad, it is probably from fermented starch or sugar. Persons with bad breath (halitosis) are probably constipated. The use of Clorets can help eliminate the odor but does nothing to eliminate the cause. Remember these things. See Cleansing the Lungs on page 102.

Pores of the Skin

People do not like to have a body odor, so now they're doing something that is extremely harmful. They're using underarm antiperspirants, all of which block free perspiration, keeping the impurities from being excreted through the pores. All they're doing is stopping the flow of perspiration, keeping it in their bodies so they don't get rid of the poisons, and therefore they're going to break down.

Under no circumstances should you use an underarm antiperspirant. It is loaded with aluminum, which interferes with the circulation of every blood vessel in your body. We see this in the alteration of the ability of your body to take minerals from the bloodstream and get them into the cell to work properly. One thing that most people do not realize is that you urinate just as much as you perspire in one year. As you sit, you are perspiring. You may not realize it, but you are. That is why it is so necessary that we get enough fluids into our system to work on a daily basis. See Cleansing Through the Pores on page 102.

Kidneys

The third avenue that we have to think about is the kidneys. The kidneys must eliminate wastes and toxic products, but a tremendous strain is put on them in the toxic person. The kidneys are vital. That's why we do our standard types of urinalysis so we know what is going on. The microscopic portion of that is even more important than the actual amounts that tell you you might have a little albumin coming through with the ketones or the acetones, these are little things that we constantly look for. **Now any of you who may have any difficulty urinating, such as burning or itching after urination, it means one thing. You are too alkaline (the urine pH is too high).**

You see, all of these diseases in the genital urinary tract come when your body is too alkaline. Test the pH (that's your acid-alkaline balance) with a little litmus paper when you have these kinds of irritations; you will always find the pH to be above 7. A pH of 7 is neutral; normal should be on the acid side between 5 and 6. That is where we want to keep it. Here's another secret. If you have an itch anywhere on your body, you are too alkaline. It is very important to understand this. In all degenerative diseases that I have been able to find since I got into this research business, the people are too alkaline. See Cleansing the Kidneys on page 103.

Bowel

The big one, of course, is the bowel. The villi of the bowel must be clean with no materials or excessive mucous adhering to the bowel wall. These block absorption and elimination of wastes from the tissues into the bowel. **The most important thing is that you definitely have a bowel movement on a daily basis.**

An absolutely normal daily bowel movement is 1" in diameter, and it should be at least 18" long, whether you go once, twice or three times during the day. Now take a look at it; you should always take a look after you have had a bowel movement. If you don't have that one incher – if it starts getting smaller and smaller – what is it? You've got allergies. That causes the swelling of the mucous membranes in your rectum and up in your nose; the two ends of the tract is where you get it. That's where allergies hit you. See Cleansing the Bowel on page 103.

And where do you go from there? What causes it to shrink up? You see, when that fecal mass comes down and hits that swollen mucous membrane, you have a bunch of hemorrhoids. The other little thing I should tell you is don't read when you go to the toilet. You don't have any support down there and it all drops down and you have more hemorrhoids. When you have the urge to go, go in and get your business done; get off the hopper and get out of there in a hurry.

Cleansing the Lungs

Four steps are important to cleansing the lungs. First, put yourself in a private, healthy environment with clean air; then follow the steps as listed below.

1. Place the tip of the tongue at the base of the teeth, roof of mouth.
2. Breath in totally through the nose.
3. Let out 3/4 of the air with with an explosive HA! sound.
4. Without breathing in, expel more air with the HA! sound.
5. Again, without breathing in again, empty the lungs of the remaining air with a final, explosive HA! sound

Repeat this exercise as needed, several times during the day (without startling anyone)!

Cleansing Through the Pores

A sufficiently acidic pH in bath water can neutralize the charges around the pores of the skin and allow a free flow of substances in and out of the skin. To take advantage of this situation to cleanse through the pores, do the following.

1. Fill your bathtub with as hot a water as you can lie in.
2. Before getting in, carefully add two cups of household bleach (do not get the straight bleach on your skin or in your eyes or mouth).
3. Stir the water slowly for a few seconds to ensure that the bleach is diluted properly.
4. Get into the tub and lie in this mixture for 15-20 minutes.
5. Rinse off in a shower.

Take one such bath each day for seven days; the second week, every other day; the third week, every three days; then every four days; then every five days. When you are taking this bath once a week, remain on that schedule. If you begin to have problems with dry skin, discontinue the bath until your skin returns to normal and decrease the frequency of the bath.

Cleansing the Kidneys

Soluble toxins that are eliminated through the bowel are also eliminated through the kidneys. Basically, whatever works to detoxify the bowel will also detoxify the kidneys, but the high concentrations of these toxins can cause discomfort and damage. **What we are looking for is an acid pH of the urine, along with dilution of the toxins to minimize pain and harm to the kidney structures.**

Avoid milk and tap water, but **drink plenty of distilled water, adding apple cider vinegar to acidify the urine. Cranberry and black cherry juices help to create an acidic urine pH.** Avoid common over-the-counter pain killers and prescription drugs such as Librium and Valium. Millions of prescriptions are written in the United States for these; they are numbers one and two on the list of all prescribed items, and all they do is destroy your liver and your kidneys. Long-term use of pain killers also causes vascular disease.

Cleansing the Bowel

In the 5th century BC, Herodotus wrote: "The Egyptians clear themselves on three consecutive days, every month, seeking after health by emetics and enemas for they think that all disease comes to man from his food." So as you can see, the objective is to maintain a free flow of good quality foods and water through the body.

Deep breathing of fresh air, drinking of distilled water, frequent cleansing, and proper dietary habits are essential. A good habit to develop is to eat one or two tablespoons of raw, unprocessed bran daily. Be sure to drink plenty of water with it; otherwise, constipation could set in. **Do not use the cereal forms of bran**; these have been infiltrated with sugar and other chemicals.

Now, if you are not feeling good or, for example, if you feel as though a cold is coming on, don't wait for it to get there. Catch it! That's why I say we predict life. Don't wait until you get sicker; we want to predict what is going to happen to you if you don't take care of yourself. So you're going to have to think, "How am I going to detoxify myself to get all of this out of me?" Several digestive tract detoxification procedures are outlined below.

Vigorous Laxative

A laxative taken by mouth is sometimes called a physic. Take two tablespoons of Fleet's Phospho-Soda in a glass of cold water. Follow this with a glass of hot water. This flushes the gallbladder and liver; the bile activates the bowel within 15 minutes to two hours. If the constipation is severe, it may take a dose every two hours, up to a maximum of three doses, until you get results.

While you are waiting for the laxative to take effect, take a lemon juice enema. It is prepared by putting the juice of a freshly-squeezed and strained lemon into two quarts of warm water. This solution will dissolve excess mucous in the bowel. Use the recommended enema technique described below.

Mild Laxative

Drink a quarter cup of aloe vera gel (not the juice) twice a day. If constipation is severe, the gel can be taken in prune, cranberry, or apple juice. What aloe vera does by mouth is empty the gallbladder and the liver to bring out the poisonous material. The bile activates the intestinal tract in a normal way, and the aloe vera helps to heal as it's going through.

The desirable reaction is a liquid stool for 10 days. If this is not obtained, use three or four ounces twice a day. Taper off to a loose but formed stool by reducing the morning amount by 1/3 every three days. Once you have the cleansing effect, keep at it. If there are food allergies, the digestive membranes will be swelled. The aloe vera gel will help heal these and reduce the swelling.

Herbal Laxatives

Not being an expert on herbs, I will not comment on their use. There are some good herbal cleansing remedies, but they should not be used indefinitely. Consult a competent herbalist.

Editor: For information, see the website of Dr. John Christopher at http://www.drchristopher.com/.

Recommended Enema Technique

Developed all of the way back In 1931, during my internship at the hospital, the proper technique in taking a cleansing or retention enema is as follows. Lie flat on your back. Make sure that the enema bag is never higher than 12" above your abdomen, preferably 10".

Cleansing Enema

For a cleansing enema, take two quarts in never less that 20 minutes, preferably 30 minutes. The slower the better. If you hit a fecal impaction or a gas pocket, it'll dilate the bowel and cause pain. When you do that always just grab hold of the tube and squeeze it and just hold onto it while the peristaltic activity works on that fecal impaction. Or if it's a gas pocket, you will find all of a sudden the peristaltic action will move it, and you will hear the gurgling as the water comes in, the pressure goes off, the pain goes out, then you can continue it until you get the whole two quarts in. If you do it that slowly then you can hang up the enema bag, and walk around for five minutes before you have to expel it.

Do not use the inferior Fredger enema cleansing enema technique, where you put it in and hold the bag up as high as you can. All that happens is a rectal dilatation, but you never get an enema. It never gets cleansing up into the colon. And when you get done and let the water out, the pressure is so great you can't hold it in.

You see, the higher you put the bag and the more force you use in an enema, the more you dilate the rectum and throw it into spasm. Actually, a person can hold three quarts, so two is not too much to ask for. If it hits a fecal impaction or a gas pocket, you immediately get the dilatation of the colon and it produces pain. If it does, pinch the tube, wait until the peristaltic action goes to work on it, and the first thing you know, it loosens up, the pressure comes down, the rest of the water goes in very easily, and you can release the pressure on the tube to let the rest of the water get in there. If you have done it slowly enough, you don't have any pain so you can get up and walk around a bit. Then sit down on the toilet and expel it. That is the proper method of taking an enema.

Retention Enema

For a retention enema, the amount we use is usually one pint. The idea with a retention enema is to keep it inside the digestive tract as long as it's possible. In other words, if you can absorb a whole pint, that's great. If you can't and it finally gets to where the peristaltic activity is pushing it down into the rectal fossa to where you get the reflex, then you better get on the toilet quickly and get rid of what is left unabsorbed. It is appropriate to take a cleansing enema first and then take a retention enema. One can make an enema out of any of the following mixtures.

Aloe Vera Cleansing Enema

We try to start patients off in the morning, usually with the aloe vera gel enema to get the bowel open; we use it most of the time. They have pretty good bowel movements, and we get an acceptable level of cleanliness. Then we follow it up with a vitamin C or coffee enema. We've tested about 15 different companies and found Lily of the Desert to be the best gel.

Preparation

The mixture is four to eight ounces of aloe vera gel diluted with water to a total of two quarts.

Technique

Use the recommended cleansing enema technique, as described above. Our bowels are shaped with villi on the inside. If you have anything stuck in between the villi, you can have three bowel movements a day and still be constipated. Aloe vera helps to grease the track as it goes down, and therefore allows the normal enzymatic activity of each of these villi, with their digestive enzymes, to digest the food. Therefore it allows the food to come through in a normal and natural way with no problems. If hemorrhoids are present or the rectum is otherwise inflamed, put two ounces of the gel in a baby syringe and administer it rectally at bedtime. Retain this material overnight.

Vitamin C Retention Enema

Any degenerative disease state needs a lot of vitamin C. Cancer, diabetes, arthritis – all of them are related to one another; there's only a little variance in the cell chemistry and in what you have to do to get them straightened out. We're finding on the arthritics we're treating some excellent results by giving two and three of these vitamin C enemas on a daily basis.

A naturopath spoke at a Cancer Control Society meeting in Los Angeles one year. He said that he was using five vitamin C enemas with a cancer patient and nothing else. The medics took him to court for practicing medicine without a license. He decided that he would go to court rather than sign an edict, which they were trying to get him to do out of court. He got into court and explained that he was allowed to give vitamin C by mouth, so why wasn't he allowed to give vitamin C by rectum? He won the case, making the medics look pretty silly. As a result of it all, he was able to lecture about vitamin C enemas in curing cancer all by themselves, and the medics could not do anything about it, because he had already been tried and found not guilty. I do not recommend vitamin C enemas alone in treating cancer.

Preparation

Make a solution of 4,000 mg of ascorbic acid to one pint of water.

Technique

Again we use the recommended technique. This is not a cleansing enema, but a way of infusing a large amount of vitamin C into the system. Retain this solution so as much of it can be absorbed as possible. Many persons experience a shift from alkaline to acid urine; this is desirable. Taking the amounts of vitamin C recommended by Pauling (50-60 gm daily) by mouth may not be practical. Using the enema form of administration, one may take as much as 10 gm.

Coffee Retention Enema

The coffee enema was popularized by Dr. Max Gerson in his work on cancer. However, it is now used in association with a wide variety of degenerative disease conditions. Coffee is something that we put in the wrong end. You have no business putting it in your mouth, it should only be used for enemas. Coffee by mouth is a diuretic; it is hard on the kidneys and helps to deplete the body of potassium and the B complex vitamins. Actually, the toxic material in coffee is the oil. As mentioned above, oils are fats are subject to rancidification. This occurs quickly after the beans are roasted and ground, and these rancid oils upset the liver and kidneys.

Preparation

The proper technique in the use of coffee enemas is to start with unground coffee beans. When you grind the coffee beans, the oil that's in the coffee bean immediately starts turning rancid. So when you make coffee and add more heat to it, you make it more rancid. When you drink it, the rancidity of that coffee oil is very detrimental to you.

Take a tablespoon of coffee beans to a cup and a half of water. Do a slow boil for 10 minutes; in other words don't put the flame up real high, just a low flame, just so you see it boiling for 10 minutes. Then drain the liquid off of the coffee beans so you only have the liquid coffee. Then you add to that (it's usually that cup and a half that'll boil down to a half a cupful, so you end up with about one cup). Add three cups of warm water to it and then take your coffee enema.

Technique

Again use the recommended technique, but with a retention enema. This is not a cleansing enema. What it does is provide caffeine to stimulate the emptying of the gallbladder and the liver and help you detoxify yourself. It also stimulates the adrenal glands and the setting up of your cortisone preparations. They are your anti-inflammatory agents, and that's what the coffee enemas are for. In the coffee work of Dr. Gerson, you are asked to take five of these every day so you're running about every three hours to take one as long as you possibly can.

We have developed one that I think is working better today. We have found that, if we alternate using 8,000 mg of ascorbic acid to a pint of water with the coffee enemas every three hours – first coffee, then the vitamin C, then coffee, vitamin C, coffee. By using it in this method, we are today getting better results in detoxifying and stimulating the cancer people. It brings them out of it faster than any other way we know. It does beautiful work.

Other Supplements

You can make a solution of the desired number of units of vitamin A, vitamin E, coenzyme Q, or any other oil-soluble vitamin preparation in one pint of water and administer them in a retention enema. This is a way of infusing these substances directly into the system. Retain this solution so as much of it can be absorbed as possible.

Fasting (Not Eating)

I am not a believer in any form of fasting. I am one who is a great disbeliever in our day and age that fasting should be used. I have seen too many of my friends die of congestive heart failure as the result of a 12-day fast!

When I talk to a lot of these people who are great believers in fasting, most of them have the same idea that the object is to change their alkaline bodies to an acid and head them in that direction and this is why we run into all of these problems, charley horses in a heart muscle, for instance, that kills you. **Consequently, if you must fast, I recommend that you go to an institution that is familiar with fasting. Do it under supervision; do not do it at home.**

Fasting Alternative (Quick Grapefruit Fast)

Because of the dangers of fasting, we decided to develop some methods to offset the risks. We devised an alternative method that is equal to a 12-day fast; we do it all in one day. **It is what I call a one-day grapefruit fast.** Buy sixteen (16) grapefruit and a bottle of betaine-HCl and pepsin tablets. Peel the grapefruit and leave the white on it; that is where the bioflavonoids are contained. Eat four grapefruit (everything but the seeds) and take three of the betaine-HCl and pepsin tablets four times during the day (8:00 AM, 12:00 noon, 4:00 PM, and lastly at 8:00 PM). This is your entire diet for the day (16 grapefruit and 12 betaine hydrochloride and pepsin tablets), and you had better drink plenty of water! The more toxic you are, the more strongly will adverse reactions set in.

Usually about 3:00 PM you're not sure you want to look another grapefruit in the eye because it's going to start pulling the poison out of your system so much that you're going to start feeling so toxic that you just don't feel like trying to eat another one of those grapefruit. At this particular time, take a lemon enema to clean yourself out. When you do that, it will be simple to eat the four grapefruit at 4:00 PM in the afternoon and again at 8:00 PM that night.

At about 9:00 PM, you will feel very bad. However, this is to be expected and should simply be tolerated; the bad feelings will pass. Another lemon enema will aid in getting the toxins out of the body more quickly. But believe you me that cleans you out. We have a lot of families today that are doing this one Sunday a month; the whole family gets into it. We do this even on hypoglycemics, the worst type. We've done it on diabetics. We have no problems with it, but on these we would rather use the slow aloe vera gel method.

For additional nutrition, take a teaspoon and just peel the white out of the peel and eat it. That's where the rest of the bioflavonoids are; that's part of your natural vitamin C complex, called civatemic acid. It is made up of ascorbogen from which ascorbic acid comes. Bioflavonoids, folic acid, rutin, and vitamin K are part of this C complex. When we use anything like ascorbic acid or sodium ascorbate, we always use a tablet of the natural C complex to get the catalytic activity of the natural synergistic factors to make the ascorbic acid or the sodium ascorbate work.

By the end of a day of eating the pulp of the grapefruit, the teeth may become sensitive. This is found in some patients, especially if they are too low in calcium. If this is the case, you must be careful of citrus; the older you get the less oranges you want to eat. All oranges are picked green and dyed to make you think they are ripe but they are not.

Fasting Alternative (Slow Aloe Vera Method)

The slow method involves the use of aloe vera gel. We prefer Lily of the Desert brand. This method is the easy one. For 10 days we want a liquid stool, so we have the patient drink two ounces (a quarter cup) of aloe vera gel morning and night. This type of gel is thick, like gelatin just before it gets a little hard. That's the way it comes in the bottle. If you have a little trouble swallowing it, add a little cranberry juice or apple juice to it, then you will have no problem.

If two ounces isn't enough twice a day to get that liquid stool, take three or four ounces. In other words, build up to a half a cup twice a day because we want that liquid stool for 10 days. If you're so toxic and so loaded with poison that the half a cup twice a day does not give you a liquid stool, then you had better take a good dose of castor oil and really flush yourself out. Then go back to the two ounces of the aloe vera morning and night.

After 10 days of the liquid stool, cut it back to where you have a loose but a formed stool. Cut out 1/3 of whatever the amount is that you take on the morning dose first, every three days, so at the end of nine days, you're finished with the one in the evening. You might bring it down to where you're only taking a teaspoonful; you never know, every person is different. We have some people that have to take two ounces morning and night just to have the loose but formed stool because we are that much different in our individuality. But whatever the amount is to get that loose but formed stool, that is the amount we want you to stay on for never less than three months. That's the slow time, all of the way through.

I have taken this for as much as 16 consecutive months just to find out, because I have heard of so many detrimental things if you continue to take it over a long period of time. I saw no detrimental effects whatsoever as far as my own health was concerned, because I'm pretty sensitive to such things.

Colonic Irrigation

A lot of people don't understand what a colonic irrigation is. It is a glorified enema. Instead of using two quarts of water, you use from five to 30 gallons of water. But you want to be very careful where you go to have colonic irrigations. If you really want to do something in your offices, put in a colonic irrigator. If done correctly, colonic irrigations are probably the finest detoxifying agents that we have. **They are absolutely the finest therapy I know for high blood pressure; with colonic irrigations, you don't need anything else. To me a Dierker Colonic is, by far, the ideal one.** I do not like gravitational types because you have to depend upon a sick bowel to tell you how much pressure you have before you try to expel it.

The following illustrates my point. One Friday night in my office, a woman came in, and we had her history. She was having all of these headaches and feeling pretty punk. I took her blood pressure her diastolic was 260, her systolic was so high above 300 I couldn't register it because at 300 it was still going "boom, boom, boom." All you do when you're having that thing happen is say, "Please God get her out of here before she has a stroke or a heart attack." Sure, she'd been taking drugs for this and had gotten absolutely nowhere, and it just kept going up.

I called the woman that did all of my colonics for me. I knew that my Elizabeth Sweicker was playing bridge with her sister which they had done every Friday night for 25 years. I said, "Elizabeth, will you give up your game tonight and give this woman a colonic irrigation? Let's save her life." She said, "Send her over." She had a Dierker Colonic machine, which I preferred. She said, "Okay, send her on down to the office and I'll take care of her." We sent her down. My technician couldn't even get a colonic started; the lady was so badly impacted that it took three enemas before the colonic could be started. The technician worked on her for a total of three hours, sent her over to the hotel, saying, "You be back at 7:30 tomorrow morning." She came back at 7:30 AM and was given another one for a whole hour. The technician said, "Come back at 11:30 AM." She came back and received another one.

I got there about 12:30 p.m. and took her blood pressure; it was 140/80. I sent her home, telling her, "I want you to go to a chiropractor and have two colonics a week for the next four weeks, one colonic per week for the next four weeks, and then one a month. Please have him take your blood pressure and write me a letter, telling me what it is each time you go." Well, like so many good cooperating patients I didn't hear from her for six months. Then she wrote me the following, "Dear Doctor Ellis: I don't need you or any other doctor. I have never felt this good in my whole 65 years of living. My blood pressure today was 120/60." That is the absolute perfect of all blood pressures because that means your pulse pressure is also 60, which is what it should be. I never did see that woman again!

Editor: The Dierker closed system colonic machine is no longer being manufactured under that name. Some used units are available on the internet. The reader may refer to the International Association for Colon Hydrotherapy publication, *Colon Therapy, 2 Edition*, found at https://www.cga.ct.gov/2013/phdata/tmy/2013SB-00873-R000220-International%20Assoc%20for%20Colon%20Therapy%20(I-ACT)-TMY.PDF.

No Detoxification is Complete Without This!

So many people have indecisions, fears, anxieties, irritabilities. and tensions. The worst one of all to get out of the system is hatred. If you project these things through a negative attitude toward people, you get back with interest what you give!

Look for the good in everything, no matter how bad it may seem at the moment; because when you go back and realize what had happened to you years later, you will find out that it was the finest thing that ever happened to you. If you keep in a positive realm within the mind, you will be able to accept the next opportunity that comes along.

What you must do more than any one thing is to start projecting love! If you still have a negative mind, you are going to miss all those opportunities. You're not going to get anywhere. The one thing that you have to do to get rid of all of these negative factors, and especially hatred, is in the spoken word, not in actions. For instance, if you husbands didn't say "I love you" to your wives when you got up this morning, if you wives didn't say "I love you" to your husbands, if you parents didn't say "I love you" to their children and if your children haven't been taught to say "I love you", you have started your day wrong.

One of the hardest things I find with people is to get out this spoken word – to talk and give love to other people. The Bible taught me to love my neighbor as myself. I'm going to start you on the right road now. When you encounter someone, shake his or her hand and say, "God loves you, and so do I!" That's your detoxification plan in a hurry!

7 Nutritional Supplements

Today, because of processing, bleaching, and canning of foods, we find very few foods that are of top quality and contain all of the nutrients that a person (especially one with vicarious eating habits) needs on a regular basis.

Although it is possible to get all of the vitamins, minerals, and protein that you need from a perfect diet of natural, high-quality foods, very few people are ever able to maintain such a diet. Therefore, it is usually necessary to take supplements to make up for the lack of food quality.

It is also possible to overdo supplementation. Some doctors prescribe from 400 to 800 vitamin and mineral pills a day. They are overstimulating their patients to the point of inhibition. They are getting some symptomatic changes in the patient where they might feel better for a while, but they usually end up in trouble later on. That's not what we want.

Let's talk about various nutritional supplements to the diet and how they are used, limiting the types to the following.

- Vitamins
- Minerals
- Emulsified Vitamins and Coenzymes
- Digestives
- Glandulars (Protomorphogens)
- Adjuncts
- Herbs

Vitamins

A vitamin is an organic (carbon-containing) compound essential for normal growth and good health. They may be fat- or water-soluble and are required in small quantities in the diet, because they are not synthesized by the body in sufficient amounts. Rather, they are synthesized by bacteria in the digestive system and contained in foods. Vitamins act as coenzymes that regulate metabolic processes but do not provide energy (as do sugars and fats) or building blocks (as do proteins). Deficiencies of vitamins produce specific disorders.

Everyone has what Dr. Roger Williams of the University of Texas calls *biochemical individuality.* That means that there is a world of difference between you and, say, your brother or sister. You may need twice the quantity of one nutrient, yet less than half the quantity of another, compared to your relatives. This is not theory; it is fact. **No one can set a maximum or minimum daily requirement of any nutrient. To do so is to thoroughly ignore the principle of biochemical individuality.**

Fat-soluble Vitamins

Fat-soluble vitamins require dietary fat to facilitate absorption. They are stored in the liver and in body fat and used as needed. Ingesting more fat-soluble vitamins than you need can be toxic, causing side-effects like nausea, vomiting, and liver and heart problems. These include those listed in Table 4, with actions and dietary sources indicated.

Table 4: Fat-soluble Vitamins

Name	Actions	Dietary Sources	Comments
Vitamin A (Retinol, Retinal, Retinoic Provitamin A, Carotenoids)	Antioxidant, benefits the eyes and vision, and in the development of bones, including the teeth. In addition, vitamin A aids immune function against infections and development of cancers.	Dark-colored fruits and vegetables; dark leafy greens, fish liver oil, egg yolk, butter, liver, beef, and fish	Synthesized in the body from carotenes present in the diet.
Vitamin D (Dihydrotachysterol, Calcitriol, or Ergocalciferol)	Offsets skeletal disease through promotion of calcium absorption, prevents abnormally low blood calcium levels that can then lead to tetany.	Fish liver oils (especially cod, salmon, mackerel, herring, and orange roughy), cereals, and sunlight	A severe vitamin D deficiency can cause myopathy, which can cause muscle weakness and pain.

Name	Actions	Dietary Sources	Comments
Vitamin E (Alpha-tocopherol)	Antioxidant, protecting cells from free radicals formed during energy metabolism. Because of its general action in the body, vitamin E may offset damage to nervous, circulatory, digestive, respiratory, and glandular tissues, but not be clearly associated with a particular disease.	Cereals, leafy green vegetables, seeds, and nuts, avocado, dark green vegetables, oils (safflower, corn, sunflower, wheat germ), wheat germ	An excess may cause muscle weakness and gastrointestinal disorders. Requirement is increased with increased intake of polyunsaturated fats.
Vitamin K (Koagulationsvitamin)	Coagulant, active in preventing coronary artery disease, osteoporosis, possibly valuable in offsetting dementia, insulin sensitivity leading to diabetes, and certain types of cancer.	Dark green leafy vegetables, cabbage, cauliflower, cereals, fish, liver, beef, and eggs	Synthesized by intestinal bacteria

With the emulsions of both vitamin A, and E, you get more activity than with the non-emulsified types. So, you use these in very small amounts. The vitamin E that we use is 35 units. You would use only about three drops a day. You get 300 times the activity as you would with any other vitamin so you don't have to take too much of it.

Water-soluble Vitamins

Water-soluble vitamins are not stored in your body and must be replenished daily. Your body takes what it needs from the food you eat and then excretes what is not needed as waste. All B vitamins help the body convert carbohydrates into glucose, which the body uses to produce energy. These B vitamins, often referred to as B-complex vitamins, also help the body metabolize fats and protein.

Editor: Dr. Ellis did not customarily use individual vitamins and minerals for their singular pharmacological effects in treating specific conditions. Rather, he used them in what he believed was an appropriate combination to support the general health of an individual patient under his care. For more information, refer to the WebMD website: http://www.webmd.com/drugs/index-drugs.aspx.

Dr. Royal Lee, founder of Standard Process, split the vitamin B complex into two groups. One of these is the B complex, consisting of the odd numbered ones to 25 – B1, B3, B5, etc. Using a complex of this type does a much better job than if a single vitamin were used by itself. When using the whole B complex, the toxicity is avoided.

If there is a high blood urea nitrogen (BUN) and a low bilirubin – a test that indicates a thick bile – never give a B complex. This is like the basis of car oil. As an example, in cold weather you would never put a 100 weight oil in your car and expect to run it at 100 mph right away. It'd give you problems. So you put a 10 weight oil in. Bile should flow like a 10 weight oil. So you thin the bile first, and this is done with vitamins A and F, along with beet juice extract (as found in Standard Process AF and BetaFood); thin the bile to let it flow. Then use B complex to keep it going.

The water-soluble vitamins are listed in Table 5, with some actions and dietary sources indicated. All B vitamins help the body to convert food (carbohydrates) into fuel (glucose), which is used to produce energy.

Table 5: Water-soluble Vitamins

Name	Actions	Dietary Sources	Comments
Vitamin B1 (Thiamin)	Offsets conditions such as Beriberi, lung congestion, heart failure, burning of the toes and feet, leg cramps, and muscle wasting.	Whole grains, liver, nuts, seeds, eggs, lean meats, legumes, beans, organ meats, peas, whole grains	The requirement is related to carbohydrate intake. When too much B1 is taken by itself, it becomes toxic to the human body, causing headache, insomnia, irritability, contact dermatitis.
Vitamin B2 (Riboflavin, old term: Vitamin G)	Offsets conditions such as jaundice, anemia, anorexia/ bulimia, cataracts, loss of cognitive function, depression, migraines, weakness, sore throat and tongue, cracks in the corners of the mouth, blurred vision, and light sensitivity.	Whole grains, enriched grains, and dairy products (not allowed in the Ellis plan)	Most people in a stress pattern are highly nervous and irritable, so we use vitamin B2. It is destroyed by sunlight.

Name	Actions	Dietary Sources	Comments
Vitamin B3 (Niacin, Niacinamide)	Niacin is commonly used as a vasodilator. Offsets high cholesterol. Because of its vasodilating ability, it is used in combination with other modalities for treating a variety of conditions, including poor circulation, migraine headache, dizziness, diabetes, skin conditions, pellagra, schizophrenia, dementia, chronic brain syndrome, depression, motion sickness, alcohol dependence, edema, and many others too numerous to list here.	Meat, fish, poultry, whole grains, avocado, eggs, fish (tuna and salt-water fish), lean meats, legumes, nuts, potatoes, poultry	An excess can cause liver damage and skin irritation. It is synthesized in the body from tryptophan.
Vitamin B5 (Pantothenic Acid)	Offsets osteoarthritis, acne, alcoholism, allergies, baldness, asthma, attention deficit-hyperactivity disorder (ADHD), autism, burning feet syndrome, (PMS), enlarged prostate, and a host of other conditions too numerous to mention here. Gives protection against mental and physical stress and anxiety. It is applied topically for itching skin.	Meat, poultry, whole grains, avocado, vegetables in the cabbage family, eggs, legumes, lentils, mushrooms, organ meats, poultry, white and sweet potatoes	Large daily doses of pantothenic acid can cause swelling of the ankles, wrists and face, with itching and local sensitivity, depression, and joint pain. Too much B5 can adversely affect the body's ability to metabolize protein, an increase in blood triglycerides, and calcification in the arteries and blood vessels.

Name	Actions	Dietary Sources	Comments
Vitamin B6 (Pyridoxine)	Pyridoxine is needed for normal brain development and function, and helps the body make the hormones serotonin and norepinephrine, which influence mood, and melatonin, which helps to regulate the body clock. Offsets anemia, heart disease, clogged arteries, PMS, morning sickness, depression, Alzheimer's disease, attention deficit-hyperactivity disorder (ADHD), and many others too numerous to list here.	Soy products, avocado, banana, legumes, beans, meat, nuts, poultry, whole grains	An excess may cause peripheral nerve damage. Requirement is related to protein intake.
Vitamin B7 (Biotin)	Biotin is used to support adrenal function, to help calm and maintain a healthy nervous system. Offsets hair loss, fatigue, depression, nausea, muscle pains, and anemia.	Cereal, egg yolk, legumes, nuts, organ meats (liver, kidney), pork, yeast	High levels of pantothenic acid, some anti-seizure drugs, and smoking can affect the levels of biotin.

Name	Actions	Dietary Sources	Comments
Vitamin B9 (Folic Acid)	Folic acid is important for the production and maintenance of new cells, prevention of anemia, proper brain function and mental and emotional health. It aids in the production and repair of DNA and RNA. Folic acid also works closely with vitamin B12 to help make red blood cells and help iron work properly in the body. It works with B6 and B12 to control blood levels of the amino acid homocysteine.	Leafy vegetables, asparagus, broccoli, beets, yeast, beans (cooked pinto, navy, kidney, and lima), lentils, oranges, wheat germ	It can mask a deficiency of B12.
Vitamin B12 (Cyanocobalamin)	Vitamin B12 helps in making DNA and red blood cells. Offsets the effects of a damaged stomach lining, pernicious anemia, Chron's disease, celiac disease, bacterial or parasitic growth, heavy drinking, immune system disorders, such as Graves' disease or lupus, and long-term use of acid-reducing drugs.	Fish, poultry, meat, eggs, organ meats (liver and kidney), shellfish	Absorption requires intrinsic factor produced by the stomach. It is found only in foods of animal origin, so strict vegetarians and vegans must take supplements.

Name	Actions	Dietary Sources	Comments
Vitamin C (Ascorbic Acid)	Ascorbic acid is a powerful antioxidant that fights free radicals. It helps the body form and repair numerous tissues in the body and protects against heart disease, scurvy, high cholesterol and high triglycerides. It offsets fatigue, muscle weakness, joint and muscle aches, bleeding gums, and leg rashes.	Citrus fruit (tree-ripened), such as oranges and grapefruits; red, yellow, and green peppers, broccoli, brussels sprouts, cabbage, cauliflower, potatoes, spinach, strawberries, tomatoes	Can cause diarrhea and oxalate kidney stones. It can be destroyed by cooking in the presence of air and plant enzymes released by cutting and grating. Watch for inflammation of the intestine. Drink plenty of water.

I read in the *British Medical Journal* that prolonged usage of 2,000 mg of ascorbic acid per day for a two-week period will impair the neutrophilic action of the WBCs. I haven't seen this on the rechecks of our patients, because we're now using as high as 16,000 mg per day in cancer patients, in those where we're expecting cancer, and in those with degenerative diseases.

I use natural vitamin C complex 4,000 mg (a teaspoonful) four times a day, at each meal and at bedtime. If taken by mouth, always take the natural vitamin C complex for each 1,000 mg of ascorbic acid or sodium ascorbate. Of course, other factors in the formation of arteriosclerosis and atherosclerosis must be taken into consideration. Vitamin C is an oxidizer and an acidifier, and one of the reasons people get diarrhea from taking ascorbic acid by mouth is that they were so highly alkaline when they took an extra amount of the ascorbic acid – the acid factor. They get a big change in body chemistry. That's what creates dehydration, pulling the fluid into the bowel. You can clear up more diarrheas by taking a physic and an enema than any other method that I know of.

Fillers

Many companies use starches and sugars for their fillers. These detract from or may even neutralize the effectiveness of the supplement. Biotics Research Corporation uses sprouts – peas and lentils. To the liquid used in sprouting, they add certain vitamins and minerals, which are then incorporated into the sprouts. After several days, the sprouts are dehydrated at 89° F, ground up, and used as fillers for their tablets. The catalyst effect is fantastic, and we get better results using their products.

Minerals

Minerals are nutrients found in the earth or water; they are absorbed by plants and animals for proper nutrition. Minerals are the main component of teeth and bones and help build cells and support nerve impulses, among other things. Minerals are customarily classified into two groups, nutritional (macrominerals and trace minerals) and toxic. Every mineral in large excess is toxic, but those in the toxic group have virtually no effect except toxicity.

Minerals are vital, because they make the enzymes in every cell and every function that takes place within your body. So if you don't have those minerals in their proper ratios to one another, they'll never work. Vitamins are the catalysts that make the minerals become enzyme systems, so if you don't have those balanced properly, it is impossible for them to become enzymes. There is only one-quarter ounce of vitamins in a 160-pound person, but it is the ratios of these, one to the other, that make all of these coordinate into a healthy individual.

Sometimes, a mineral level is fairly closely related to current dietary behavior, such as the scarcity of zinc, which is seen commonly in vegetarians. Sometimes, the influence is roundabout, such as the tendency of people who do not get enough of the vitamin B complex to develop scarcities of sodium and potassium. Some tissue minerals are high when the body is losing them or transporting them to another location, such as the excess seen in osteoporosis. Some minerals interfere with other minerals, such as excessive selenium causing a scarcity of copper.

The subject of minerals is one vitally important to each of us. Let's lay some groundwork. Each of the minerals we require is equally capable of combining in the digestive tract with some other material to form an inassimilable compound. Even calcium can combine with phytates from whole grains or oxalic acid from spinach to form compounds that the body cannot use. **Consequently, mineral nutrition is never just a simple matter of numbers.** For instance, if we lack chromium we may not notice the lack for many years until we develop maturity onset diabetes. A good book on mineral metabolism is *The Trace Elements and Man* by Henry A. Schroeder, M.D.

It is important to know exactly which amino acid is best suited for a particular mineral and how to chelate it exactly as nature does it. Anything less than natural will also be less than ideal for the purpose. That is why certain companies come out on top with all of their products. Especially good is Miller Pharmaceutical Co.; also good is Biotics Research Corporation. So when dealing with minerals, be aware of all of these facts.

How to Take and Not Take Minerals

It is important to learn how the minerals blend (not interfere) with each other, so you can get them into your body without wasting them. There's no testing method that we know of to determine this. Depending on what we find in a hair mineral analysis and bloodwork, along with knowing what the ratios are to one another, we can determine which minerals to give someone and when to take them. Certain minerals, we have found, have no best time to take or not take, such as potassium.

Do not try to take all of your minerals at the same time, such as are found in dolomite. Dolomite is loaded with aluminium and lead to very high toxic amounts. I really believe that using dolomite killed my good friend Jerry Rodale, the head of *Preventiion* magazine, who had a massive heart attack while appearing on the Dick Cavett Show. The program was recorded but never shown to the public.

Some months before that, I had gone up to his office with my medical lab assistant; I took my centrifuge and other equipment with me and walked in. I said, "Jerry, in your last article, you're talking about how good you were and what good shape you are in, but you refuse to let a doctor do any blood work to find out whether or not you are in good shape. I am going to take your blood and process it in front of you."

He was in excellent shape; then he went on this dolomite kick. In all of his articles, he started pushing it. I still say this is the thing that killed him because of the accumulation of aluminum and lead, throwing his minerals out of balance. It also contains cadmium, chromium, and certain types of nickel that can give you metal poisoning. All of this can create a spasm in the muscles and in the heart. You see, you can have a charlie horse in any muscle, including the heart, just the same as you can have one in your leg. Yet, when you are autopsied, nothing is found to be wrong with the heart.

Mineral Summaries

The following tables list information about various minerals. Macrominerals (Table 6) and trace minerals (Table 7) are important and beneficial to body functions and should be taken, when necessary, to supplement deficiencies. Toxic metals (Table 8 and Table 9) are dangerous to body functions and should be avoided. The toxic metals are listed in this chapter to help the reader understand possible interactions with the beneficial minerals.

Table 6: Summary of Macrominerals

Macrominerals	
Name	**Notes**
Calcium	**Take upon waking on an empty stomach with betaine hydrochloride or acidic juices (cranberry or black cherry). Do not take at the same time as magnesium or manganese.** Calcium is absorbed from the upper parts of the small intestine. The amount of absorption depends on the acidity of the intestinal contents and the amount of phosphate present. Calcium salts are soluble in acids. Calcium, along with protein, phosphorus, and magnesium are important to the formation of bone. The remaining 1% of the calcium in the body is essential for blood clotting, blood pressure stabilization, normal brain function, glucose metabolism, and contraction of muscles.
Magnesium	**Take at suppertime. Do not take at the same time as calcium.** Magnesium is needed for more than 300 biochemical reactions in the body. It helps to maintain normal nerve and muscle function, supports a healthy immune system, keeps the heart beat steady, and helps bones remain strong. It also helps to regulate blood glucose levels and aid in the production of energy and protein. One can for a long time be nervous, irritable, or easily fatigued with no awareness of a deficiency of magnesium and potassium. Magnesium is commonly administered as a sulfate; but the absorption is 2.6 times as great when in the amino acid chelated form.

Macrominerals	
Name	**Notes**
Phosphorus	**Take half way between breakfast and lunch and lunch and supper and sometimes as an aid to digesting carbohydrates. Do not take at the same time as calcium.** Phosphorus is a major component of bone, but it also combines with lipids to make phospholipids, a major structural component of all cell membranes, or walls, throughout the body. Phospholipids in brain cells control which minerals, nutrients and drugs go in and out of the cell. Phosphorus is required for energy production and storage, helping the body change protein, fat, and carbohydrate into energy. As a component of DNA and RNA, phosphorus is also involved in the storage and transmission of genetic material. It activates enzymes, hormones, and cell-signaling molecules through phosphorylation. Phosphorus also helps to get oxygen to tissues and buffers a normal pH.
Potassium	**Take at no particular time.** Potassium, along with sodium, maintain heartbeat and nerve function. They also regulate hydration in accordance with the adrenal hormone, aldosterone. The potassium level rises from kidney disease, use of diuretics, and the use of aldosterone supplements, causing muscle weakness, tingling, and even cardiac arrest. A potassium deficiency is more common, with similar symptoms to that of an elevated level, such as kidney malfunction, vomiting, and dangerous heart arrhythmias. Along with a supplement, eat ripe bananas, avocados, and parsley.
Sodium	**Provided by salt-containing foods.** Sodium and potassium are electrolytes that work together to carry electrical charges in the body, facilitating muscle contraction and nerve cell transmission. They maintain normal water balance in the body, thereby keeping control of the body's blood volume and blood pressure. If either blood volume or sodium levels get too high, the kidneys are stimulated to excrete excess sodium, returning blood volume to normal levels. It is recommend that people limit sodium intake to 2,400 mg, but most Americans consume 4,000-6,000 mg a day.
Sulfur	**Usually provided by a protein source.** Sulfur is a component of four amino acids: methionine, cysteine, cystine, and taurine and is highly concentrated in the protein structure of the joints, hair, nails, and skin. It is also important in the production of insulin, which is rich in sulfur-containing amino acids. Certain conditions, such as arthritis and liver disorders, may be improved by increasing the intake of sulfur, which is found in good quantity in sulfur-rich foods, such as eggs, legumes, whole grains, garlic, onions, brussel sprouts, and cabbage. Deficiencies occur only with a severe lack of protein.

Table 7: Summary of Trace Minerals

Trace Minerals	
Name	**Notes**
Boron	Arthritis and osteoporosis are managed by using boron, and it helps to relieve menopausal symptoms. It is believed to improve the body's ability to absorb calcium and magnesium. Boron is used for building strong bones and muscles, increasing testosterone levels, and improving thinking and muscle coordination. Boric acid is used to kill yeast that cause vaginal infections.
Chromium	Chromium helps insulin transport glucose into cells, where it can be used for energy. Chromium also appears to be involved in the metabolism of carbohydrate, fat, and protein. It may play a role in the management of type 2 diabetes. Low chromium levels may be associated with increased risk of glaucoma. Chromium slows the loss of calcium, so it may help prevent bone loss. Chromium has a toxic form that is chemically different from its nutritional form. If the measured level of chromium is low, there is a scarcity (not necessarily a deficiency) of the nutritional form. If the level is high, there may be an excess of either form.
Cobalt	Although commonly used in electroplating and the production of alloys, cobalt is an essential trace dietary mineral for all animals, being the active center of coenzymes called cobalamins, the most common example of which is vitamin B12. Cobalt is beneficial to the circulatory system, and, along with iodine and copper, improves light sensitivity, reducing glare, and improving vision.
Copper	Copper has 5.8 times better absorption as an amino acid chelate (5.8 times as much as copper carbonate, 3 times as much as copper oxide, and 4.1 times as much as copper sulfate). Copper is essential as a trace dietary mineral because it is a constituent of the respiratory enzyme complex cytochrome c oxidase. In humans, copper is found mainly in the liver, muscle, and bone.

Trace Minerals	
Name	**Notes**
Germanium	We have noticed that germanium promotes more efficient use of oxygen in the body. The main effect of germanium is to increase the oxidative index of blood and body. Studies on germanium therapy for cancer were done by Dr. Asai in northern Japan. Germanium can easily cure blue lips. The lips start to get pinker and pinker. Other food sources of germanium are ginseng and garlic; they are both very high. Garlic caps from Japan are most effective. Take them 30 minutes before meal. You know, everybody goes to Lourdes, France to be cured at the church. During all of these years, the church received all of the credit, but, you have to stay there a certain number of days and drink the water. It was found that germanium is in high concentration in the water; therefore, the cures actually result from the water and germanium rather than from the church.
Iodine	Iodine is not only required for proper function of the thyroid, other tissues absorb and use large amounts of iodine, including the breasts, salivary glands, pancreas, cerebral spinal fluid, skin, stomach, brain, and thymus gland. Iodine deficiency in any of these tissues may cause dysfunction of that tissue. **Take only a few drops in juice. Take care not to overdose; there are many recommendations about dosage, but one indicator of excessive intake is development of a sore throat, independent of a cold or other infection.** The following symptoms may point to insufficient intake of iodine in the diet: dry mouth, dry skin, lack of perspiration, reduced alertness, nodules or scars in the muscles, along with pain, such as fibrosis or fibromyalgia. **Editor:** See the article *The Silent Epidemic of Iodine Deficiency.* October 2011, by Nancy Piccone at http://www.lifeextension.com/magazine/2011/10/the-silent-epidemic-of-iodine-deficiency/Page-01.
Iron	Iron gives black stools when it is not absorbed; it also causes constipation. If properly chelated; you never see black stool or constipation. **It is best to take iron tablets before bed**; you will have more absorption and the stomach will be less irritable at that time. Avoid taking vitamin E with iron, as they neutralize and are not absorbed. (If the stool is black and tarry; blood is present; if it is black with its usual consistency, iron is usually present).
Lithium	Commonly used for its mood altering pharmacological effects. Lithium is used to treat manic depression with its hyperactivity, poor judgment, sleep deprivation, aggression, and anger.

Trace Minerals	
Name	**Notes**
Manganese	Manganese is found mostly in the bones, liver, kidneys, and pancreas and helps the body form connective tissue, bones, blood clotting factors, and sex hormones. It also plays a role in fat and carbohydrate metabolism, calcium absorption, and blood sugar regulation. Manganese is also necessary for normal brain and nerve function. It is a cofactor of the antioxidant enzyme superoxide dismutase (SOD), which fights free radicals. Low levels of manganese in the body can contribute to infertility, bone malformation, weakness, and seizures. Too much manganese in the diet could lead to neurological disorders or poor cognitive performance. A proper level of manganese may offset osteoporosis, arthritis, PMS, diabetes, and epilepsy. **Take at lunchtime. Do not take at the same time as calcium.** Dietary sources of manganese include nuts and seeds, wheat germ and whole grains (including unrefined cereals, buckwheat, bulgur wheat, and oats), legumes, and pineapples.
Molybdenum	Molybdenum deficiency results in high blood levels of sulfite and urate. Dietary molybdenum deficiency from low soil concentration of molybdenum has been associated with increased rates of esophageal cancer in China and Iran. Because it is an antagonist of copper, molybdenum can prevent plasma proteins from binding to copper, increasing the amount of copper excreted in urine. A congenital molybdenum cofactor deficiency disease, seen in infants, results in interference with the ability of the body to use molybdenum in enzymes. It causes high levels of sulfite and urate, and neurological damage.
Rubidium	Rubidium has no known biological role and is non-toxic. However, because it is chemically similar to potassium, we absorb it from our food, and the average person stores about 1/2 gm.
Selenium	Commonly used in the glass and photocell industries, selenium is involved in some health conditions – such as HIV, Crohn's disease, and others that are associated with low selenium levels. People fed intravenously are also at risk for low selenium.

Trace Minerals	
Name	**Notes**
Vanadium	Vanadium is used to make alloys for jet engines, in bonding titanium to steel, and with gallium to form superconducting magnets. Vanadium pentoxide is used in ceramics and as a catalyst for the production of sulfuric acid. In the body, vanadium is used to treat diabetes, low blood sugar, high cholesterol, heart disease, tuberculosis, syphilis, a form of tired blood (anemia), and water retention (edema). It is also used for improving athletic performance in weight training and for preventing cancer.
Zinc	**Take before or with a meal, depending on need. Do not take on an empty stomach to avoid nausea.** If we lack zinc; wounds take longer to heal; men may not notice the deficiency until they develop prostate problems. Zinc has 2.3 times better absorption as an amino acid chelate than as zinc sulfate. Typically, amino acid chelated zinc is retained twice as well as zinc fluoride. Important also is which amino-acids are used to form the chelate. Zinc and cadmium occur naturally in the earth. Zinc in the diet can prevent the assimilation of cadmium.
Zirconium	Zirconium is used to protect alloys from corrosion. Although it has no known biological role, the human body contains, on average, 250 mg of zirconium. It is used in medicine to offset hyperkalemia. High blood potassium levels are associated with cardiac arrhythmias, conduction system abnormalities, and increased mortality. In acute hyperkalemia. Zirconium cyclosilicate rapidly lowers potassium levels, thus delaying or potentially averting the need for emergent dialysis.

Table 8: Well-researched Toxic Minerals (Metals)

Toxic Minerals (Metals)	
Name	**Notes**
Aluminum	Aluminum plays no biological role, but it is found in nature in large amounts. Aluminum hydroxide is used in some antacid preparations, but the aluminum is not converted into a product that can be eliminated from the system. We can pick up the level in a hair analysis. We also find aluminum in canned foods, foods wrapped in aluminum foil, in aluminum utensils, and in antiperspirants. These are the biggest sources, stay away from all of them. Once the aluminum is in the system, it can be removed using methionine, alginates, and a lot of vitamin C.
Arsenic	Arsenic is found in some skin lotions, hair dyes, medicines, water, seafood, some fruit, and in cigarette smoke. If found in the body, it is usually in the liver, bones, and hair. In cancer, there is an increased amount in the blood. Aside from the tars, arsenicals, etc. in cigarette smoke, the most important substance (which we are never told about) is sulfuric acid, used in the manufacture of the cigarette paper. Lung cancer is going up rapidly in females who smoke. One cigarette will destroy more vitamin C than you can eat in one day.
Cadmium	Zinc and cadmium occur naturally in the earth. Zinc in the diet can prevent the assimilation of cadmium. Too much cadmium is an important cause of anemia and emphysema; it also causes high blood pressure, arteriosclerosis, and heart disease. Poisoning results from ingestion of fumes. Other sources are: oyster, cigarettes, gasoline, rubber tires, heating oils, steelmaking, and lead and copper processing. We are putting six million pounds into our atmosphere each year.

Toxic Minerals (Metals)	
Name	**Notes**
Lead	Lead and cadmium are toxic elements usually found in smokers. Sources of lead include toothpaste, hair dyes, airplane exhaust, alloys, asphalt, air conditioners, automobile exhaust, auto heaters, batteries, bone meal, building debris, ceramics, charcoal, coal-gas, cosmetics, dolomite, dust, dyes, fertilizers, gas burners, gasoline, leaded glass, hair shampoos, hair rinses, hair sprays, linotype, some milk, minerals, petroleum oils, paints, pencils, pesticides, pewter, plaster, poultry, print shops, printed paper, rain, road dust, rubber tires, scrap metals, smog, smoke, tobacco, forest fires, vegetables, water, water-pipes, welding, wine. Symptoms of lead poisoning include porphyria, kidney damage, a relationship to gout, memory loss, mental retardation, infertility, damage to the central nervous system, anemia, jaundice, liver malfunction, low blood levels of vitamin B6, vitamin C deficiency, pituitary damage, and reduced levels of blood proteins.
Mercury	Symptoms of mercury poisoning include pain in the left part of the chest, retinal bleeding, dim vision, film over eyes, dry eyes, grey ring around the cornea, red irritable throat, inflammation in the upper airways, pleurisy, difficulty in swallowing, severe amnesia, anxiety, irritability, difficulty to impossibility to control behavior, indecisiveness, loss of interest in life, tiredness, a feeling of being old, resistance to intellectual work, increased need for sleep, vertigo, headaches (often migraine type), facial paralysis, painful pull at the lower jaw toward the collar bone, increases salivation, a metallic taste (gallbladder), bleeding gums especially while bruising teeth, joint pain, lower back pain, muscle weakness, slow muscle action, pressure pains (needles) in the liver, asthmatic breathing, gastrointestinal irritation, eczema, needle-like sensations in lymph glands under the arm and in the groin.
Nickel	Nickel activates the enzymes arginase carboxylase and trypsin. It binds with protein to form nickeloplasmin, the function of which is not known. Nickel exposure causes formation of free radicals in various tissues in both human and animals which lead to various modifications to DNA bases, enhanced lipid peroxidation, and altered calcium and sulfhydryl homeostasis. Nickel inhibits acid phosphatase and is associated with cancer and some skin ailments. It is found in amalgam fillings, in stainless steel cooking utensils, as well as in some food and drinks, such as margarine and some decaffeinated coffees (not allowed in the Ellis program).

Table 9: Less Well-researched Toxic Minerals (Metals)

Other Toxic Metals	
Name	**Notes**
Antimony	Pure antimony is used in semiconductors, batteries, low friction metals, flame-proof materials, paints, ceramic enamels, glass, and pottery. Antimony is used as a medicine for parasitic infections, but exposure to relatively high concentrations of it can cause lung diseases, heart problems, diarrhea, severe vomiting, and stomach ulcers.
Barium	Barium is used in spark-plugs, vacuum tubes, and fluorescent lamps. It is used by the oil industry as drilling mud and by other manufacturers to make paint, tiles, glass, and rubber. Water-soluble barium compounds can be harmful to human health, causing paralyses and in some cases even death. Small amounts may cause breathing difficulties, elevated blood pressure, heart rhythm changes, stomach irritation, muscle weakness, changes in nerve reflexes, swelling of brains and liver, and kidney and heart damage.
Beryllium	Beryllium improves many physical properties when added as an alloying element to certain metals. It is used commonly in dental alloys. Approximately 35 micrograms of beryllium are found in the average human body, an amount not considered harmful. Beryllium is chemically similar to magnesium and therefore can displace it from enzymes, which causes them to malfunction.
Bismuth	Bismuth is the most naturally diamagnetic element, and has one of the lowest values of thermal conductivity among metals and is weakly radioactive. It is used in cosmetics, pigments, and a few pharmaceuticals, notably bismuth subsalicylate, used to treat diarrhea. Bismuth has unusually low toxicity for a heavy metal. As the toxicity of lead has become more apparent in recent years, there is an increasing use of bismuth alloys as a replacement for lead.
Platinum	Platinum is used to increase wear- and tarnish-resistance in fine jewelry. It and its alloys are used in surgical tools, laboratory utensils, wire, and electrical contact points. It is used in catalytic converters and in liquid crystal display glass. Platinum bonds are often applied as a medicine to cure cancer, but success is dependent upon the kind of bonds that are shaped and the exposure level and immunity of the patient. Although not a very dangerous metal, platinum salts can cause DNA damage, cancer, allergic reactions of the skin and the mucous membrane, damage to organs, such as intestines, kidneys and bone marrow, and a loss of hearing. It can also potentiate the toxicity of other dangerous chemicals in the body, such as selenium.

Other Toxic Metals	
Name	**Notes**
Silver	Silver is used in electrical contacts and conductors, specialized mirrors, catalysis of chemical reactions, and in photographic film and X-rays. Silver is also used in food coloring. Dilute silver nitrate solutions and other silver compounds are used as disinfectants and microbiocides (oligodynamic effect), added to bandages and wound-dressings, catheters and other medical instruments. Silver is used in water purifiers to prevent growth of bacteria and algae in filters. Silver plays no known natural biological role in humans and is not toxic to humans, but most silver salts are. In large doses, silver and compounds containing it can be absorbed into the circulatory system and become deposited in various body tissues, leading to argyria, which results in a blue-grayish pigmentation of the skin, eyes, and mucous membranes.
Strontium	Strontium burns in air, and because of its extreme reactivity with oxygen and water, this element occurs naturally only in compounds with other elements. It is kept under mineral oil or kerosene to prevent spontaneous ignition and oxidation. The primary use for strontium is in glass for color television cathode ray tubes to prevent X-ray emission. The human body absorbs strontium as if it were calcium. However, the stable forms of strontium do not pose a significant health threat. The radioactive Sr-90 can lead to various bone disorders and diseases, including bone cancer.
Thallium	Thallium is used in photoresistors and high-temperature superconducting materials for magnetic resonance imaging, storage of magnetic energy, magnetic propulsion, and electric power generation and transmission. Soluble thallium salts (many of which are nearly tasteless) are highly toxic and were used in rat poisons and insecticides. Thallium and its compounds are extremely toxic, and should be handled with great care. People can be exposed to thallium in the workplace by breathing it in, skin absorption, swallowing it, or eye contact. Contact with skin is dangerous, and adequate ventilation should be provided when melting this metal. Man-made sources of thallium pollution include gaseous emission of cement factories, coal burning power plants, and metal sewers. The main source of elevated thallium concentrations in water is the leaching of thallium from ore processing operations. Prussian Blue dye is used to rid the body of thallium.

Other Toxic Metals	
Name	**Notes**
Thorium	Thorium was commonly used as the light source in gas mantles, but this application has declined because of concerns about its radioactivity. Thorium is still widely used as an alloying element. It is also popular as a material in high-end optics and scientific instrumentation. The chemical toxicity of thorium is low because thorium and its most common compounds are poorly soluble in water. People who work with thorium compounds are at a risk of dermatitis. It can take as much as thirty years after the ingestion of thorium for symptoms to manifest themselves. Exposure to an aerosol of thorium, however, can lead to increased risk of cancers of the lung, pancreas, and blood, as lungs and other internal organs can be penetrated by alpha radiation. Exposure to thorium internally leads to increased risk of liver diseases.
Tin	About half of the tin produced is used in solder. The rest is divided among tin plating, tin chemicals, brass and bronze, and niche uses, such as production of PVC pipe and Lithium-ion batteries. Cases of poisoning from tin metal, its oxides, and its salts are almost nonexistent, but certain organotin compounds are almost as toxic as cyanide. People can be exposed to tin in the workplace by breathing it in, skin contact, and eye contact.
Titanium	Titanium is alloyed with iron, aluminium, vanadium, and molybdenum to produce strong, lightweight, non-corroding alloys. These are used in aerospace, military, manufacturing, desalination, and agri-food. Some products are medical prostheses, orthopedic implants, dental instruments, sporting goods, jewelry, and mobile phones. Titanium is non-toxic even in large doses and does not play any natural role inside the human body. It does, however, sometimes accumulate in tissues that contain silica.

Other Toxic Metals	
Name	**Notes**
Uranium	Originally, uranium was used in glass making and in photographic chemicals. Now, the major application of uranium in the military sector is in high-density penetrators. Depleted uranium is also used as a shielding material in some containers used to store and transport radioactive materials. Uranium-235 has been used as the explosive material to produce nuclear weapons. The main use of uranium in the civilian sector is to fuel nuclear power plants. A person can be exposed to uranium by inhaling dust in air or by ingesting contaminated water and food. Most ingested uranium is excreted during digestion. After entering the bloodstream, the absorbed uranium tends to bioaccumulate and stay for many years in bone tissue because of uranium's affinity for phosphates. Normal functioning of the kidney, brain, liver, heart, and other systems can be affected by uranium exposure, because, besides being weakly radioactive, uranium is a toxic metal.

Emulsified Vitamins and Coenzymes

When you ingest the oil-soluble vitamin A suspended in an emulsion, instead of it being picked up in the portal system, it is picked up in the lymphatic system. When the lymphatics pick it up, it goes up through the cisterna chyli and empties into the inferior vena cava just before it goes into the heart. It's in the bloodstream and goes directly to the affected cell, and the cell picks it out of the bloodstream before it ever goes through on its second pass into the portal system. Then, much of the vitamin is destroyed in the liver. The cells have the first opportunity to get it.

What we're trying to do is use emulsions of oil and water. We use sesame oil in making these emulsions, and can put vitamin A and vitamin E together if we choose. **Conventional vitamin A supplements must be taken carefully.** Many references tell you to take 100,000 units of vitamin A. However, if you were to take that much vitamin A in the little gel capsules on a daily basis for 30 to 60 days, it could kill you.

In the therapy of Dr. Hans Nieper of Germany, nine million units of emulsified vitamin A have been given on a daily basis with only slight toxic effects. In cancer work, they use three million units on a daily basis. I take somewhere around 750,000 units of vitamin A every day in the emulsion form with no harmful effects. I have been on this for over a year. We're doing the same thing with emulsified vitamin E that is 300% more potent than any other form of vitamin E.

Digestive Aids

Although the main function of digestion is to convert the foods that we eat into energy, the digestive system has even more functions. It is the main area of contact with an external environment full of bacteria, protozoa, fungi, viruses, and many toxic substances. To deal with these insults, the digestive tract is infiltrated with a large number of immune cells in what is called gut-associated lymphoid tissue (GALT). This is a very important part of mucosal-associated lymphoid tissue (MALT) representing almost 70% of the entire immune system. Approximately 80% of plasma cells reside in GALT, standing by to issue an immune response to whatever antigens appear in the tract.

Although I have covered these topics previously, I would like for you to remember that the type of foods that Americans eat, the way the foods are cooked, the way in which they are combined into a meal, and the presence of stress in our everyday lives makes efficient digestion unlikely for the majority of us and creates problems for our immune systems.

Ideally, you would eat your meal in a calm environment and have plenty of time to eat slowly. Your meal would consist only of healthy raw and properly cooked foods combined and eaten together in a way that supports good digestion. Your goal would be to eat only until your hunger was satiated and no more. In other words, you would not overload your system.

If your digestive system were working at top efficiency, you would feel good after eating, you would have no symptoms of indigestion, and your next bowel movement would be well-formed and without discomfort. To understand an ideal digestive process and to indicate stages when and what digestive aids might be necessary, refer to Table 10.

Table 10: Comparison of Ideal Digestion to Need for Digestive Aids

Stage of Digestion	Location	Ideal Outcome (Simplified)	Difficulty	Digestive Aid/ Action
Mastication	Mouth	Food is converted from solid to small-particle, liquid form by extensive chewing.	Inability to chew properly, either through lack of teeth or paralysis.	None, except for blending food before consumption. Even blended material should be given an opportunity to mix with saliva.
Alkaline Hydrolysis	Mouth	Food particles are thoroughly mixed with the alkaline enzyme ptyalin (alpha-amylase) to digest starches (carbohydrates) and trigger the digestive process. Starches should be digested as completely as possible down to short-chain saccharides during this stage.	Inability to produce sufficient saliva. Undigested carbohydrates ferment and interfere with acidic environment in the stomach.	None. Although the amylase enzyme is found in enzyme supplements, taking them by mouth serves no purpose in the mouth. The enzyme should be mixed with the food before eating. Liquid phosphorus as a digestive aid is beneficial to phosphorylate sugars at the initial steps of energy metabolism.

Stage of Digestion	Location	Ideal Outcome (Simplified)	Difficulty	Digestive Aid/ Action
Acid Hydrolysis	Stomach	The alkaline bolus coming from the mouth through the pharynx and esophagus and into the stomach triggers the production of strongly acidic stomach secretions essential to the breakdown of proteins.	Inability to produce sufficient hydrochloric acid in the stomach causes protein to linger in the stomach and be subject to putrefaction.	Betaine hydrochloride tablets or apple cider vinegar taken approximately one hour after the meal to allow stomach to produce as much natural secretions as possible.
Fat Digestion and Absorption of Various Digested Materials	Small Intestine	The acidic bolus coming from the stomach passes through the pyloric valve into the duodenum of the small intestine. There it is exposed to bile that neutralizes the acid and pancreatic enzymes that digest fats, as well as carbohydrates and protein.	(1) Insufficient hydrochloric acid in the stomach cannot overcome highly alkaline bile leaking back into the stomach through the pyloric valve, causing an alkaline "heartburn." (2) Individuals without gallbladders may not have have sufficient bile secretions after a meal.	(1) Betaine hydrochloride tablets or apple cider vinegar taken at the onset of discomfort may relieve the indigestion and bitter taste in the mouth. (2) Given that hydrochloric acid secretion is complete, bile salts in tablet form may be necessary to continue the digestive process at this stage.

Stage of Digestion	Location	Ideal Outcome (Simplified)	Difficulty	Digestive Aid/ Action
Nutrient Absorption	Large Intestine	Digested materials to be absorbed, such as amino acids and simple sugars, are picked up by the capillaries of the large intestine and pass through the portal vein into the liver and on to the bloodstream. Fatty acids are taken into the lymph system through the thoracic duct and carried to the bloodstream. Water and salts are also absorbed. Appropriate bacteria act on the bolus, producing beneficial substances such as vitamins.	Disturbance of the intestinal environment can occur from improper diet, alcohol consumption, and smoking. The population of bacteria may not be optimal, allowing fermentation of carbohydrates, putrefaction of proteins, and rancidification of fats. Diarrhea or constipation may result.	The long-term solution is a program of cleansing the intestines, no more frequent than a monthly basis, treating inflammation with raw cabbage juice and/or aloe vera gel before bedtime, and repopulating the intestine with beneficial bacteria by taking high potency lactobacillus capsules (probiotics) after each cleansing.

Glandulars (Protomorphogens)

Glandulars, or protomorphogens, as Dr. Royal Lee called them, are nutritional supplements made from organs and tissues of cattle. Use of such materials is not new, as they have been used by health practitioners for over 100 years. Originally, protomorphogens were available as injectables, which were very effective, but the drug companies pressured the FDA to ban this form in the United States. Proponents of glandular therapy were forced to find another way to deliver them to the body, so they developed ingestible forms.

The basis for glandular therapy is that degeneration of an organ can be offset or reversed through ingestion of the tissue of that particular organ. Degeneration occurs when the cells of the organ are damaged and debris from the cells are released into the bloodstream. The body makes antibodies to the debris that can also attack the original organ. This is a manifestation of autoimmune disease, such as diabetes, rheumatoid arthritis, and neuromuscular disorders.

Do Protomorphogens Work?

One of the criticisms I have heard is that protomorphogens taken by mouth must be completely broken by digestive enzymes into fats, carbohydrates, and amino acids. Therefore, there would be no significant, biologically-active fragments, such as enzymes, hormones, and DNA sequences to be assimilated in the whole. To counter this notion, I recommend Dr. Royal Lee's and Bill Hansen's book, *Protomorphology.* It is a toughie and you need to be a good biochemist to understand it.

These protomorphogens work; we see them working all of the time. Most criticism comes from doctors and Ph.D.s who have no clinical practice and are just theoretical chemists. But remember, minerals make the enzyme systems, and vitamins are the catalysts that make the minerals and protein become the enzymes. There are certain minerals that will work with the protomorphogens, but again, total balancing is what we want.

Most of the time we give them to you with meals. Like Standard Process' Cardiotrophin, the protomorphogen for the heart, is given one tablet three times a day (t.i.d.). If you have a lot of spasm we'll give you their Cardio Plus that contains a lot of vitamin E2. It is an antispasmodic. People with a lot of angina pain take nitroglycerin, but if they take vitamin E2, it'll do a better job and relieve the pain. Also nitroglycerin has to be broken down in the liver, and it breaks your liver down. You protect the patient by getting them off nitroglycerine and putting them on vitamin E2. It also has vitamin B2 in it.

Editor: Directly quoting the *New York Times* article of October 18, 1994, *Hair of Dog Tried as Cure For Autoimmune Disease* by Jane E. Brody. It was reported that "researchers have modernized an ancient Chinese remedy that shows great promise for treating and perhaps preventing various autoimmune diseases, including rheumatoid arthritis, multiple sclerosis, insulin-dependent diabetes and uveitis, an inflammation of the eye that can cause blindness.

The treatment, called *oral tolerization* (a form of glandular therapy), seeks to turn off patients' rejection of their own tissue by feeding them small amounts of a protein directly or indirectly involved in the attack by their immune systems. The approach was derived from the well-established fact that people rarely mount an immune response to food. For example, patients with diabetes would be given insulin, which is produced by the pancreas; those with multiple sclerosis already are being given a protein from the myelin sheath that surrounds nerves in the brain and spinal cord and patients with arthritis are being given the joint protein collagen. The first two are administered in powdered form, in a capsule, while the collagen is a liquid given in orange juice....

Dr. Howard Weiner, an immunologist and specialist in multiple sclerosis at the Brigham and Women's Hospital and Harvard Medical School in Boston, calls oral tolerization, a form of vaccination via the gut. It stimulates the immune system in a way that helps the host suppress autoimmune disease,' he said....There appear to be no side effects.'....the technique is 'so simple and apparently so safe that it seems too good to be true.' In fact, nearly every scientist who is now working with it was skeptical at first and a few remain so, awaiting a clearer understanding of how oral tolerization works in test animals and in people.

However, when Dr. Lloyd Mayer, an immunologist at Mount Sinai Medical Center in New York, first suggested studying the technique, he said his Chinese-born graduate students told him, 'This is old hat. The Chinese were doing this 4,000 years ago. If a patient had a problem with his pancreas, he was fed pancreas, and if a patient had a

problem with his liver, he was fed liver.'

Oral tolerization takes advantage of a very basic protective mechanism built into the body: the ability to prevent attacks on the various proteins, carbohydrates and microorganisms that are consumed in an ordinary diet. Dr. Mayer explained that the intestines house 'the largest lymphoid organ in the body' and their job is to enable animals to ingest and digest food without the body launching an immunological attack against these foreign invaders."

Adjunct Supplements

An adjunct supplement is usually considered as a non-essential substance or compound added to the diet to perform a particular function or variety of functions. It is usually not taken for a single pharmacological effect. The following are examples of adjunct supplements.

Aloe Vera

Aloe vera has been used both as an anti-inflammatory to treat mildly inflamed mucous membranes of the mouth, throat, and digestive tract. It has also been shown to relieve diabetic neuropathy.

Bioflavonoids

Bioflavonoids (biologically active flavonoids) are found in plants, fruits and vegetables and are consumed by animals and humans. Bioflavonoids are beneficial in improving connective tissue, local circulation, and the collagen matrix; and in protection of collagen against non-enzymatic proteolytic activity. They are also protective against alveolar bone loss in periodontal disease. As free radical scavengers, flavonoids inhibit lipid peroxidation, promote vascular relaxation, and help prevent atherosclerosis.

Carnitine

Carnitine is found mainly in animal tissues. Lysine and methionine are needed to make L-carnitine, but the useful form is produced only in the liver, brain, and kidneys. Muscles take up carnitine from the bloodstream and contain most of the body's carnitine stores. L-carnitine transfers fatty acids to the mitochondria where they undergo oxidation to regenerate coenzyme A, a vital part of energy metabolism. Defective L-carnitine metabolism has been shown in individuals with diabetes mellitus, malignancies, myocardial ischemia, and alcohol abuse.

Editor: More information about carnitine can be found at the WebMD webpage: http://www.webmd.com/vitamins-supplements/ingredientmono-1026-l-carnitine.aspx?activeingredientid=1026.

Co-Enzyme Q10 (CoQ10)

CoQ10 is an important cofactor in the transfer of electrons in energy metabolism. It is an effective antioxidant that participates in the function of cellular membranes and stimulates the growth of new cells.

Fish Oils

Omega-3 polyunsaturated fatty acids are found in fish oils, such as those from cod, salmon, tuna, and halibut. It is also found in krill, plants, algae, and nuts. Omega-3 fatty acids are important to brain function and in normal growth and development.

One of my colleagues on the lecture circuit is Dale Alexander, whose first book, *Arthritis and Common Sense*, came out in 1950, selling more than one million copies. This and several other of his books and lectures did a lot to call people's attention to the virtues of cod liver oil, earning him the nickname, "Codfather." He refers to cod liver oil as the only perfect human machine oil that will loosen stiff joints and reverse dry skin and hair, among other conditions.

Dale was a medical technologist in the Air Force, looking for a way to cure his mother's arthritis, and happened upon a book in the Harvard Medical School titled *Cod Liver Oil*, written in 1855 by Dutch physician L. J. DeJohgh. He started his mother on daily doses taken on an empty stomach, coping with the objectionable odor and flavor by shaking up a tablespoon of the oil with two tablespoons of milk in a baby-food jar. (**No milk for you! Use an acid-forming juice, instead.**) This broke the mixture into thousands of tiny emulsified, milk-coated oil droplets, disguising its taste. After six months, they started to see beneficial results, especially in the appearance of her skin and hair.

When the oil is taken by itself, the liver, which acts like a sponge, removing vitamins A and D-3 before they can be distributed throughout the body. However, when emulsified oil is taken on an empty stomach, it goes directly into the bloodstream, passing easily to places where the active vitamins are needed.

Superoxide Dismutase (SOD)

Superoxide Dismutase is an enzyme associated with copper, zinc, manganese, and iron. It catalyzes the dismutation reaction of toxic superoxides (free radicals) to molecular oxygen and hydrogen peroxide. Three forms of superoxide dismutase are present in humans. SOD1 is located in the cytoplasm, SOD2 in the mitochondria, and SOD3 is extracellular. SOD1 and SOD3 contain copper and zinc, whereas SOD2, the mitochondrial enzyme, has manganese in its reactive centre. Manganese and zinc stimulate production of SOD.

Herbs

Herbs are plants used as flavorings and spices in cooking, but herbs can also be used as supplements for health or medicinal reasons. They are also referred to as botanicals, which are substances obtained from plants and used in food supplements, personal care products, or pharmaceuticals. Other names include herbal medicine and plant medicine.

There are many brands of herbs available, and I am not well-schooled in their use. One must be careful; some herbs can interact with certain medications, including those for high blood pressure, diabetes, and depression, as well as blood thinners and even over-the-counter drugs. **Also, do not take too many herb capsules. More is not necessarily better, and it could be dangerous. My concern is overuse of herb concoctions and the possibility of their causing regional inflammations in the digestive tract.** Therefore, consult a competent herbalist.

Dr. John Christopher is without a question the best I have ever run into in telling about herbs. And the herb movement is coming very rapidly in the United States. We have herbology societies that have meetings with one and two hundred lay people, learning how to use herbs, and they're doing a better job of treating people than a lot of doctors that I know.

Editor: The website of Dr. John Christopher is http://www.drchristopher.com/.

Some herbs that you might investigate for symptomatic relief include the following, for the indicated reasons.

- **Turmeric** – contains circumin, a powerful anti-inflammatory that may be of value in reducing the size of colon polyps and offsetting Alzheimer's disease.
- **Ginger** – prevents stomach upset from many sources that works by blocking the effects of serotonin.
- **St. John's Wort** – relieves mild to moderate depression and anxiety. It contains melatonin and increases the body's melatonin, helping to improve sleep.
- **Garlic** – contains more than 70 active phytochemicals, including allicin, which may decrease blood pressure. Garlic may also help to prevent strokes by slowing arterial blockages by reducing the body's level of homocysteine.

A Word About Homeopathy

Homeopathy is defined as the treatment of a disease by small doses of natural substances that, in a healthy person, produces symptoms of that particular disease. However, I believe that homeopathy is the use of any vitamin, mineral, or drug in small amounts. For example, instead of using 300,000 units of penicillin, which is a typical dose, use only 1/6 or 1/12 millionth of a unit.

Homeopathy has proven to me that you can use very small amounts if you know how to put supplements into the system on a proper basis. Homeopathy does a very wonderful job as an activator to what you have in your body. The goal is for the penicillin to act only as a catalyst to help the body do its own job. We are finding that a lot of the protomorphogens that we use are better in smaller dosages. In fact, if a value in the bloodwork is not too far off from desired, we may use only one protomorphogen per day. Most of the time, we use three.

8 Feet and Posture

Start with the feet, or you are defeated before you start!

I begin this chapter with one of my favorite sayings to emphasize the importance of the feet to the health of the entire body. Did you ever stop to think how important your feet are? First, you should realize that 1/4 of all of the bones of the body are located in just the two feet – 26 bones in each one! The feet represent the foundation of the bony structure of the entire body; **it is of tremendous importance that the bones be balanced properly, otherwise any discrepancy, even in one foot, creates a short leg and a resultant spinal curvature.** As a result, the vitality of the body is lowered at least 10%, based on my own research during which I treated the feet of over 100,000 persons.

Modern Shoe Construction

The shoes made today, regardless of the quality of the leather, are not constructed properly. To save money, the manufacturers have neglected to include a substantial steel shank – the part that joins and supports the shoe from midfront to heel. A strong shank is absolutely necessary to prevent the anterior portion of the calcaneus (os calcis or heel bone) from rotating downward, with concomitant internal rotation of the cuboid bone. This movement causes a depressed fourth metatarsal and an elevated fifth metatarsal.

The visual indicator of improper shoes is the relative positioning of the toes. Let the feet dangle down and look at the alignment of the toes, all of which should lie on the same plane. If they do not, the bones in the foot are out of position and need to be corrected.

Misalignment of the toes indicates that the middle of the shoe is flexing downward toward the floor with every step. The sole probably makes a quiet slapping sound. There is little or no support between the heel and the sole, and the foot becomes fatigued and painful. To treat this condition, the foot should be manipulated and the calcaneus supported by a felt pad affixed to the insole; further, wedge-soled or well-shanked shoes should be worn. Women have a more difficult time finding properly-constructed dress shoes. To acquaint yourself with possible conditions that can be caused by incorrectly-supported shoes, see Figure 3, below.

5 VITAL POINTS

Five vital points of the body that may be affected with incorrect shoe support.

1 Neck and shoulders reflect strain of carrying head erect and balanced with the rest of the body.

2 Back strain reflects the compensation for curvature of spinal column accompanying abdominal distention and shift of center of gravity.

3 Pelvic tilt out of normal position reflects equilibrium adjustments between upper and lower body portions at hip joint and sacroiliac joints.

4 Knee joints reflect the weight bearing stresses of walking and standing. Muscles and ligaments of legs are among the most powerful in your body.

5 Feet and ankles support entire body weight and improper weight thrust may result in muscle fatigue and foot discomfort.

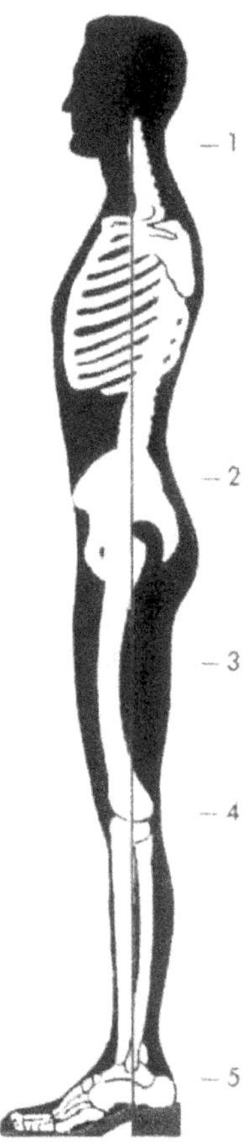

Figure 3: Five vital points chart, used by permission, Foot-So-Port Shoe Corporation.

Functions of the Feet

Let's understand something about proper functioning of the feet.

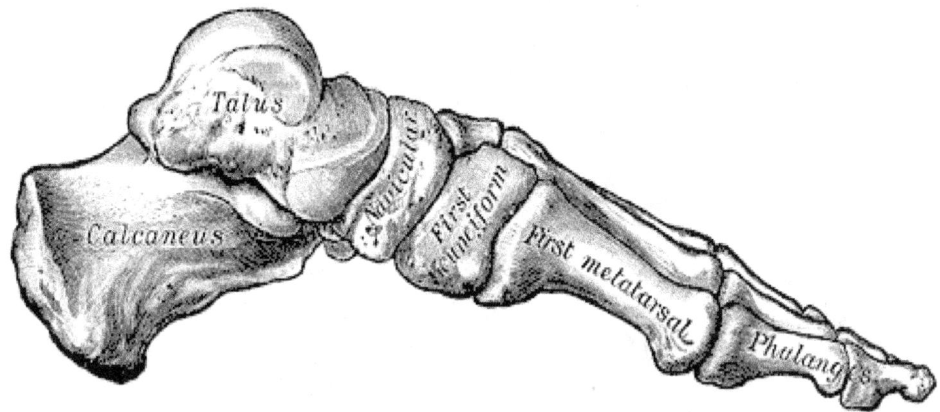

Figure 4: Left foot medial view. From *Gray's Anatomy*, 1918.

First, we should consider the os calcis, or calcaneus, better known as the heelbone. To find out if you are standing correctly, have someone look at your foot and lower leg from the back as you stand on a hard surface. If the inner side of the Achilles tendon is perfectly straight, perpendicular to the floor, this is the normal position.

The more that the Achilles tendon bows to the inside (the medial side), the weaker the foot. Contrary to what you may have been told, flat feet are the strongest feet; the higher the arch, the weaker the foot. The heelbone is the rudder of the foot. If not held in the proper position, it may rotate inward, creating a pronation, or it may drop, but this motion depends on the relative orientation of the bone directly in front of the heelbone, the cuboid.

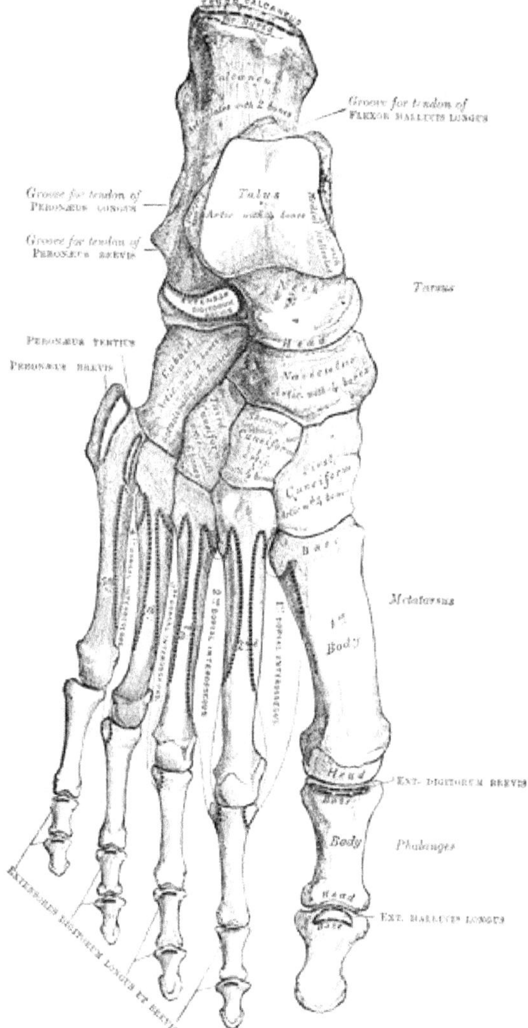

Figure 5: The right foot shown from the dorsal surface. From *Gray's Anatomy,* 1918.

I consider the cuboid to be the most important bone of the foot. This bone, at its posterior/ superior aspect has a twist facet under the os calcis to hold it in its position. The cuboid can rotate inward and downward, thus allowing the os calcis to either pronate or drop straight forward down in front. This problem can be easily seen in the walking pattern. The cuboid controls the fourth and the fifth metatarsal.

Other bones that play major roles in foot function are the navicular, or pivotal, bone; the talus; and the three cuneiforms, each of which controls a metatarsal bone. The interior cuneiform controls the motion of the first metatarsal, the middle cuneiform controls the motion of the second metatarsal, and the external cuneiform controls the motion of the third metatarsal.

Walking Patterns

In a normal walking gait, 60% of the body's weight is carried on the heel. As the weight is transferred to the toes, the load is distributed along the outer side of the foot, along the styloid process, then to the fifth toe, then to the fourth, as the foot rolls to the inside, the fifth metatarsal carries approximately 30% of the weight. Then the load is transferred to the big toe, which carries 10% of the weight. The big toe produces the greatest part of the push during forward propulsion. **If the feet slap, lacking a smooth transition of the weight from the heel to the ball of the foot, the cuboid has probably rotated inward and downward.**

Shoe Construction and Fit

Shoes are man-made contraptions. God made us to go barefoot, but with today's concrete, wood, and asphalt surfaces, there is too much potential for shock to allow it. **The rule in selecting a pair of shoes is to stay as close to nature as possible to accommodate the dimension and uninhibited motion of the foot. Don't fit your eyes; fit your feet! Think first of normal function and forget style.**

Bunions

If shoes are too pointed, too narrow, or too short, they can cause bunions (a dislocated big toe) and talar bunions (a dislocated little toe). The worst bunion I have ever seen involved the big toe being dislocated so far as to be over or under the other toes! In such a case, the best treatment would be surgery. However, the best preventive measure is wearing hose of the proper length and well-fitted shoes with low heels. It is very important that the toes be allowed freedom of motion within the shoe.

Anyone who has bunions should do the following one to three times every day. Expect the full effect not to take place for one to two years of daily application.

1. Grasp the foot, holding the first metatarsal with the base of the thumb and first finger.
2. With the other hand, grasp the big toe (or the little toe in case of a talar bunion).
3. Pull the toe away from the foot and rotate it in both directions for several minutes. This exercise does cause some discomfort because it makes the muscles and ligaments go back to work, whereas they had been relaxed. Try not to cause too much pain or inflammation.

Vericose Veins

Rotation of the cuboid is common today, because modern shoes are manufactured with flat or concave arches and without a steel shank. These deficiencies in design allow the cuboid bone to rotate inward and downward. The styloid process is out and up; the fourth toe is down; and the fifth toe is up. This is evidence that the cuboid has rotated. As this bone is also attached to muscles that run around the foot to the outside, a tightening of the musculature of the lower leg is usually experienced. This tightening leads to the development of varicose veins in the legs of many persons. It also causes the tibia and fibula to rotate, constricting the interossus membrane, which narrows the space needed for the veins of the calf to work properly. Blood is forced into the smaller external veins, producing vericosities.

Callouses

If one develops a callous on the bottom of the foot, the usual cause is the inward rotation of the cuboid, thereby flattening the cuneiforms and allowing the metatarsals to drop. The excessive amount of pressure and friction that is put on the metatarsal arch causes the callous. A callous is nature's way of protecting the tender, sensitive areas underneath the skin. The excessive amount of pressure can cause a plantar wart, a very difficult problem. Restoration of the proper relationship of the cuboid to the other bones of the foot is aided by the use of the cuboid pad. This pad is 1/8" thick, 1 1/4" wide, and from 1 1/2" to 3" long, depending on the size of the shoe. The pad should be 1/4" to 1/2" behind the heads of the metatarsals and never directly under them, and extend to just ahead of the calcaneus.

Socks and Hose

Serious problems result from the wearing of short hose. The way to test hose is to stand in your stocking feet and look at them. Unless you have excess hose extending past your toes, you are wearing them too short. Women have the greatest problem with hose, because they must wear them wrinkle-free, therefore too tight! The pulling back on the toes produces bunions and talar bunions. Short hose cause hammer toes, a condition in which the toes are flexed. The tendons tighten and hold the toes in that position so that they cannot effectively balance the body as they are called upon to carry their part of the load in walking.

Heel Height

Men should never wear a heel height exceeding 1"! A man's pelvis allows him to withstand only 1" elevation of the heel relative to the level of the ball of the foot. This revelation excludes many of the boot types, especially cowboy boots. That style of boot was developed for the purpose of keeping the foot in the stirrup – not for walking!

Men in cowboy boots and women in high heels have more severe problems with heel height. The first thing to remember is that, for every forward movement, you have a backward movement. Right? So when you get on those high heels, you raise your heels up in the air. That means one thing – you have a backward movement in the ankles. To offset that, you have to have a forward movement, so your knees go forward. Because your knees go forward, you have to have one that goes backward so your rump goes backward. When your rump goes backward, you have to have a counter movement forward, so your shoulders go forward. When your shoulders go forward, your head goes up in the air!

In my work as educational and research director for an orthopedic shoe company, I had the opportunity to participate in many different studies. In one, we varied the heel heights of womens' shoes and used X-ray photography to record the influence of these changes on the feet, ankles, knees, and pelvises. The heels were varied from 1/4" to 2" in 1/4" increments; above that, they were varied in 1" increments to 3", 4", 5", and 6". Pictures were taken of each woman's feet without shoes and with shoes of each of the heel heights. We found that the womens' pelvises can withstand up to, but not over, a heel higher than a 1 1/2" heel – what is called in the shoe business a "12-8 heel." For every 1/8" that the heel is raised above the 1 1/2" height, the pelvis is tipped forward seven degrees, and it locks. The uterus keeps going backward and ends up on the rectum, as a retroverted uterus. The locking is a result of the fifth lumbar vertrebra going so far forward that it could not regain normal motion.

If ladies are having problems with their backs or menstrual cycles, the heels on their shoes are most likely too high. Ladies wearing three-, four-, and five-inch heels will wind up with menstrual problems, most likely ending with a hysterectomy. The twisting effect also interferes with the functioning of the ovaries in producing estrogen and progesterone and throwing the cycle out of balance. Women should not wear a heel height over 1 1/2" if they want good posture, more vitality, and mental acuity.

Exercise for Weak Feet

Whenever there is a weakness, there is inward rotation of the os calcis, a condition called pronation. The more that the Achilles tendon slants toward the inner side of the foot, the more severe the weakness. This condition can be alleviated by the comprehensive exercise described below.

Before you fall asleep at night or before you get out of bed in the morning, do the following:

1. Extend both feet off the end of the bed, placing the Achilles tendon even with the edge of the mattress.
2. Flex (curl) the toes down as far as possible. Keep the toes in this position during the entire exercise.
3. Bend both feet upward, toward the shins, keeping the toes curled.
4. Bend both feet downward, away from the shins, keeping the toes curled.
5. Alternate these two movements, counting an up/down movement of both as one repetition. Do 100 repetitions. This movement exercises the arch. Anticipate that you cannot do more than 20 repetitions without the muscles beginning to cramp.
6. When a cramp develops, stop and rest.
7. Continue until the goal of 100 is reached.

When you can do 100 repetitions without cramping, you will probably discover that your feet are functioning perfectly.

Strapping the Feet and Ankles

Athletes should properly strap their feet before competition. The objective is to create pressure against the internal cuneiform, the cuboid, and the styloid process of the fifth metatarsal bone as one is walking, jogging, or running. This pressure creates an upward force to the middle and external cuneiforms and the inner aspects of the cuboid. 60% of the blood comes down the leg, under the sustentaculum tali bone (juts out) on the inner side of the ankle, and into the plantar arch blood vessels. 40% of the blood goes into the front part of the foot. The tape creates a pump action as it pushes the arch up when the foot contacts the ground and releases the arch when the foot is recovering before making contact with the ground again. An increase in circulation is afforded the entire foot and, as a result, the feet do not become tired.

Over the years, including my own stint in professional basketball, I have wrapped the feet of my own teammates after manipulation while a game was in progress! For example, using these techniques of strapping after a first half let the player participate in the second half without any further problems or complications.

Strapping the feet also helps to prevent sprained ankles. Sprained ankles involve three foot bones that are prone to becoming jammed (limitation of motion) during normal use. The most important one is the cuboid, which rotates inward and downward. The middle cuneiform is a triangular bone that becomes a wedge. As the foot spreads, the middle cuneiform lowers to a point between the internal and external cuneiforms and locks the two in place. The third jam occurs where the tibia inserts forward of the talus.

To check this relationship, try to put your finger in a depression, or hollow spot, on the top of the talus. If the tibia has moved too far forward, you cannot get your finger into the depression. In some cases the tibia goes into a stuck position. The position of the displaced bones causes the slapping of the foot during walking, and the ankle is not given its desired range of motion. The foot plainly cannot operate properly!

Those of us who believe in the benefits of manipulation are far superior in helping patients with sprained ankles than those who are not inclined to use manipulative techniques. These three bones must be put back into their proper relationship so that they can move normally. If they are never put back, one will have a chronic foot and/or ankle problem for the rest of his or her life.

Foot Strapping Method

To strap the feet, use non-waterproof adhesive tape. Application is rather simple and can be done by the performer without the aid of a trainer or doctor. Use two strips of non-allergenic, non-waterproof adhesive tape 1 1/2" wide and of sufficient length to encircle the foot and overlap on the dorsal surface (instep). Follow these directions:

1. Place the first strip on the bottom surface of the foot so that the front edge of the tape is slightly in front of the head of the fifth metatarsal. Make sure that there are no wrinkles in the tape.
2. **Bring the tape up on the outside, over the instep**, pulling it taut (not tight; do not stretch the skin). The only tape that is put on tight is that which directly contacts the sole.
3. **Bring up the tape on the inside, overlapping the tape from the outside** and pulling it taut, as well. Relax the tape and let it literally fall over itself, following the contour of the foot and overlapping itself.
4. **Place the second strip overlapping the first strip by 1/8" uniformly all the way around.** Apply it in the same way as the first strip. These two strips should cover the posterior transverse arch and the posterior metatarsal arch.
5. After competition, remove the tape by loosening the end of the tape that was last applied and drawing it back over itself in the direction that it was applied.

Ankle Strapping Method

This method is used to keep the foot in the proper lateral position by preventing the foot from inverting and everting, while allowing the foot to flex and extend normally. The limitation of lateral motion prevents the sprain from taking place. Replace the tape every 24 hours to avoid irritation and possible blistering. Use two strips of non-allergenic, non-waterproof adhesive tape 2" wide and approximately 28" long. Follow these directions:

1. Apply the tape approximately 12" vertically, up the outside of the leg.
2. **Turn (evert) the foot to the outside and pull the tape underneath the foot and around to the inner side.** Press the tape, making sure that there are no wrinkles on the bottom.
3. When you have the foot in that position, **turn the entire foot to the inside (invert) as far as it will go.**
4. **Pull the tape around, letting it wrap around and adhere to the leg** in an easy manner. Let it fall into place and adhere to the inner side of the leg vertically, until it reaches approximately 12" above the ankle.
5. **Place the second strip of tape vertically, across the forward part of the tibia,** overlapping the first tape.
6. **Turn the foot to the outside (evert), pull the tape taut on the outside**, and apply it to the bottom of the foot. Press the tape, making sure that there are no wrinkles on the bottom.
7. **Turn the fore part of the foot to the inside (invert)** and let the tape run up vertically and adhere to the leg as before.

Additional tape may be applied over these strips for additional support.

Anatomical Short Leg - A Major Problem

In the late 1930s, I was part of a study of children of the Three Rivers, Michigan school system. Further, I was involved in a similar study of mentally deficient children in a special school in St. Louis, Missouri. The children of grades 1, 3, 5, 7, 9, 11, and 12 were checked on three consecutive years with a posture check machine, while the teachers kept track of the IQ scores. **These studies revealed that 62% of all of the students we checked had an anatomical short leg, meaning that one leg was at least 1/8" shorter than the other.** Corrections of these deficiencies raised the IQ scores an average of 10%. Uncorrected deficients tended to have more irritations in the feet, legs, and spine than those with legs of equal lengths. As recent as 1980, researchers at the Michigan State Osteopathic College reported that 60% of the persons that they checked had an anatomical short leg. **Of course, we are talking about a true, structurally short leg, based on the length of the bones and not on any muscular tension that may give the impression of a short leg.**

The lumbar vertebrae will rotate in a direction toward the anatomical short leg. However, if there has been some type of accident that has twisted the spine, the rotation may be in the opposite direction. This is why it is necessary to take a standing postural X-ray in an anterior-posterior plane, as well as in a lateral plane. It may be advisable to use a larger plate so that the plate extends approximately 2" below the acetabulum.

Our own research, described above, revealed that the greatest irritation was caused by a difference in leg length of 1/8" to 3/16". Differences in this range cause an imbalance at the base of the sacrum, creating a twist in the entire pelvic girdle. I have a 1/4" buildup on my right side because my right leg is a 1/4" shorter than my left. As long as I wear this, I don't have any back pain. If don't put it on my shoe, I use 10 times more energy every day than I should be using. It is very vital that you find somebody that can do this type of X-ray work.

To correct the rotation, it is necessary to add a lift, or shim, under both the sole and heel of the anatomical short leg. Unfortunately, over the years, we have heard so many so-called authorities — even some of my colleagues — state that all one needs is a heel lift. Nothing could be further from the truth. If we raise the heel without raising the sole, the spine is thrown into a torsion that is worse than would happen if no lift had been added at all! Therefore it is imperative that both the sole and heel be lifted by the same amount.

9 Common Health Issues

Editor: This chapter contains remarks made by Dr. Ellis about various health issues and how he preferred to address certain conditions. **No opinion contained herein, regardless of how thoughtful it seems, constitutes a complete method of treating a particular disease or condition.** Dr. Ellis emphasized that no one should expect nutritional modalities to act like drugs in giving immediate relief for a condition or render a decisive pharmacological effect. **It is imperative that anyone with a serious disorder seek a thorough evaluation by a trusted medical professional and follow sound medical advice resulting from the evaluation.**

This chapter contains thoughts on several common health issues, their significance, and what may be done to offset them.

"Acid Indigestion"

See Ulcers on page 174.

Aluminum Toxicity

Aluminum hydroxide is used in some antacid preparations, antiperspirants, and in baking powder, but the aluminum is not converted into a product that can be eliminated from the system. We can pick up the level in a hair analysis. We also find aluminum in canned foods, foods wrapped in aluminum foil, and in aluminum utensils. These are the biggest sources, stay away from all of them.

Antiperspirants that contain aluminum block the third passage of elimination of poisons out of your body. If you've got body odor, it's because your bowel is not working properly and it's kicking the poison out of your pores. If you have bad breath (the fourth passage of elimination), most of it comes from the undigested food in your stomach. You can get breath odor from periodontal diseases and gums, but it's minor compared to the amount caused by the gut. Once the aluminum is in the system, it can be removed using methionine, alginates, and a lot of vitamin C.

Arthritis

Arthritis occurs when the body attempts to maintain a proper level of blood serum albumin, the protein that normally covers joint surfaces. when the albumin level drops, protein is pulled into the bloodstream from the joint. The calcium that is left behind lays down a rough surface on the bone, and it becomes irritated during movement. If the albumin loss continues, a chronic painful arthritic condition results. **Cortisone relieves arthritis because it makes the body draw albumin from the muscles to raise the bloodstream concentration and to serve the joints. The joints, so supplied, show a decrease in irritability and inflammation until cortisone's effect wears off and the supply of looted protein from the muscles is cut off.** The first step in stopping protein thievery is to have ample, assimilable protein in the diet. Digestion of protein must be efficient and complete. Supplement with calcium, magnesium, manganese, phosphorus, and protein.

One of the good things for the pain of arthritis is to take a potato, cut it in half, take a teaspoon and scrape it and eat the scrapings. It'll take your pain out of an arthritis. But if you cut a piece out and eat the potato, it does not work; you must scrape it with a teaspoon.

Arthritis (Reactive)

Reactive arthritis was once called Reiter's Disease. See the Editor's note under Osteoporosis.

Back Pain (Lower Back/Anatomical Short Leg)

Low back pain is one of the most common complaints that a practitioner hears. It may originate from a number of causes, with a multiplicity of associated symptoms.

Causes

I can safely say that the majority of patients with low back pain have had other conditions associated with the primary complaint. These include:

- **Physical stress on the spine** with muscular imbalances and postural defects resulting from an anatomical short leg. See Feet and Posture on page 141.
- **Irritation of the internal organs and tissues** served by the nerves emanating from the lumbar and surrounding areas. Such irritation is commonly initiated by a toxic bowel. Avoid alkaline-forming foods (raise urine pH) in favor of acid-forming ones. See Detoxification on page 99.
- **Protein insufficiency**, with resultant hypothyroidism, immune deficiency, lack of muscular tone, and inefficient mineral transport through the bloodstream. See Protein Nutrition, Protein Intake on page 52.
- **Mineral imbalances** brought about by inattention to proper dietary habits and vicarious patterns of supplementation. See Food and Diet on page 59 and Nutritional Supplements on page 111.

- **Inflammation and infection** of the prostate, uterus, bladder, etc., with accompanying alkalinity of the body fluids and regional hypoxia (poor oxygenation) within the affected tissues. See Protein Nutrition, Acid-Alkaline Balance on page 56

Anatomical Short Leg

Studies show that 60-62% of the population has an anatomical short leg, meaning that one leg is at least 1/8" shorter than the other. Uncorrected deficients tend to have more irritations in the feet, legs, and spine than those with legs of equal lengths. Two conditions commonly encountered are generalized lower back pain and sciatica.

The one and only way to determine an anatomical short leg is in a standing position, as follows.

1. Take your clothes off and stand in front of a full-length mirror. If a hip is high on one side, a shoulder is high on one side, or if one breast is lower on one side, you've got a curvature in the spine that probably is caused by an anatomical short leg. Sixty-two percent of the hundreds of persons we tested in the 1930s had an anatomical short leg.
2. Put your thumbs on the crest of your ilia (outermost part of your hips) in exactly the same place on both sides, making sure that your feet are even with each other and squared to the mirror. If your legs are the same length, a line drawn between your thumbs should be perfectly level. The difference in the distance between your thumbs and the floor are indicators of the difference in the length of your legs.

A postural doctor, especially a good osteopath or chiropractor, will do a standing X-ray front to back through an anterior/posterior lateral from the side of the lumbar, spine, and pelvis. Then he or she can measure the base of the sacrum to see how much it takes to get it back into a horizontal plane. That represents the thickness of the lift you apply to the sole and heel of the shoe on the short side.

What do you need to do about it? **To correct the rotation, it is necessary to add a lift, or shim, under both the sole and heel of the anatomical short leg.** Unfortunately, over the years, we have heard so many so-called authorities – even some of my colleagues – state that all one needs is a heel lift. Nothing could be further from the truth. If we raise the heel without raising the sole, the spine is thrown into a torsion that is worse than would happen if no lift had been added at all! **Therefore it is imperative that both the sole and heel be lifted by the same amount.** I estimate that persons with uncorrected anatomical short legs use 10 times the energy to accomplish the same tasks as if the problem were corrected.

Do not be fooled if a doctor checks your leg length while you are lying on a table, manipulates you, and claims to have corrected the short leg. He is not only fooling you; he is fooling himself! It is not possible to correct the length of leg bones through adjustment of the spine.

Blood Pressure Elevation

The common treatment for elevated, or high, blood pressure usually involves the long term use of diuretics. The first thing diuretics do is eliminate potassium from the system. You see, sodium is high on the inside of a blood vessel, potassium is high on the outside of a blood vessel. Nerves are just the opposite. Potassium is high on the inside of the nerve; sodium is high on the outside of the nerve. In the bloodwork, we use a ratio of sodium to potassium (Na/P) between 28/1 and 30/1. A ratio above or below that range means that you have broken down the nerve centers of the body. So it is vitally important that we understand what we are doing with sodium and potassium.

When you don't keep the levels so that the ratio stays within the range, you are going to break down and get worse. I recommend treatment of an elevated blood pressure with colonic irrigations – two a week for four weeks, one a week the next four weeks, one a month thereafter. We have not had any problem bringing down blood pressure so far. The ideal is approximately 120/60.

Breast Feeding

When you have a child, the most important thing, even before you cut the cord, is to have the child suckling the mother's breast. If not, it does not get the enzymes, and the Lactobacillus acidophilus bacteria that makes the baby's digestive system work the rest of his life. This is the most important fluid that you will ever put in your mouth. Breast feeding should be continued as long as the mother can tolerate the teeth. Two years is the end of it. That is when the digestive enzyme rennet leaves the stomach, and the child then has no business touching any milk product, including mother's milk after this age.

Some bottle-fed babies have been found to have no production of hydrochloric acid between the ages of 2 and 5 years, but it occurs commonly during the early teens to early 20s. **Why can't some women breast feed? Imbalance, not only from a hormonal standpoint but also from mineral and vitamin. We've had very little trouble if we have seen these women early.** Those ladies with small breasts can be helped; we use the mammary protomorphogens along with a regular program that we've developed (**Editor:** The program is not defined herein.). There is another product called Fortil, made by Standard Process that may be able to enlarge the breasts. One of the things in it is made from the leaves of Spanish moss, or Tillandsia (from Florida); this is the highest source of vitamin E we know of.

There was once an article titled, *Inability to Love is Linked to Breast Feeding Neglect*. I can't remember the author's name or the source, but I would like to expand on it. I have already told you that the human baby is the only one who cannot get to the breast of its mother by itself. So that child, after the cord is cut and is put into a crib right away, is neglected, because the mother did not love it enough to put it on her breast; the child knows it. The child who is suckled says, "Hey man, this shows you love me so I'll help you by sucking on your nipple to help you shrink your uterus so that you won't need a shot in the tail to stop you from bleeding when that placenta comes out."

I worked with the Pathfinders group in Dallas; they are taking care of these so-called "hyperactive children." All of these kids were bottle-fed babies. They have been neglected right from birth, and they are the ones who, in their teens, cause most of the trouble between children and parents. Think about yourselves, were you breast- or bottle-fed? This idea of early rejection has very deep psychological impact. Often, you have to reach 30 or 40 years of age to realize that your parents were really wonderful people.

Breast Tumors

Women with breast tumors should get out of synthetics and nylons, because many of these tumors are nothing but congested milk ducts, and the surgeons want to do a radical mastectomy. Bruises will produce congested milk ducts. If they are only congested milk ducts, you can use castor oil packs, and there is evidence that supplemental iodine is helpful in treating breast lumps. The best iodine to use is Formula 636, or Atomidine, sold in health food stores in a dropper bottle.

Cancer

I am an advisor to more than 300 doctors, and I guess I'm supervising about 200 cancer patients. In this cancer work, the first thing we do is blood, hair, and urine analysis to find out where we're going. We do an anthrone test, which is also known as the Navarre test, or Beard test; it checks for human chorionic gonadotropin (HCG). It does show a lot of false positives if the testing routine is not followed properly. So we make sure that an instruction sheet is given and how many days it might take to get ready before the urine is taken so that we know we get an accurate sample.

This sample is then divided in a V-shaped cruet with the fluid added first and then the urine. The faster it sets up a white ring on the bottom, the more cancer there is in the body. I'd say that its 95-98% accurate. The amount we find determines how we might treat a cancer patient. In fact, M. D. Anderson Hospital in Houston is now using it, and they are one of the groups that fought this for many years.

I don't know of a single method that will cure all types of cancer. On most of these patients, we use about three different things and, as long as we use them together, we get somewhere. B17 (Amygdalin, Laetrile) should be legalized, if for no other reason than it is the best pain reliever in cancer patients that I know of. It's better than demerol, Darvon, or morphine. I think Dr. Philip Benzan of Washington Courthouse in Ohio has the highest cure rating with B17 by itself, and that's about 18%. Studies on germanium therapy for cancer were done by Dr. Asai in northern Japan. Dr. Asai showed us case histories and slides from 30 patients, each having been given less than two months to live, but who were all completely cancer-free after a month of treatment.

Most cure rates are down around 10-12%. Even those from Mexico are doing about the same. A lot of these organizations will say to use only B17, which we don't want. But a cancer patient also requires a very specific diet that, for the first month, allows no proteins, because we want to get away from putrefying protein. All people that I know with cancer cannot digest meat properly, so it putrefies and causes cell degeneration. They need HCl, trypsin, and chymotrypsin, in addition to a disciplined, targeted regimen. So these must be supplied, as determined by the hair, blood, and urine and so we know what and how much to use, and when.

Then we have Mitozyme, and we cannot get Dr. Lester Wesners to give us its analysis. But our analysis tells us it has a great deal of thymus in it, which of course, is one of the biggest activators of the immune response against any disease. The other thing that holds people back is that a six-week treatment is fairly expensive. But on many of these cancer patients, it does a fantastic job. However with the materials in it, you cannot use pancreatic enzymes or vitamin C, which is pretty tough on the patient. So on many of these patients, we have gone along about six to 12 weeks, either one or two rounds.

Editor: As of 2016, the product name Mitozyme is registered in India by Southern Petrochemical Industries Corporation Limited and is described as being a "Concentrate versatile enzyme preparation developed exclusively to reduce wrinkles and growth marks, imparts appreciable softness and smoothness to the leather." **It is doubtful that it is the same product mentioned in the text by Dr. Ellis.**

Then we take them off that and put them on our method with the Wobe Mugos proteolytic and pancreatic enzymes. That is the name of the German product. Here, we use Retenzyme and Intenzmye made by Biotics Research Corporation. These enzymes, by the way, if taken when an injury occurs, like a sprained ankle in sports (take five Intenzyme tablets), cut out most of the pain and swelling in about 24-48 hours. The trypsin and chymotrypsin neutralize the inflammation and swelling in the system, which has been documented with football players. We use 17 germanium tablets along with it.

I worked with the Brozny-Levinsky Clinic in Pittsburgh using Mycorrhiza. They were put out of business but came back with it as a food supplement. It does work with some people, and we have found that it works in conjunction with other things, but not too much. I worked with Dr. Bill Coate in Detroit in 1936-37 until the 1940s, when he was put on trial. We worked with glyoxalide and parabenzoquinone. Parabenzoquinone is the finest antibiotic I have used in all my years of practice and is far superior to penicillin, erythromycin, acromycin, paramycin, or any of the other mycins. One shot intramuscularly in the buttocks can usually knock out any infectious disease in the body.

Glyoxalide was synthesized by William Frederick Koch (1885-1967). It is taken intramuscularly in the buttocks. Glyoxalide increases the oxidative index of the body. It is number one on my list for treating cancers of all types. Then again, you have a specific diet that must be followed with no proteins or tomatoes. Koch taught me in his clinic, where he was treating 30-40 cancer patients of various types a day.

Glyoxalide works on a cycle of three; every three days you should have a reaction like a cold or you feel a little more tired than you were the day before, or the day after. A woman in California with cancer had to go to bed on the 21st day; she had such a reaction; on the next day, she couldn't believe how good she felt. I'd told her that anything that divides by three will give a reaction. When you multiply it in the multiples, you will get an even bigger reaction. The biggest reaction is on the 27th week. I don't know why, but this was the published routine. However if you don't get a reaction on that day then you should get another Injection of glyoxalide, to keep it in the same routine. Combined with the diet, you can get better results than anything else that I know of. To Dr. Virginia Livingstone, the Progenitor cryptocides is a microorganism found in all people with cancer, and, in her opinion, it is one of its basic causes.

Editor: See *Virginia Livingston, M.D.: Cancer Quack or Medical Genius?* by Alan Cantwell, M.D., reprinted by permission of the author in Additional Reading on page 361.

As of 2016, it is possible to determine an individual's genetic propensity to develop certain types of cancers. The reader is encouraged to review the following website that discusses genetic tests for breast cancer: https://www.knowbrca.org/Learn/brca1-and-brca2-gene-mutations and the following website that discusses genetic tests for prostate cancer: http://time.com/4395658/aggressive-prostate-cancer-test/.

Castor Oil Versatility

Castor oil is used commonly as a laxative. However, the use of castor oil packs in any area of the body is helpful to relieve pain. Put castor oil on the affected area and cover it with a towel and apply a heating pad. Congested milk ducts in the breasts call for castor oil packs. A good book about using castor oil packs is *The Palma Christie* by William MacCary M.D. See also Eye Inflammation (Blepharitis) on page 160.

Cholesterol Elevation

Cholesterol is manufactured in the lining of the intestinal tract and liver mainly from starches, sugar, and dairy. Less than 15% is ingested, so beware of TV advertising. To lower cholesterol, eat eggs daily – a fine source of protein – just remember that under the shell is the enzyme avidin, which on exposure to the air, immediately destroys the biotin and pantothenic acid in the egg. So, I recommend that you eat eggs soft boiled for at least 30 seconds to destroy the avidin. You can eat six eggs per day and never worry about cholesterol. Supplementation may include niacin, vitamin C, and vanadium.

Chron's Disease

Chron's disease is an inflammatory bowel disease in the form of colitis. Again, you have to go with the digestive enzymes and use aloe vera gel to do the healing. The aloe vera taken by mouth does an excellent job. Raw cabbage juice (without the pulp) and lactobacillus tablets are of great help, as well. **Do not eat the cabbage pulp; it can kill you!** You may mix the aloe vera gel into the cabbage juice, or you can drink the aloe vera with cranberry or prune juice in the daytime.

If you do not have a juicer, take 1/4 head of cabbage and put it in a blender. Add one quart of distilled water, put the lid on the blender, and blend it on a high setting until the particles are as small as you can get them. Strain the mixture, discarding the pulp (again, do not eat the pulp), and store the juice in a glass bottle with a tight lid; it is very aromatic, to say the least! Drink eight ounces of this at bedtime, preferably on an empty stomach to protect the lactobacillus organisms from digestive juices.

You can also use highly concentrated chlorophyll; made from buckwheat, available from Standard Process, and the protomorphogens of the GI tract. Take each one 30 minutes before each meal; you can also use comfrey and pepsin or Hydrozyme from Biotics Research Corporation. The healing properties of these is great! Sulfa drugs are very harmful. They work for only four days, and then make your infection worse.

Colds and Flu

Whenever you have the first sign of a cold or flu, you're not up to par, you're sort of listless, and you're tired, we recommend a cleansing enema to flush putrefied, fermented, and rancid substances from the bowel. These devitalize a person, are easily eliminated, and prepare the bowel to absorb beneficial nutrients. You do this by getting from the drugstore Fleet's Phospho-Soda. On the label they tell you to take two teaspoons and a glass of water. I will tell you to take six teaspoons or two tablespoons in a glass of cold water due to the fact that this is a salt and it goes down a whole lot easier in cold water. After you put that one down, follow it with a glass of hot water as hot as you can drink it.

This is a flushing mechanism. This will flush your gallbladder and your liver and then the bile will activate your bowels completely from your stomach right on through, and especially as it gets into the small intestinal tract and empties your gallbladder of bile. Then the bile activates it in a normal and natural way. It will operate somewhere between 15 minutes and two hours. While you are waiting, take a lemon enema; that's the juice of a freshly squeezed and strained lemon in two quarts of warm water.

Deodorant Interference

What can you use for a deodorant? That's easy, don't have constipation. Because if you don't have constipation, you don't have a body odor. Why do you need any kind of deodorant; even talcum powder just blocks the pores, and you must keep them open to get rid of the extra poisons in your perspiration. The poisons should have come out of the bowel and the kidneys first. When it doesn't, it gives you a body or breath odor. Whatever you do, don't use antiperspirants that contain aluminum, because they block the third passage of elimination of poisons out of your body.

Depression

How does one combat depression? Well, the first thing anyone should do is learn how to live on a positive realm. Always look for the good out of everything, regardless of how bad it seems. Next, do the blood, hair, and urine analyses and find out where the discrepancies and metal poisonings are. When you get rid of these, there doesn't seem to be any more problems with these kinds of people. One of the things you want to realize with this type of disorder was shown in the work of Dr. Alexander Schauss, who worked in the prison systems. He found that murderers and rapists are hypoglycemic. Hypoglycemia, low blood sugar, is probably one of the most common diseases that exist today. We teach doctors that can't make a diagnosis to write down hypoglycemia, and they will be right 90% of the time. It is the greatest masquerader of all diseases that we know of.

Editor: Dr. Alexander Schauss wrote a book titled *Low Blood Sugar and Antisocial Behavior.* He explains how sugar can cause a whole range of behavioral symptoms, "from depression and hyperactivity to acting out behaviors that may be extremely asocial." Dr. Schauss uses case histories, graphs and illustrations to show the connection between food additives, food allergies, alcoholism, junk food, and environmental pollutants and how all of these contribute to the development of crime.

Diabetes

Anybody with a high blood sugar level should always check zinc, chromium, potassium, and protein to give the body the opportunity to let the glands do their job. With respect to thyroid, if you don't check the amount of inorganic iodine and the amount of protein, which are the two things blended together by the cells of the thyroid to produce thyroxine; you will never learn anything about thyroid function. The ideal ratio is 3:1. Anything over 4:1 gives hyperactivity of the thyroid gland and highly nervous, irritable factors. The same can occur even though you could have an absolutely perfect T3, T4, T8, T9, or Protein Bound Iodine (PBI). Supplement to the deficiencies of minerals and ensure optimum protein assimilation.

Disc Degeneration

You may have disc lesions that you will never know, because they never hit a nerve root. If the rupture is through the anterior side, you never know it because there's no nerve there. We can detect it by sclerotherapy, using a 6" needle going in from the side, and directly through the disc area, using dyes and X-ray. We inject a sclerosing material and heal that ruptured disc on the inside. Then we pull it out on the outside capsular ligaments.

Once, I had a patient with a torn back, taking sclerosing treatment. I was using magnesium, but low back pain kept recurring. We started him on manganese, and this time, when he came back from his treatment, he had no more problems. Manganese is the catalyst that makes calcium, magnesium, and phosphorus do their job on the muscle and ligamentous integrity of the body. All you need is one tablet of manganese at lunch time. If you supplement yourself in calcium and magnesium, you should take calcium at or before breakfast and magnesium at dinner time.

Exercise Precautions

If you go jogging, you must make sure that you keep your body perfectly straight. If you bend forward as you jog your heart keeps hitting against your chest wall and can be damaged. The men who are now jogging, standing in upright positions, instead of bending over like so many of them do, are getting better results and have more vitality than they did previously. **Some authors like Dr. George Goodheart tell you that you shouldn't jog at**

all; walking exercise is all you need. In a good exercise, your heart should beat from 100-120 beats per minute over a long period of time. So, we used to tell that walking fast, swimming two miles a day, or riding a bicycle 10 miles a day will do the same thing from the standpoint of body functioning.

One thing that jogging does is destroy the protein metabolism in your muscles, and walking does not. That's why most of the long distance runners are on the thin side; they are utilizing and burning that protein out of their system, and it isn't replaced as much as it should be. Olympic team members were not allowed to touch a milk product for 48 hours before competitions, because they found out that it slowed them down too much. Actually they should never touch it an any time. To help with oxygenation of tissues and endurance, we recommend adding octacosanol to the diet, which is contained in high concentration in Viobin Wheat Germ Oil and in Biotics Research Corporation's Bioctasol Forte.

Editor: See the following link to Dr. Thomas K. Cureton's work about the use of wheat germ oil in physical training: https://catalog.hathitrust.org/Record/001556016?type%5B%5D=author&lookfor%5B%5D=%22Cureton%2C%20Thomas%20Kirk%2C%201901-%22&ft=

Eye Inflammation (Blepharitis)

For blepharitis, put one drop of raw castor oil in the eyes, four times a day. These drops burn but should be continued, because as the treatment progresses, the pain gets less and less. This could be a form of allergy, so the treatment should be continued as needed; otherwise, it can be discontinued until the next time it is necessary. We have also used the castor oil to dissolve cataracts inside the eye, using one drop four times a day.

If you wear contact lenses, get some pure castor oil and place one drop in your eyes each night before you go to bed. Close it and don't rub it. This is probably the finest healer for the conjunctiva of your eye and removes all of the irritating factors that you might get from your contact lens. Automobile mechanics or anybody working where dirt can fall into the eyes should always keep a dropper bottle of castor oil around. It is thick and stops the itching; everything rolls over to the inner corner of your eye, and it is very simple to take it out with a handkerchief.

Fasting and Congestive Heart Failure

I do not believe in fasting because unloading so much poison out into the system can create a "charley horse" in the heart muscle. One of my closest friends was George Tong. He invented the Tong Table, a really fine manipulative table. George ran the biggest health food store down in St. Louis, Missouri.) We were at an osteopathic convention when he said, "I'm going home to go on a 12-day fast." I said, "After you get through with this convention and the food that you've been eating, you'd better not do It. You will get congestive heart failure and die." That's exactly what he did. He went home, fasted, and died on the twelfth day.

I have seen this happen too many times, and that's the reason why I still say that I would rather use our other methods of detoxification, like the A and E emulsions, along with aloe vera gel. I'd rather use this slow method than a fast method. To detoxify quickly, do what I said is the equal of a 12-day fast by using sixteen grapefruit and hydrochloric acid tablets. See Fasting Alternative (Quick Grapefruit Fast) on page 108.

Fluorescent Lighting Precautions

Overhead fluorescent lights cause your brain to deteriorate. It also lowers the resistance mechanisms of your body, so don't stay under florescent lighting. I attribute the harmful effects of fluorescent lights to radiation or to the spectral balance. If you must work under these lights, wear a visor and consume foods and supplements rich in antioxidants.

Fluoride Toxicity

The federal courts in Pennsylvania and Illinois have already decided that fluorides cause cancer. I received word on toothpastes containing fluoride. They also cause cancer in your cheeks and gums. I just hope that all of these companies, the dental health associations, and the Public Health Service wake up to how dangerous fluoride is. Fluorides displace iodine in the tissues and destroy the production of hydrochloric acid in your stomach. Drink distilled water and supplement to your mineral deficiencies. Long-term consumers of fluoridated water should check the inorganic iodine and total protein levels and supplement accordingly.

Whoever tried to get anybody to start fluoride rinsing in a school is plain stupid; using fluoride rinses in schools is stupid. If you don't speak out against using these, you don't love your children. Let me just tell you about one instance.

A dentist took on a little three year old boy with no cavities. During the boy's first visit, the dentist insisted on using fluoride gel. After treating him, he told the little boy to rinse, which he did and then swallowed the mixture. Either the doctor, the nurse, or his dental assistant apparently didn't stay long enough, and the three year old didn't know enough to spit it out. He got sick immediately.

The doctor didn't know what to do, so he sent him over to the emergency room at the hospital. The child sat for one hour before he was taken in, even though he was acutely ill. When he did get in, those treating him didn't know what to do either. He was in there for two hours before he died. The parents sued the hospital and the doctor and collected $750,000 for his death.

I lectured for the Canadian Dental Association, and they kicked me out because of my stand against fluoridation. Before I said anything about fluorides, I asked the 400 doctors sitting in front of me how many of them carried malpractice insurance for fluoride poisoning? Not one hand went up. I then asked how many of them kept the antidote for fluoride poisoning in their offices. No hands went up. I said. "Man, I thought I was sticking my chin out to talk about this before you. Look what you do every day if you use fluoride in your office, and you don't know what to do if someone gets poisoned by it!"

I didn't tell them what the antidote was. I finished my talk and left 20 minutes at the end of my two hours for questions. How many people right away asked me what is the antidote for fluoride poisoning? Absolutely none. The funny part about it is that the one thing I say is the greatest single cause of disease in the human is milk. All you have to do is drink a glass of milk if you have fluoride in your stomach.

Food Allergies

The top five allergenic foods are milk products, chocolate, wheat, corn, and beef, in that order. **Peanut allergy is the leading cause of anaphylaxis and death due to food allergy.** We can add to that the coal tar products – synthetic vitamins, and we can even get into it as far as metal poisonings creating an allergic reaction. The allergen swells the mucous membranes, and creates an irritation in the nose and throat area. That makes the area wide open for pollen or dust to have easy access for more irritation, because these areas are already swollen and irritated.

There are several things that help get rid of allergies. First, eliminate from your diet the things that produce allergies. Use bee pollen to stop allergies. It contains 20 of the amino acids (including all eight essentials), vitamins, and minerals. A natural antihistamine with beef liver extract is often helpful. Standard Process has a product called Antronex, containing the Japanese yakatron beef liver extract. Take one of these pills three times a day, and you will see improvements; discontinue treatment when no longer necessary.

Food Poisoning

For suspected food poisoning, hydrochloric acid is the antiseptic in the stomach. The best treatment is large doses of betaine HCl or apple cider vinegar. It either lets food progress along the tract or causes vomiting. If antibiotics are used, always follow up with Lactobacillus acidophilus and bifidus to reestablish the desired bowel flora. These bacteria help digest the fiber and avoid constipation. The emulsified vitamins A and E are helpful. Because hydrochloric acid and pepsin can destroy many protomorphogens that we ingest, select those that are prepared to withstand the acid medium until they pass into the small intestine.

Foot Strains and Sprains

There are three bones in the ankle that are always rotated and stuck; the most important one is the cuboid. The second most important is the middle cuneiform, and the third is the tibia; it always rotates posterior on the talus. **All three must be manipulated. These must be treated as soon as they occur and strapped with no inversion or eversion of the foot.** Then, one can be put back on his or her feet with no problems. Balance Is important, and if this injury is not treated, there will be a chronic ankle problem for life. Also use pancreatic enzymes to take out the inflammation and swelling.

Gout

Uric acid causes gout. People with gout are usually very low in potassium, the neutralizer for uric acid in the body. They are also very low in hydrochloric acid, and pepsin. Pork products are loaded with uric acid; they also have nitrites, nitrates, and nitrosamines, which are cancer agents. Also, don't eat sardines, because the DNA mixes with uric acid and makes the hands and feet swell. In addition to the hydrochloric acid and pepsin, use one teaspoon daily of Carbamide by Standard Process.

Hands (Cold Hands)

The hands falling asleep is an indication of a potential heart attack. The other indication is a low thyroid functioning. Cold hands and feet need ribonucleic acid, called RNA potassium, and betaine hydrochloride. These are the factors that you must put together, and you can get rid of your cold hands and feet. The only counterindication to the use of RNA is a possible rise in uric acid.

Healing of Tissues

If you are having a hard time healing, or if you are going in for surgery, take vitamin T (sesame seed factor) because it will aid in the healing process by encouraging platelet formation. Vitamin E will help to keep platelets from sticking together and aggregating. The night before surgery, have them give you a bottle of amino acids with 3,000 mg of vitamin C. We have had hundreds of patients doing this. We have no shock, no pneumonia, and they are up on the same day of surgery. Their stitches are out on the fourth day, and they go home on the fifth day.

For example, there was a woman with a tumor on her left breast. It was 10" long, 3" in diameter, and it weighed 10 pounds. It took us three months to find a surgeon that would only remove the tumor, nothing else. Before surgery, he gave her Aminosol, which is the name of the amino acid supplement, plus 3,000 mg of vitamin C. We saw that we were doing so well that the next morning, as soon as the surgery was over we gave her the second bottle, the third one that night.

This surgeon is still pulling his hair out, because that breast was in such good condition that, after cutting a 3" hole, he was still able to pull the skin together without skin grafting. Her stitches could have come out on the fourth day, but he was so scared about taking them out that he waited four more days. Eight weeks from the day of surgery, this woman was back at work.

The following lists conditions and supplementation that may restore normality to the indicated tissues. However, it is always better to determine the need for minerals based on comprehensive testing, rather than overloading an individual with minerals that may not need to be taken.

Skin conditions, including fungus (such as athletes foot), warts, etc.: Supplement with zinc, copper, and cobalt.

Nasal congestion, sore throat and mouth (including cold sores): Supplement with cobalt, manganese, magnesium, iodine, vitamins B1 and B6, emulsified vitamins A and E, and tryptophan.

Fractures: We use 20 cc of 2% magnesium chloride solution IV once weekly, with vitamin and mineral supplementation that includes copper and cobalt.

Immune system support: We use calcium lactate, vitamin F, thymus, vitamin C, and proteins.

Cardiovascular integrity: Supplement with sodium, potassium, calcium, magnesium, zinc copper, molybdenum, chromium, vanadium, manganese, iodine, and cobalt

Heart "Attack"

A true heart attack involves a problem within the heart itself. However, many deaths attributed to heart attacks may not be true heart attacks at all. Let me ask you an important question, What room in the house has the highest frequency of deaths due to heart attacks? It is the bathroom! Are you surprised? Because most people have their heart attacks within two hours after a meal; what happens is that they are not digesting their food so they get a gas pocket, either in the stomach or the transverse colon. Persons suffering from pain go to the bathroom to get an alkalizer. What happens then? After taking the alkalizer, gas in the stomach increases, causing an increase in upward pressure, stopping the diaphragm from working properly, creating severe pressure on the heart, and producing a cardiac spasm. This spasm can be so great that it can kill before relief of pressure can be obtained. When the person dies, the heart comes back to normal; they do an autopsy and can't find anything wrong with the heart.

If you ever get a chest pain up on that side, head for the kitchen and take some apple cider vinegar — one or two tablespoons in a small amount of water. Always use apple cider vinegar and drink it. If the pain is due to the gas pocket bottling up and producing a charlie horse, that acetic acid will break that bond, and you won't have a charlie horse any more, the vinegar relaxes it. It is one of the easiest tests you can give on a heart attack. **But, if that pain persists beyond five minutes you had better get somebody to get you to a hospital because you are having a heart attack.**

We were up at Denver, Colorado at the Brown Palace Western Research Laboratories; this company put on the finest seminars I have ever attended. It is the company that had an attorney come in to teach us how to handle the FDA agents when they come into our offices. Anyway, this doctor attendee had gone up to the hospitality room and had a couple of whiskies; then he went down and ate a big smorgasbord dinner. When he got finished, he went bank up to the hospitality room, eating potato chips and roasted nuts and having more alcoholic beverages.

I had gone downstairs and was walking around. All of a sudden, the elevator doors opened, and a wheelchair came out carrying the doctor, all ashen gray. Well, everybody knew he had a heart attack but me, so I sent a kid after some apple cider vinegar, but telling him to get what he could. I intended to put a couple of tablespoons in a glass of water and give it to him before the ambulance got there. So he went out, and the only thing he could get was white vinegar. There are two things I know that white vinegar is good for; one is if a cat or dog comes around and puts spots on your rug it is the best thing in the world to clean it up, and the other is for a women to take douches with.

Anyway, we gave it to him and we got about 3/4 of that glass into him before they got him into the ambulance. It took about 15 minutes to get him to the osteopathic hospital. By the time they got him to the hospital, all of his aches and pains were gone out of his chest. They took him into the emergency room and did an electrocardiogram on him; it was completely negative. Because of the severity of the pain he was talking about, they kept him overnight. The next morning, they did another electrocardiogram, and it was still negative so they discharged him.

I didn't see him when he first got back, so at noon, we had another smorgasbord, and this doctor ate the same type of foods all over again. He had listened to what I had told him the night before, and of course, I went up to him and told him I was sure glad to see him and that I was glad it wasn't a heart attack. He said, "Don't tell me it was that damn vinegar that kept me from having a heart attack." I said, "Well if you are that stupid, it is alright with me if you have another one; just eat that junk on your plate and you will have another one."

This sort of bothered him, because he came up to me later and said, "You know, you are pretty irritating when you say things like that." And I said, "The hardest thing a person has to do is face the truth face to face, and that's what hit you, because you knew I was telling the truth." He went home and did some thinking on it and decided he had better do what I had told him to do. Within a month he was feeling better than he had in ages.

Heartburn

See Ulcers on page 174.

Hemorrhoids

A hemorrhoid or pile is nothing more than a varicose vein in the rectum. To relieve hemorrhoids, use aloe vera gel. Take a baby syringe containing two ounces of aloe vera gel. People that have hemorrhoids or piles should inject that solution into their rectums before they go to bed at night and let it stay there, soothing and shrinking the tissue.

Iodine Deficiency

The thyroid is not the only tissue that needs iodine; it is needed by breast, salivary, pancreas, brain, spinal fluid, skin, stomach, and thymus tissue, as well. There are two popular sources of iodine: kelp capsules and iodine solutions. There is only one kelp that anyone should use today and that comes out of Norway and it is pretty hard to get. There's plenty of American kelp, but it is pretty bad. You're also unable to ascertain with kelp the amount of iodine that your thyroid needs. Kelp, when you analyze it, varies so tremendously. I've found problems from the use of kelp. So we just tell people not to use It.

We would rather they use the Formula 636 (Atomidine). That way we know exactly what we're dealing with. You might use from one drop per week to one drop or even more per day. If a sore throat results, discontinue until the condition goes away, then resume at a lower dosage. There is evidence that supplemental iodine is helpful in treating the enlarged prostate and breast lumps. Atomidine is sold in health food stores in a dropper bottle.

Kidney Stones

A kidney problem signals a bowel problem, because most of the body's poisons are supposed to be going into the bowel. When the bowel can't handle these poisons, they go to the kidneys. This insult is in addition to what the kidney itself has to do. Most of these are caused by the urine being too alkaline, again a lack of hydrochloric acid and pepsin. The sodium and potassium must be in balance to make the kidneys work properly. The pH is very important because most kidney infections or diseases occur in an alkaline urine.

Any pains in the kidneys, ureters, bladder, and urethra are more severe when the urine is alkaline. Many times, you can relieve such pain with just a couple of teaspoons of vinegar. You might need to form antibodies to fight the infections, and then acidify them. You can clear up most of them in this manner.

For calcium stones, we use phosphorus and magnesium, dissolving the calcium stones and enabling them to be passed. We then use a big dose of olive oil or castor oil. The hardest ones to clear up are uric acid stones, which can form in the kidneys or gallbladder. They can be removed surgically without having to take the kidney or gallbladder out.

To lessen the chance of developing stones, the vegetables In salads, such as cabbage, cauliflower, spinach, and tomatoes, should always be eaten raw; never cooked. They are all high in oxalic acid, which interferes with calcium metabolism. The only fruit that leave an acid residue are prunes, plums, cranberries, and rhubarb. Rhubarb should be eaten raw because of its oxalic acid content. All other fruits leave an alkaline residue (make the urine alkaline). When you eat alkaline fruit, it is much better to eat them as a snack individually between meals, at least three hours after protein.

Knee Joint Deterioration

What can be done for the deterioration of the knee that is causing pain and fluid buildup? The first thing would be to examine it for a rotation of the tibia on the femur. I did this for one of the football players for the Buffalo Bills. They asked me to take a look at it. This player had been in constant pain for two years and yet was playing football. He came over to my hotel room. When I travel, I always carry my portable table with me. I set it up, put him on the table, and there was this rotation. So, instead of coming through even when he turned, it would hit and irritate. He started getting an inflammation in the knee.

I pump handled it a little while and stretched the cartilages that had not been operated on, because he had had two operations on one knee, and one on the other. It took me about 10 minutes of doing this on the two knees on each side. I got him up, and we walked up and down the room. He said, "I can't believe it, I am walking for the first time in two years with absolutely no pain." We recommend using emulsified cod liver oil on a long-term basis. See Arthritis on page 152.

Liver Toxicity

Let's go over how to detoxify the liver. Number one, take vitamin A, vitamin F, and beet juice extract from Standard Process 30 minutes before a meal. This will thin the bile and let it flow. That's the easiest and fastest way to get it out. The use of aloe vera gel by taking two to four ounces every day gives you the opportunity of healing the gastrointestinal tract, and making it flow better. Coffee enemas do the same thing. But probably the great thing you need the most is hydrochloric acid, and pepsin within the stomach. Because if you don't have sufficient amounts of hydrochloric acid, the liver does not do its job. Neither does the bile come out of the gallbladder as it should.

Chew your food thoroughly to take the strain off your liver and intestinal tract, because if you don't have enough enzymes, you're going to putrefy the protein and ferment the starches and sugars. The end products have to be filtered through the liver, and if you don't have sufficient digestion, you are going to clog the liver. Let's predict, prevent, and keep out of trouble from the start. If a cleansing is necessary, follow the appropriate procedures given in Detoxification on page 99.

Lupus and Other Autoimmune Conditions

We have had some success with lupus, but not total success. We use the same type of treatment as for malignant conditions. See Cancer on page 155 and the Editor's note on page 136.

Menstrual Problems

Many women with menstrual problems have a cholesterol level that is too low. They are treated by having them eat more fats; their ovaries produce more hormones and get rid of dysmenorrhea or menopausal hot flashes. In our diet, we require both saturated and unsaturated fats. Foods to eat are fish (as recommended previously); olive, safflower, and sunflower oils; nuts; and seeds. Cook meat at 138° F, and the saturated fats will still be fine.

Ladies wearing three-, four-, and five-inch heels will wind up with menstrual problems, most likely ending with a hysterectomy. The treatment for the resulting dysmenorrhea is to decrease the heel height and use what we call a knee to chest breathing exercise, which lets the uterus go forward again. Another way to get the uterus to go forward is to get pregnant and, immediately after delivery, have the mother sleep face down.

Supplementation

I use Vitaminerals formulas 2BG and Number 16. Vitaminerals 2BG has double the amounts of D complex with its mineral synergists and also contains vitamins A, B, C, and F with their mineral synergists. Number 16, a polymineral, has 34 minerals in it, and two tablets are suggested per meal.

Editor: The Vitamineral (VMMedical) Company website is currently http://www.vmmedical.com/.

Knee to Chest Breathing Exercise for Dysmenorrhea

Women have a constant small opening that runs through the vagina and cervix into the uterus, then through the fallopian tubes and up into the abdominal cavity. The objective of this exercise is to get air to suck in and out of this opening, allowing the fallopian tubes to open up. The action causes the uterus to tip over to a forward position.

Directions:

1. Start out with the woman on her back with her knees bent and feet flat on the floor.
2. Bring one knee to the chest and hold the position for 15-30 seconds. Breathe deeply, allowing the abdomen to move freely.
3. Return to the starting position.
4. Repeat the movement with the other leg.
5. Perform this exercise 2-4 times with each leg.

Metal Jewelry Irritation

Wearing metal jewelry next to your skin is harmful, and the most harmful place to wear metal is the midline of the body; this is especially true for glasses. The presence of metal upsets the electrical field of the body. One half of your brain has a positive magnetic charge, the other half a negative magnetic charge. If you have metal in the middle line you neutralize brain function. If you have a big belt buckle in the midline, being the location of your solar plexus, it destroys the function of the nerves of the solar plexus. So never wear metal on the midline, put it on one side or the other.

Now one thing we know, if you put on certain things like copper bracelets or anklets it can be good for you, or it can be harmful to you. **One should do a hair analysis to find out what minerals are imbalanced in the tissues before attempting to wear a copper bracelet.** If you have too much copper in your system and put a copper bracelet on, it will break down your brain, your nerves, and your blood vessels. It is important that you neutralize, normalize, and make everything in balance; then you will not have any problems.

Multiple Sclerosis

One of the things we have found in most multiple sclerosis cases is metal poisoning, with aluminum being number one on the list. We try to neutralize these metals, using octacosanol, superoxide dismutase (SOD), and catalase. These have been used very successfully.

There was an experienced physician in a veterans hospital who took six of the M. S. cases and used octacosanol, superoxide dismutase, and catalase; he was getting very good results. What do you think happened? They transferred him out of the division so he couldn't touch the cases any more. That's what you run into with the kind of medicine we see from the American Medical Association. If you take SOD straight it does form peroxides. But if you use catalase to neutralize the peroxides, it's a very excellent product. We use it to normalize cell development and cell function. Catalase is found in all normal cells, but most people don't have enough, so we give it to them to rebuild the cell structures.

Muscle Pulls (Charlie Horses)

You can put double-wide pieces of non-waterproof tape above and below a pulled muscle to keep the pull from spreading. During walking or running, the tape becomes a massaging agent. You may expect the pull to become smaller at the end of the activity.

Always remove the tape in the evening; this is especially important in persons with fair skin. Do not have any tape on for more than 48 hours. Check the blood calcium level, the calcium/phosphorus ratio and the level of manganese in the system, if possible.

Osteoporosis

Someone asked me, "What would you advise the older ladies with osteoporosis to do?" We suggest doing 44 blood tests, 19 metals in the hair, a standard urinalysis, and the patient's seven-day diet. Then we analyze and correlate the results to find out what may be causing the osteoporosis, among many other possibilities. Osteoporosis comes from a lack of the balance of the minerals, mainly calcium, magnesium, manganese, and phosphorous. It also is a hormonal insufficiency; thus you see this in the older people. If you don't have sufficient hormones, it is one of your biggest problems in rheumatoid arthritis, along with imbalances of those four minerals. It is the variance of the ratios among each of these that helps to produce this type of disease.

Editor: John D. Carter, MD is the Director of Clinical Research for the Division of Rheumatology at the University of South Florida. His primary research focuses on Chlamydia-induced Reactive Arthritis. **Chlamydia trachomatis is the leading sexually-transmitted bacterial infection in the United States and can cause a serious form of arthritis (reactive arthritis, or ReA) in some individuals**. Chlamydial infections can also exist in a persistent state that has been linked to not only ReA, but also other potential diseases. It is believed to play a role in some of the adverse effects that occur with certain treatments for other types of arthritis. Practitioners treating arthritis, osteoporosis, and spondylitis should review the following of Dr. Carter's publications.

Carter JD, Valeriano J, Vasey FB. *A Prospective, Randomized 9-Month Comparison of Doxycycline vs. Doxycycline and Rifampin in Undifferentiated Spondyloarthropathy - with Special Reference to Chlamydia-Induced Arthritis. Journal of Rheumatology.*

31(10):1973-80, 2004.

Carter JD, Valeriano J, Vasey FB. *Antimicrobials for the Treatment of Chlamydia-Induced Reactive Arthritis. Annals of the Rheumatic Diseases.* 64(3):512-3, 2005.

Carter, JD, Espinoza LR. *The Interplay of Environment and Host Response in Reactive Arthritis: Can We Intervene? Future Rheumatology.* 1(6):717-27, 2006.

Parasites

Ninty percent of people have parasites. The feeling is almost like the flu. Again we go to blood work to determine whether parasites are present in the system. The following story will illustrate what I am trying to tell you.

I had a radiologist call me from Atlanta, Georgia. He said, "Doctor for two years I have been trying to find out what is wrong with me. I weighed 190 pounds, and now I weigh 100. I have been to the best doctors in this entire area trying to find out what is wrong with me. Nobody knows what it is. I was just talking to a friend of yours, and he says you are the best diagnostician in the country and that I'd better call you on the phone." I said, "Well doctor, I imagine your being a doctor yourself that you have done some blood chemistry work; let's start with your CBC, the complete blood count."

White blood count: normal is 5-10,000, ideal 7,500; his was 3,200. His red cell count was down to 3,200, this means that he was anemic. Hemoglobin for men should be between 15 and 16; his was 13.2. The hematocrit, which indicates the volume of a red blood cell, was also pathologic; the cells were too small. The normal count for eosinophils is 1-3, he had 70. Then we looked at the count, and I asked what was it four or five? He said, "Five."

I said," I know what's wrong with you. You have got parasites, microorganisms, or worms." He said, "But doctor, I had a stool culture, and they didn't find anything." I said, "Doctor, do you think that worms can be only in the intestinal tract?" He said, "Yes." I said, "Man, you have got a lot of studying to do." We find these in the brain, in the muscles, heart, tissues; you name it, and we have found them. You are loaded with them."

Chickens and turkeys that are raised on wire are loaded with a microorganism called Progenitor cryptocides (see Additional Reading). These are part of the microorganisms we are talking about. So, always check whether the chicken or the turkey that you are about to buy were raised on the ground. If not, don't buy them.

We can get rid of these microorganisms in several ways. The fast way, which can also cause reactions, is to take a half a teaspoon of confectionary sugar. On this, put six drops of turpentine and swallow it. Man, does it react. Do this at night, then the next morning either take a dose of Fleets Phospho-Soda or a couple teaspoons of castor oil, and some prune juice; then you don't taste it at all. That will really take them out of your system in a hurry.

There is a milder way of doing this. Standard Process has two things one can use. The first is called Zymex II, and the second is called Multizyme. We use Zymex II more than we use anything. Take three of them four times a day for three weeks, and then you cut them to one three times a day for another month. We usually get rid of the parasites in that period of time.

Prostate Problems

Supplemental iodine is helpful in treating the enlarged prostate, as well as other prostate conditions. The best iodine to use is Formula 636 (Atomadine), sold in health food stores in a dropper bottle. You might use from one drop per week to one drop or even more per day. If a sore throat results, discontinue until the condition goes away, then resume at a lower dosage.

Psoriasis

Psoriasis is cholesterol coming out of the pores of your skin. Lower your cholesterol and you'll find it's what we are doing today with emulsions of RNA-DNA, hydrochloric acid, and the pancreatic enzymes, we are clearing up probably most of these in 6 to 8 weeks. Apply Borage oil topically.

Sciatica

See Back Pain (Lower Back/Anatomical Short Leg) on page 152.

Shoulder Pain

When I went over to see the Buffalo Bills football team, I treated six of them, including one of their officers, who said, "What do you do for shoulders, I can't get my arms up any higher than this." I said, "Jump up here on this table." This guy had an anterior third rib out in the front. The one on the left side controls 16 organs, and 22 muscles. The one on the right side, 8 organs, and 22 muscles. I fixed this rib first. Then, I did the pump handle on his elbows and then his shoulders. I corrected the acromio-clavicular lesion, that's where the collar bone is in the shoulder joint.

Then I did the one on the other side, and said, "Would you mind raising your arm." Well I thought his eyes were going to pop out, because his arms went straight over his head. He said to the trainer, "If he wants to treat anybody down here, let him treat him. He knows what he's doing." So I didn't have any trouble. Where we see rib and disc lesions all of the time is with an anatomical short leg. It causes a twist in the knee, the back, or the shoulders as well as up into the head. It also can give you headaches. Take trypsin and chymotrypsin supplements to reduce inflammation.

Skin Conditions

To keep the skin nice and flexible; take vitamin A and E emulsions each day. Routinely do blood analysis and hair mineral analysis every year and supplement for deficiencies. The emulsions, along with Lactobacillus acidophilus and bifidus, draining the liver and gallbladder, and stimulating the adrenals, produce anti-inflammatory agents. With proper diet, the skin condition should clear up in six weeks. Add the thyroid protomorphogen (Standard Process Thyrotropin) to clear up psoriasis; remember that thyroid function and cholesterol levels are inversely related. People with skin diseases must be detoxified, according to the protocols listed in the chapter titled Detoxification. The key is to keep your body balanced. Postural balance is of key importance too. Add omega 3 oils to your diet.

Stroke

The main cause of strokes is arterio- or atherosclerosis. One of the important factors are the triglycerides – today considered more important than cholesterol. Oranges will raise triglycerides faster than anything else I know of. Other foods that cause a rise in blood triglycerides are processed starches, sugars, and milk products. These must be avoided. Treatment and physical therapy will be tailored to the patient, based on the severity of clinical symptoms. Adjuncts to treatment may involve lowering triglycerides with vitamin C, thinning the blood with HCl in the diet, dilating the blood vessels with vitamin B3, and strengthening the vessel walls with vitamin E, but care must be taken not to interfere with prescribed medications.

Sunburn (Tendency to Sunburn)

I believe that the tendency to sunburn is influenced by the level of calcium in the body. Brunettes are low in calcium, and blonds and redheaded persons are especially low. Supplement calcium if you have a tendency to burn and not tan well. Use all sensible precautions to avoid too much exposure to the sun, and keep in mind that you can burn just as severely on an overcast day.

Teeth Fragility and Pain

To have good teeth, start early in life, stay away from all starches, sugars, and milk products. One of the worst cavity producers is cheese. One of the most severe causes of migraine headaches that we know of is the phenylethylamine in cheese. Taken together, all milk products are the single greatest cause of disease in the human body that I know of.

Painful teeth need magnesium, zinc, iodine, and methionine. Along with these trace elements, methionine can cause the gums to grow back along the tooth and maintain a very tight attachment at the gingival margin. It was shown by Dr. Ralph Steinman many years ago how completely permeable the teeth are to iodine.

Dental Caries (Cavities)

In 1919, Melvin E. Page, D.D.S. began practicing dentistry in Muskegon, Michigan and soon became known as a top prosthodontist. He noticed that it was necessary to remake the classic dentures for many of his patients within two and a half years. Their jaw bones would resorb under the dentures and bridges. To learn why his patients' mouths deteriorated, Dr. Page ran more than 2,000 blood chemistries. **He found that no absorption of bone and no**

cavities occurred when the blood calcium to phosphorus ratio (Ca/P) was in a proportion of 10 to 4, or 2.5:1. Dr. Page also found that the blood sugar level should be at 85, plus or minus 5 (Sclavo test) and that resorption of bone would stop when the Ca/P ratio was restored to 2.5. He also cautioned against eating white sugar and refined carbohydrates and drinking milk. He advocated the use of vitamin and mineral supplements and the avoidance of chemical additives and preservatives in foods.]

Editor: Thanks to the International Foundation for Nutrition and Health for the information about Dr. Page. For further information about the IFNH, see http://ifnh.org/product-category/educational-materials/pioneers-of-nutrition/dr-melvin-e-page.

Environment of the Mouth

The mouth should be isoelectric, meaning there should be no electrical current activity occurring within. The presence of mercury amalgam fillings allows such activity to occur. Major acupuncture circuits go through the teeth as follows:

- The upper and lower central lateral incisors relate to the kidney and urinary bladder.
- The cuspids relate to the liver and gallbladder.
- The lower molars and upper premolars relate the the large intestine and lung.
- The lower bicuspids and upper molars relate to the spleen, pancreas, and stomach.
- The third molars relate to the heart and small intestines.
- Each tooth is also related to the function of nine muscles.

When electrical conductivity occurs across the teeth, all of the endocrine glands are affected adversely. Also, it has been shown that mercury leeches from amalgam fillings over time, subjecting the individual to varying degrees of mercury toxicity. Symptoms of mercury escaping from tooth fillings may include the following.

- Sensitivity or allergy to any metal, food, detergent, pollen, etc.
- Metallic taste in the mouth
- Burning sensation in the mouth
- Increased flow of saliva
- Gum disorder or disease
- Frequent unexplained fatigue
- Headaches
- Ringing or noise in the ears
- Cold hands or feet
- Skin rash or dermatitis
- Any change in health after dental work
- Nervous disorders in any part of the body, such as numbness, tingling, shaking, or trembling

Thyroid Deficiency

You can be harmed by taking synthroid; it is a synthetic thyroid, as is proroid, neither of which we recommend. If you are going to use thyroid itself, I would use only as a last resort. We would prefer to let the gland do its own job. We would rather use the protomorphogens of Standard Process or the neonatals of Biotics Research Corporation. The regrowth factors are made from thyroid; you use it with iodine and protein because these are the two ingredients that make thyroxine. In doing this, we are able to build the patient's thyroxine to where it belongs, and in doing so, promote normal thyroid functioning. See Iodine Deficiency on page 165.

TMJ (Temporomandibular Joint, Jaw) Pain

The temporomandibular joints are directly in front of the ears. 43% of the nervous system is connected to the TMJ. Likewise, the teeth and entirety of the mouth receive an abundant nerve supply out of proportion to the rest of the body. The teeth are related through meridians and nerves to the 12 cranial nerves, and each tooth is directly or indirectly related to a specific organ of the body. So, it is not surprising that fillings can cause neurologic allergies or irritations to all 12 of the cranial nerves.

Symptoms of irritation of the TMJ may include the following.

- Pain in the ears, including the middle and inner ear, earache, and tinnitis
- Backaches, scoliosis, neck problems, headaches, sinusitis
- Weak muscles and disequilibrium
- Pain in the shoulders
- Leg length abnormalities
- Stomach, small intestine, and endocrine abnormalities

Tranquilizer Precautions

If you want to use wonderful tranquilizers, take magnesium and vitamin B6. They are the finest tranquilizers we have ever used. They are so superior to librium or valium. Last year there were 22 million prescriptions written for valium and librium in the United States. Number one and number two on the list of all prescribed items, and all they do is destroy your liver and your kidneys.

Ulcers

Your stomach, lined with a mucous membrane, is made to hold an acid. No one has an overabundance of stomach acid; it is likely that no one has enough. See *Acid Indigestion: Myth and Mysteries, Time Magazine*, Friday, Aug. 28, 1964. **This article documents that there is no such thing as an overacid stomach.** When you age, you start losing hydrochloric acid, nature has its own way of compensating for it by regurgitating the concentrated, highly alkaline bile back into the stomach.

How They Develop

Bile burns mucous membranes and produces a gastric ulcer. If you lack hydrochloric acid in the stomach, bile will be regurgitated into the stomach. The average stomach withstands a pH of 2. The mucous membranes are made to withstand acids. Bile is highly alkaline and burns worse than acid. The constant reflux of bile causes gastritis and finally an ulcer. When we stop the bile reflux by taking hydrochloric acid, the ulcer has an opportunity to heal. Alternately, the constant irritation can lead to oversecretion of hydrochloric acid. After the food leaves the stomach, extra acid continues to be produced. The mucous membranes of the duodenum normally withstand alkalis, not acids. This hypersecretion of hydrochloric acid produces a duodenal ulcer.

A person who has had a gallbladder removed has a constant flow of bile and must be very careful about what he eats. Otherwise that bile, with no food coming through, will irritate and cause a gas problem, duodenitis, or jejunitis. Also, taking too much aspirin is one of the best ways I know to get a gastric ulcer. Being an achlorhydric, I have had to be very careful about what foods and supplements I take, so I can stay alive. If I were unable to do this, I would be in real trouble. Achlorhydrics are absolutely fit candidates for cancer. Their alpha-2-globulin and pancreatic enzyme levels are abnormal.

If a gastric ulcer is removed surgically, the problem that caused it remains. I have seen cases of gastrectomy where two-thirds of the stomach is removed from an achlorhydric. However, two months later the problems recurred. These people may not have as much acute pain, but only the symptoms have been removed. People having recurrent ulcers and on a Sippy diet (milk products) can develop new types of ulcers.

The article, *The Incidence of Coronary Heart Disease in Patients Treated with the Sippy Diet, American Journal of Clinical Nutrition*, 15:205, 1964, explains how the Sippy diet uses milk, cream, butter, eggs, and mild cheeses to treat ulcers. It is the biggest cause of strokes, and heart attacks that we know of. It never cures the ulcer, but it just creates enough mucus to cover the crater. You get rid of the symptoms, you don't feel as much pain, and you think you have done pretty good.

In one case, we had to remove the stomach of a man who had had nine ulcers. We dissected it, and right beside each area of scar tissue was a new ulcer. He had hemorrhaged so badly that we couldn't do anything else but operate. When this man healed, the first thing I had to do was teach him how to balance his lack of hydrochloric acid for the rest of his organs to work properly.

How They Can Be Healed

Ulcers are easy to clear up; I've cleared up more ulcers by giving patients hydrochloric acid and pepsin to help digest their food than any other method I've ever used. We use Standard Process comfrey and pepsin. **The only thing I can tell you is that aloe vera gel is a great treatment for ulcers**, and we give patients a teaspoonful at a time, every three or four hours, and we do get healing.

Pepsin is the main stimulator for the cells to make more acid. When we feel the tissue has healed sufficiently, we switch to hydrochloric acid therapy. This is how I healed my own duodenal ulcer. I have tried the same technique on others, and I have never had to resort to surgery.

Another good treatment for ulcers is to take a four- to six-ounce glass of raw cabbage juice (fresh, not canned); drink this every couple of hours all day, consuming the juice within seven minutes of extraction; the enzymes will heal the ulcer (believe me, it has a horrible aroma). Eat bland foods along with it. Do not eat the cabbage pulp itself, it could kill you!

If you do not have a juicer, take 1/4 head of cabbage and put it in a blender. Add one quart of distilled water, put the lid on the blender, and blend it on a high setting until the particles are as small as you can get them. Strain the mixture, discarding the pulp (again, do not eat the pulp), and store the juice in a glass bottle with a tight lid; it is very aromatic, to say the least! Drink eight ounces of this at bedtime, preferably on an empty stomach.

You can also use highly concentrated chlorophyll made from buckwheat, available from Standard Process, and the protomorphogens of the GI tract. Take each 30 minutes before each meal; you can also use comfrey and pepsin or Hydrozyme from Biotics Research Corporation. Ulcers in the digestive system should heal themselves within six weeks.

Vaccination Precaution

I do not recommend vaccinations; they are not necessary, unless you want some degenerative diseases to appear in life later on. The National Health Federation has a kit that will show to you, and all authorities, that vaccinations are not necessary, and they do more harm than good. I'll tell you one thing that you learn about vaccinations like small pox. This has always been interesting to me. We haven't had it in our country for a good many years.

Weight Control Problem

With regard to the diet for obese patients, there seems to be a lot of confusion about low calories and low carbohydrates. **When you want to count calories, whatever your perfect weight is, you need 10 times the amount of calories per day.** For instance, if you weigh 150 pounds, you need 1,500 calories per day to maintain that weight.

People go to Weight Watchers and take a 500-calorie diet, thinking that they will lose weight automatically, but they will lose it at the expense of their health. **Balance your diet, staying away from the extra starches and sugars and milk products, they're the biggest ones that give you weight. If you eat raw green and yellow vegetables, rare meats, raw nuts, and seeds, this will automatically balance your diet. If you're overweight, you will lose. If you're underweight you will gain.**

Sources of proteins? Meat, fresh eggs, fish, and gelatin are your best sources of protein. The fish is the top of protein that you can buy; I recommend salt water fish. The only thing that you have to watch in salt water fish is the potential for lead and mercury poisoning that you can detect with the hair analysis.

Do not touch bottom fish; that includes lobster, shrimp, crabs, oysters, clams, etc. You can eat fish that remain close to the surface, such as tuna, salmon, sardines, etc. If you eat a can of sardines every day, it's one of the greatest helpful protein you can eat. But these are short sardines from Norway, which are loaded with natural DNA. Most of the sardines that you get are wider and longer, but they are actually herring. Now we get the natural DNA and RNA from herring sperm.

This is the poor man's cell therapy that rebuilds cell structures in the body. The only contraindications for the use of RNA-DNA is a high uric acid count in the blood, which may cause the hands and feet to swell up. What is involved in gout besides uric acid? Gout results from the inability to digest protein. Low potassium is another factor. it is the neutralizer of uric acid in the body. Supplementing hydrochloric acid and potassium can reestablish the balance.

Yeast Infections

One other thing, especially in women that we check, and that is for budding, yeast in the urine. We are seeing more and more yeast infections in women. And for the women: get away from the synthetics and the nylons especially with panty hose because they are one of the greatest mediums you have for growing a yeast infection within the vagina because they don't breathe.

Withdraw sugars from the yeast; this is best done with the healthy diet described elsewhere in this book. There are some effective herbal combinations that discourage the growth of yeast, and the lactobacillus is desirable to repopulate the intestine with beneficial bacteria that can out compete the yeast.

10 Comprehensive Assessment and Plan

My father (Humphrey A. Ellis, mechanical engineer and inventor) taught me one thing as a young man, and I will tell it to you, because I think it's been one of the most important things that was ever told to me. He said, **"Son, regardless of how ignorant a man is, he usually knows one thing, and it pays you to listen to it."** Think about that for a minute. Don't condemn anybody for what they are. Even the worst man that's out of business will know one thing, and you can learn what that is. If you can do this with a hundred people who have failed, then correlate these hundred ideas together, you can have a million dollar idea as far as your future is concerned, because it's the correlation of ideas that counts.

This chapter will help you learn how to put a collection of patient information together into a comprehensive plan to restore the health of the patient and, hopefully, to engage the patient sufficiently to make him or her responsible for maintaining a high level of good health. I think that we are curing most patients if we get them before the point of no return. Where that is I don't know, but I want to know what a patient's deficiency patterns are, and then I'm going to go to work on them and see what I can do in rebuilding them.

Since I am an osteopathic physician and surgeon, I have been fortunate to have had the best of both worlds – the ability to manipulate the skeletal system and the ability to utilize laboratory testing – in order to provide this systematic, comprehensive patient care. **As a counselor to hundreds of physicians worldwide, I use four categories of information in my patient analysis.** These are:

- A blood chemistry profile of 44 tests, consisting of the SMAC, CBC, T4, protein electrophoresis, and an atherogenic index
- A standard urinalysis
- A diet diary, including a record of everything a patient eats and the way the foods are prepared for a period of one week
- A hair analysis of 19 minerals found in a sample of a patient's hair

Using such information, a practitioner can get a good impression of the underlying physiological problems associated with the overt symptomatology and restore homeostatic balance. **These analyses are time-consuming, and the practitioner who undertakes them must have studied a great deal.** Although much of the information exists in scholarly journals and texts, insufficient emphasis has been placed on the use of these tests for routine patient care. In addition, the normal ranges for individual tests are far less important that the ratios of the resulting levels to each other.

The Evidence

Let's think about the heart, for instance. Millions of people have died from what was believed to be heart attacks; at least, that is what appeared on their death certificates. But before you can treat a heart case, you have to solve their liver problems; because every single heart case you will ever run into starts with a liver problem. Therefore, I advise all of you to become friends with undertakers!

Why? You won't be signing too many death certificates, I hope. I think, in my 46 years as a doctor, I've only signed 12, so I was pretty fortunate. But I made a lot of friends with undertakers, so I have the opportunity, if they have an unusual case that they are going to do an autopsy on, to go in and watch the autopsy and take their subject's case history. What did the death certificate show as cause of death? What were the contributing factors?

In one undertaking establishment, we observed 16 consecutive cases, all of that had been under therapy for a heart condition; all of the death certificates stated that they had died from coronary attacks. Under the guise of embalming them, we cut their hearts every way you can think of, opened up every coronary vessel; we found absolutely no pathology in any one of the 16. But yet, when we took specimens from the various organs, the one thing we did find was that their livers were practically non-functioning. Now, when you tell this to a cardiologist, he'll laugh at you. The same thing applies to the lungs; you must detoxify these patients, because the lung is the fourth avenue of elimination out of your body. If you do not detoxify the body, you are not going to straighten out the lungs.

The Inspiration

To me, blood chemistry became very, very apparent, early in my life, that there was something we had to find out about the quality of the blood so we could supply the cells of the body with the ingredients necessary for them to work.

Our use of the blood chemistry in the way that I describe was inspired by the University of Illinois College of Medicine's research report on protein metabolism. I got an invitation for a seminar to be held between Christmas and New Year's in Dallas, Texas. I had just finished 15 years as Educational Research Director for an orthopedic shoe company (Musebeck). In fact, the occasion was a chance conversation, involving one of the presenters, Dr. Ransom Dinges, a member of the Board of Osteopathic Registration of the State of Illinois. I was passing by and overheard him talking to another doctor, apparently from his home state. He said, "I understand you are in the Research Department." "That's right!" the doctor replied. Dr. Dinges asked, "Have you been doing any research lately?" The doctor said, "Yes, we finished the greatest thing we've ever turned out at the University of Illinois." "What's that?" Dr. Dinges asked. He replied, "On protein metabolism."

Dr. Dinges got a copy of that report, and this is what he gave us at the seminar. It rang a bell with me that this is the way we had to go into blood chemistry – to find out first what protein metabolism is doing. So, I took a week off and went over to Dr. Dinges' office in Orangeville, Illinois. Now, here was a man in a town of 489 people that had over $100,000 a year practice. He was that good. He was also the finest teacher I have ever had the privilege of standing in front of.

Between us, we developed a 14-test blood chemistry profile to get started; and all it took us was a couple of months to realize that 14 tests were not going to be enough, so we started doing 28 tests, which is the typical panel used by most doctors today. We found out that wasn't enough. Now we are up to 44. So you see, we just keep advancing with what we're learning and doing. Over the years, as new information about these tests becomes available, we change the names and normal values. Later, we take a close look at the meaning of each test, adding material that you usually cannot find in textbooks.

RANSOM LORAYNE DINGES, D.O. was born on July 20, 1907 in Clarno Township, Green County, Wisconsin. He graduated from Kirksville College of Osteopathic Surgery in 1934 and practiced medicine in Orangeville, Illinois until the time of his death in 1965.

He was President of the Illinois Osteopathic Association, and many young physicians had their knowledge extended by Dr. Dinges in his office in Orangeville after they finished their internships.

He traveled extensively, teaching Food Education throughout the United States. In 1954, he compiled a book entitled *Food Education Booklet* for physicians to use in their practices to educate their patients and to assist in their treatment. It was revised in 1957, and it is still available from Amazon.com.

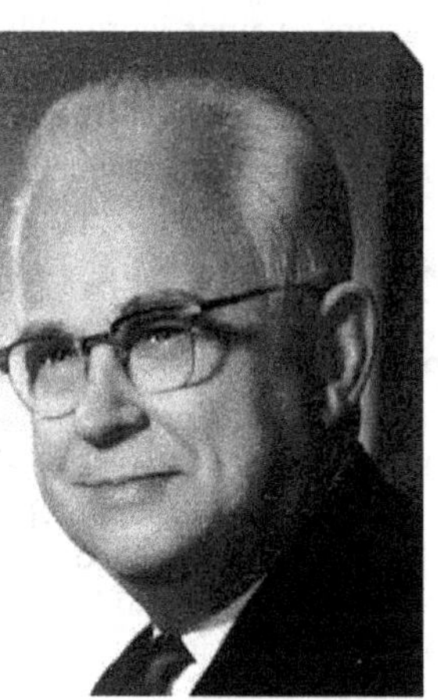

Blood Chemistry, Health, and Death

I have done now better than 25,000 patient blood chemistries. Out of these 25,000, I have found only five that had an adequate level of protein in their bodies, according to my adjusted working normal values of total protein 7.4, albumin 5.2, and globulin 2.2, with a better than 2:1 ratio. Five out of 25,000 people! Now you know why I say that we don't find healthy people anymore.

An interesting outcome involving blood chemistry occurred only four times during my career. These cases involved very sick patients, and all of their blood chemistry values from the laboratory were within 5% of the accurate working normals that I prefer to use. When this happens, you may assume that the patient will probably be dead within seven days. My last case like this was when I was practicing in Tarentum, Pennsylvania.

This lady had a tumor about as big as a fist on her right leg, she couldn't bring it up, she had to leave it outside the bed. She also had a heart condition plus diabetes, very bad: you could smell the acetone, it almost knocked me over when I walked in the room. She was the mother, and her family insisted that I do blood work on her. When the results came back, I showed the family all of these test results and explained how normal everything seem to be.

I advised them to put the mother in the hospital and just keep her comfortable, because she was probably going to be dead in seven days. Oh, they couldn't see this. But, I could have gone ahead and sold them a couple of hundred dollars worth of supplements and tried to do something, but I did not. I said, "I don't want to waste your money; I don't want to waste my time having her come, here. Put her over in the hospital." The chief internist at the hospital called me the next day and said, "I understand that you have a scientific method for determining the status of death." I replied, "No, nothing like that. But if you have a piece of paper and a pen handy, I'd like to give these to you." I gave him a sheet with my working normals on it and explained what we were doing. I also told him what the patient's values were. When we got finished, he said, "Well doctor, I think this is the best array of tests that I have ever seen put together. When you show these normals and explain what this patient is doing, I'm going to agree with you, because in checking the patient on our way, I would still say you're right." Actually, she died on the fifth day.

Obtaining a Good Blood Specimen

Proper preparation of the patient is absolutely essential if the physician is to obtain reliable results. Therefore, your instructions to the patient must be specific, leaving nothing to the imagination. I have seen dozens of tests performed on an improper specimen only to have the added expense of repeating the laboratory procedure. Couple this with the necessity of the patient being inconvenienced and having to have the skin punctured a second time; the embarrassment can become great! In short, make sure the specimen is perfect on the first attempt; this is the professional way!

Chemistry tests usually require that the patient fast for eight to ten hours prior to the test. The best time for the tests is in the early morning, because this lessens the period of waiting time before a meal. The specimen can be taken, and the patient can have breakfast.

It's very important that blood work be done on a fasting blood. Chemistry tests usually require that the patient fast for eight to 10 hours prior to the test. At least five tests are destroyed by drinking fluids before the blood is drawn. So we always try to get it done at 8:00 or 8:30 in the morning, with nothing to eat or drink after midnight, with the exception of a very small amount of water. This precaution assures accuracy of the blood count. The specimen can be taken, and the patient can have breakfast.

Postprandial blood – blood taken after a meal – is not suitable for analysis. Likewise, one must not have consumed alcohol for a similar time period before the blood is drawn. Always ask the patient if he has eaten before drawing the specimen. If he has eaten, do not attempt to draw the specimen; send the patient home and try for a fasting specimen the next day. Some laboratories suggest that, if the patient wants to have the test performed anyway the words "non-fasting" should be indicated on the form. This may be a possibility, however, for good results and dealing with the nutritional profile detailed in this book, non-fasting specimens are not suitable. Note that fasting does not mean that the patient may not drink water, on the contrary, dehydration can alter test results from the actual values, so water is permitted.

Another factor that may affect test results is exercise. Even though moderate, exercise can elevate blood glucose, lactic acid, proteins, and some of the enzymes found in muscle, such as creatine phosphokinase (CPK). Emotional stress can cause an elevated value for white blood cells and serum iron. Changes in adrenal activity and consequent concentrations of body fluids (dehydration) can elevate the eosinophil count and the serum iron level, as well as protein lipids (in the form of lipoproteins), triglycerides, and red blood cells.

One of the real good lab books that I've run into is the Quick Reference Laboratory Manual for the Physician. This is probably the best one for the price that I've seen anybody put out. The address is The Medical Service Company of Arizona, P.O. Box 26146, Phoenix, Arizona 85068.

Comprehensive Profile (Editor's Comments)

The following pages contain some actual worksheets that Dr. Ellis completed for patients referred to him by physicians; the names have been concealed to protect the privacy of both physician and patient and to comply with federal law. Dr. Ellis did not perform these analyses for the general public, rather he supported approximately 300 licensed health care professionals worldwide, under whose licenses he could work legally. His conferrals were directed to the doctor, nurse, etc. who was responsible for managing the patient and the suggested plan.

Once, a person who had heard Dr. Ellis on a radio program wanted to travel to Texas to be treated personally, but Dr. Ellis issued the following message in a letter.

> 10/19/82, "Greetings. In response to your letter. Your son is not accurate in his statement as to our blood, hair, urine, and diet. The Comprehensive Profile group of tests (44 blood tests, 19 minerals [from the] hair, a standard urine analysis, and your 7-day diet) are done by your local cooperating health doctor. The doctor sends a copy to me with a 90-minute tape cassette, a self-addressed, stamped mailing address, and a check for $40.00. I do the analysis, put the report on tape, and send it back to the doctor. He then has you listen to the tape and follows the program I've placed you on. Have your doctor contact me on how to proceed. Health, happiness, and blessings, William A. Ellis, D.O."

What Is Missing

No clinical examination notes submitted by doctors requesting Dr. Ellis' analyses were found in his files. Dr. Ellis' routine was to send all submitted materials back to the cooperating doctor, keeping only his worksheets. **Therefore, no clinical exam notes can be provided that correspond to the example worksheets in this chapter.**

It may be fortunate that clinical examination notes are not provided, because Dr. Ellis wisely preferred that his students meld his or her own, first-hand observations with what he taught to validate the opinions in their own minds. In that way, conclusions remain the health professional's responsibility, based on careful study of Dr. Ellis' teachings, his or her own experience, first-hand knowledge of any patients subjected to analysis, and knowledge of the ingredients contained in the nutritional modalities indicated on the analyses.

Notes About Example Worksheets

Figure 6 shows a blank worksheet typical of the one used by Dr. Ellis in organizing test results obtained from the laboratory and annotating other pertinent information. Except for Figure 7, all patient and physician identifying information has been removed, in compliance with federal privacy regulations. **The information contained in these profiles is presented only for the purpose of study by licensed health practitioners; no expressed or implied conclusions are given other than those written on the forms by Dr. Ellis himself at the time he was performing the analyses. No further explanation is given about the patient information, because to do so would presume more than what Dr. Ellis intended.**

Several nutritional products are listed by Dr. Ellis on these example profiles; most are still manufactured, although some of the names may have been changed. Some may no longer be available and are candidates for substitution; see Appendix D: Vendors. Again, no specific brand or product recommendations are made in addition to those of Dr. Ellis. **If a licensed health practitioner administering Dr. Ellis' plan desires to substitute familiar, trusted brands for those recommended by Dr. Ellis, he or she may be assisted by the brand conversion charts provided by most vendors for that purpose.**

Figure 7 depicts Dr. Ellis' actual, completed COMPREHENSIVE PROFILE worksheet, namely, the first CBC and blood chemistry analysis that Dr. Ellis performed for the Editor (for which I give myself permission to publish). Dr. Ellis' preferred norms and ratios are indicated in either parentheses or bold writing, while the normal values for the Atherogenic Index have been transferred from a chart.

The Sedimentation Rate is written in the first space under the caption, NORMAL RANGE. In the first column captioned DATE, Dr. Ellis has written the values that appeared on the laboratory report, while in the second column captioned DATE, he has inserted his comments about how my test values compare to the laboratory's or his preferred ranges and means. Sometimes, Dr. Ellis designated values within the laboratory's normal range as hi or lo, as found in the Calcium, Phosphorus, and Uric Acid levels. At the bottom of the page, between his name and address and the instruction, SPECIMEN REQUIRED, he has written significant notes about my urinalysis.

At the top right of the page, Dr. Ellis has written his conclusions from the analysis. The meaning of the abbreviation DDSLKP is unknown. Below these notes, under REMARKS, he listed recommendations for nutritional supplementation to correct the physiological conditions responsible for any diagnostic indicators and for the abnormal values shown on the CBC, blood chemistry, and urinalysis. Standard medical abbreviations for dosage are given. Abbreviations for products used in this column are shown in Table 11. Information from a hair analysis or a test such as an EKG would have been considered, but notated separately.

All other analyses provided as examples in this chapter were done by Dr. Ellis in the same way as the Editor's. Notice that, in some of the subsequent examples, several normal ranges have been altered to reflect the values used by the individual laboratory. Table 11 also indicates Dr. Ellis' rationale for recommending a listed product.

Table 11: Typically Recommended Products (See also **Vendors** on page 415)

Abbreviation	Meaning	Dr. Ellis' Rationale
Aloe Vera Gel	Lily of the Desert	A preferred drink for reducing inflammation and normalizing the digestive tract.
Biotics	Biotics Research Corporation	Integrating neonatal glandular products into his programs, along with individual mineral supplements, CoEnzyme Q, SOD, and Vitamin A and E emulsions.
Enzyme	Enzyme Process	Long-term familiarity with products; used enzyme and glandular combinations frequently, such as Libec.
RF #2	Research Formula #2 (now labeled Life-Mate, from Natural Wonders)	A multiple supplement that Dr. Ellis used with almost every patient to start a program, possibly because of its long list of ingredients.
Standard	Standard Process	Long-term familiarity with products; often used their glandular products and combinations, such as AC Carbamide.

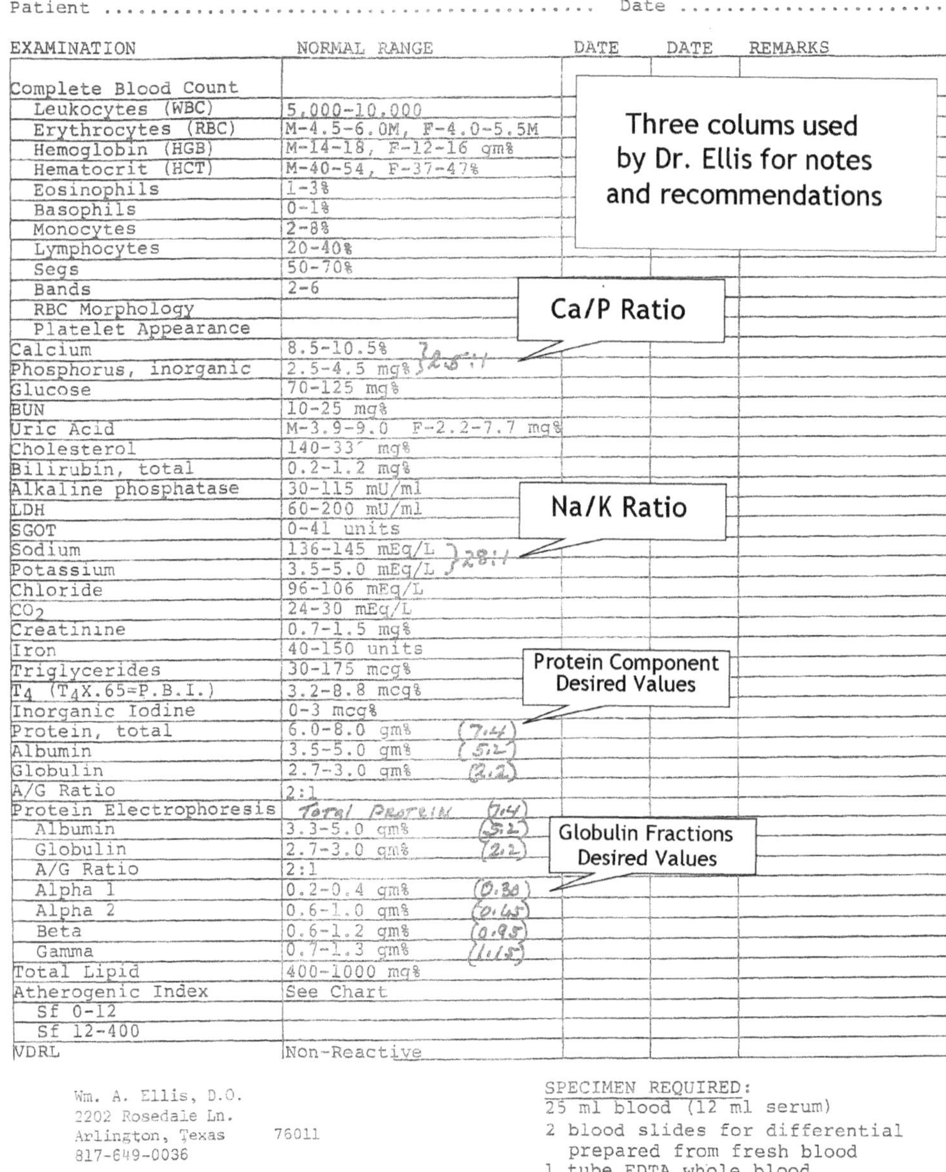

COMPREHENSIVE PROFILE

Patient .... Date ....

EXAMINATION	NORMAL RANGE	DATE	DATE	REMARKS
Complete Blood Count				
Leukocytes (WBC)	5,000-10,000			
Erythrocytes (RBC)	M-4.5-6.0M, F-4.0-5.5M			
Hemoglobin (HGB)	M-14-18, F-12-16 gm%			
Hematocrit (HCT)	M-40-54, F-37-47%			
Eosinophils	1-3%			
Basophils	0-1%			
Monocytes	2-8%			
Lymphocytes	20-40%			
Segs	50-70%			
Bands	2-6			
RBC Morphology				
Platelet Appearance				
Calcium	8.5-10.5% }2.5:1			
Phosphorus, inorganic	2.5-4.5 mg%			
Glucose	70-125 mg%			
BUN	10-25 mg%			
Uric Acid	M-3.9-9.0 F-2.2-7.7 mg%			
Cholesterol	140-33´ mg%			
Bilirubin, total	0.2-1.2 mg%			
Alkaline phosphatase	30-115 mU/ml			
LDH	60-200 mU/ml			
SGOT	0-41 units			
Sodium	136-145 mEq/L }28:1			
Potassium	3.5-5.0 mEq/L			
Chloride	96-106 mEq/L			
CO_2	24-30 mEq/L			
Creatinine	0.7-1.5 mg%			
Iron	40-150 units			
Triglycerides	30-175 mcg%			
T_4 (T_4X.65=P.B.I.)	3.2-8.8 mcg%			
Inorganic Iodine	0-3 mcg%			
Protein, total	6.0-8.0 gm% (7.4)			
Albumin	3.5-5.0 gm% (5.2)			
Globulin	2.7-3.0 gm% (2.2)			
A/G Ratio	2:1			
Protein Electrophoresis	Total Protein (7.4)			
Albumin	3.3-5.0 gm% (5.2)			
Globulin	2.7-3.0 gm% (2.2)			
A/G Ratio	2:1			
Alpha 1	0.2-0.4 gm% (0.30)			
Alpha 2	0.6-1.0 gm% (0.65)			
Beta	0.6-1.2 gm% (0.95)			
Gamma	0.7-1.3 gm% (1.15)			
Total Lipid	400-1000 mg%			
Atherogenic Index	See Chart			
Sf 0-12				
Sf 12-400				
VDRL	Non-Reactive			

Wm. A. Ellis, D.O.
2202 Rosedale Ln.
Arlington, Texas 76011
817-649-0036

SPECIMEN REQUIRED:
25 ml blood (12 ml serum)
2 blood slides for differential
prepared from fresh blood
1 tube EDTA whole blood

Figure 6: Blank blood profile form used by Dr. Ellis

COMPREHENSIVE PROFILE

Allergies
Periodontal Disease
Gout – arthritis
early poor care – nerve
[illegible]

Patient Robert Strickland (38) .... Date ....

EXAMINATION 6/2/83	NORMAL RANGE	DATE	DATE	REMARKS D.D. SCKP.
Complete Blood Count	Sed Rate 0-7	10		GU – mild infection
Leukocytes (WBC)	5,000-10,000	5900		
Erythrocytes (RBC)	M-4.5-6.0M, F-4.0-5.5M	5360000		
Hemoglobin (HGB)	M-14-18, F-12-16 gm%	16		RF # 2
Hematocrit (HCT)	M-40-54, F-37-47%	46.9	Lo	
Eosinophils	1-3%	6	hi	Standard
Basophils	0-1%	0		Cataplex 1pc
Monocytes	2-8%	7		Phosfood 5D BID
Lymphocytes	20-40%	34		Thymex 1pc.
Segs	50-70%	52	Low.	Sympl M 1pc
Bands	2-6	3		ac each 1t
RBC Morphology		N		
Platelet Appearance		ad.		
Calcium	8.5-10.5% 3.25:1 3.4/1	9.6	Lo	
Phosphorus, inorganic	2.5-4.5 mg%	2.8	Lo	
Glucose	70-125 mg%	87		Enzyme
BUN	10-26 mg%	8		add. – 2 QID
Uric Acid	M-3.9-9.0 F-2.2-7.7 mg%	6.6	hi	
Cholesterol	~~140-335~~ mg% / 120-220	238		
Bilirubin, total	0.2-1.2 mg%	0.9		
Alkaline phosphatase	30-115 mU/ml	105		
LDH	60-~~200~~ mU/ml 230	170		
SGOT 35 (0-45)	0-41 units	20		Berberis
Sodium	136-148 mEq/L 28:1 32.4/1	146		Lacto 2-3 ac
Potassium	3.5-5.0 mEq/L	4.5		[illegible] 2-2 tpc
Chloride	96-106 mEq/L	107		[illegible] 2 pc.
CO_2	24-32 mEq/L	28		1-2 [illegible]
Creatinine	0.7-1.5 mg%	1.0		[illegible]
Iron	40-150 units	133		
Triglycerides	30-196 mcg%	71		
T_4 (T_4X.65=P.B.I.)	3.2-8.8 mcg%	6.4		
Inorganic Iodine	0-3 mcg%			
Protein, total	6.0-8.0 gm% (7.4)	7.40		
Albumin	3.5-5.0 gm% (5.2)	4.60	Lo	200 mg C. QID
Globulin	2.7-3.0 gm% (2.2)	2.80	hi	
A/G Ratio	2:1	1.6/1	Lo	[illegible]
Protein Electrophoresis	TOTAL PROTEIN (7.4)	7.40		
Albumin	3.3-5.0 gm% (5.2)	4.00	Lo	
Globulin	2.7-3.0 gm% (2.2)	3.40	hi	
A/G Ratio	2:1	1.16/1	Lo	
Alpha 1	0.2-0.4 gm% (0.30)	0.30		
Alpha 2	0.6-1.0 gm% (0.65)	0.80	hi	
Beta	0.6-1.2 gm% (0.95)	1.10	hi	
Gamma	0.7-1.3 gm% (1.15)	1.30	hi	
Total Lipid	400-1000 mg%	618		
Atherogenic Index	See Chart 69	52	– 17	
Sf 0-12	347	382	hi	
Sf 12-400	243	76	Lo	
VDRL	Non-Reactive	NR		

yellow Clear 1.023 5.0 neg
occ epith
few Bacteria

Wm. A. Ellis, D.O.
2202 Rosedale Ln.
Arlington, Texas 76011
817-649-0036

SPECIMEN REQUIRED:
25 ml blood (12 ml serum)
2 blood slides for differential
prepared from fresh blood
1 tube EDTA whole blood

Figure 7: Blood chemistry analysis of Robert Strickland performed by Dr. Ellis

COMPREHENSIVE PROFILE

Patient Female Age: 44 .... Date ....

(BP) 6/12/85

EXAMINATION	NORMAL RANGE	DATE	DATE	REMARKS
Complete Blood Count	Sed Rate 0-20	6		
Leukocytes (WBC)	5,000-10,000	8,900		
Erythrocytes (RBC)	M-4.5-6.0M, F-4.0-5.5M	4,140		
Hemoglobin (HGB)	M-14-18, F-12-16 gm%	12		
Hematocrit (HCT)	M-40-54, F-37-47%	36		
Eosinophils	1-3%	1		
Basophils	0-1%	1		
Monocytes	2-8%	6		
Lymphocytes	20-40%	43		
Segs	50-70%	44		
Bands	2-6	1		
RBC Morphology	atypical lymphs	4		
Platelet Appearance		adq.		
Calcium	8.5-10.5%	9.0		
Phosphorus, inorganic	2.5-4.5 mg%	2.6		
Glucose	70-125 mg% 65-110	88		
BUN	10-26 mg%	7		
Uric Acid	M-3.9-9.0 F-2.3-7.0 mg%	4.3		
Cholesterol	140-335 mg% 220	145		
Bilirubin, total	0.2-1.0 mg%	0.3		
Alkaline phosphatase	30-115 mU/ml	33		
LDH	90-200 mU/ml 225	112		
SGOT	0-41 units	16		
Sodium	136-145 mEq/L	137		
Potassium	3.5-5.0 mEq/L	4.2		
Chloride	96-106 mEq/L	107		
CO_2	24-30 mEq/L	28		
Creatinine	0.5-1.5 mg%	1.2		
Iron	40-150 units			
Triglycerides	30-175 mcg%			
T_4 (T_4X.65=P.B.I.)	3.2-8.8 mcg%			
Inorganic Iodine	0-3 mcg%			
Protein, total	6.0-8.0 gm% (7.4)	6.5		
Albumin	3.5-5.0 gm% (5.2)	3.9		
Globulin	2.7-3.0 gm% (2.2)	2.6		
A/G Ratio	2:1	1.5/1		
Protein Electrophoresis	TOTAL PROTEIN (7.4)	7.2		
Albumin	3.3-5.0 gm% (5.2)	3.9		
Globulin	2.7-3.0 gm% (2.2)	3.3		
A/G Ratio	2:1	1.2/1		
Alpha 1	0.2-0.4 gm% (0.30)	0.3		
Alpha 2	0.6-1.0 gm% (0.65)	0.9		
Beta	0.6-1.2 gm% (0.95)	0.9		
Gamma	0.7-1.3 gm% (1.15)	1.3		
Total Lipid	400-1000 mg%			
Atherogenic Index	See Chart			
Sf 0-12				
Sf 12-400				
VDRL	Non-Reactive			

Wm. A. Ellis, D.O.
2202 Rosedale Ln.
Arlington, Texas 76011
817-649-0036

SPECIMEN REQUIRED:
25 ml blood (12 ml serum)
2 blood slides for differential
prepared from fresh blood
1 tube EDTA whole blood

Figure 8: Blood chemistry analysis of a 44 year old woman

COMPREHENSIVE PROFILE

tient Male Age: 42 .... Date ....

AMINATION	NORMAL RANGE	DATE	DATE	REMARKS
mplete Blood Count	Sed Rate 0-7	7		
Leukocytes (WBC)	5,000-10,000	8700		
Erythrocytes (RBC)	M-4.5-6.0M, F-4.0-5.5M	5,260,000		
Hemoglobin (HGB)	M-14-18, F-12-16 gm%	17.5	hi	
Hematocrit (HCT)	M-40-54, F-37-47%	49.8		
Eosinophils	1-3%	1		
Basophils	0-1%	1		Standard
Monocytes	2-8%	0	Lo	
Lymphocytes	20-40%	38		
Segs	50-70%	58		
Bands	2-6	2		
RBC Morphology		N		
Platelet Appearance		ad		
lcium	8.5-10.5%	10.3	hi	
osphorus, inorganic	2.5-4.5 mg%	2.6	Lo	
ucose	70-125 mg%	88		
N	10-26 mg%	8	Lo	
ic Acid	M-3.9-9.0 F-2.2-7.7 mg%	6.5	hi	
olesterol	~~140-33~~ mg% 170-270	196		
lirubin, total	0.2-1.2 mg%	0.9		
kaline phosphatase	30-115 mU/ml	65		
H	60-200 mU/ml 230	217		
OT 24 (0-45)	0-41 units	16		
dium	135-145 mEq/L	142		
tassium	3.5-5.0 mEq/L	3.9		
loride	96-106 mEq/L	99		
2	24-32 mEq/L	28		
eatinine	0.7-1.5 mg%	0.8		
on	40-150 units	135		
iglycerides	30-150 mcg%	192	hi	
(T_4X.65=P.B.I.)	3.2-8.8 mcg%	7.9	hi	
organic Iodine	0-3 mcg%			
otein, total	6.0-8.0 gm% (7.4)	7.80		
bumin	3.5-5.0 gm% (5.2)	4.8	Lo	Aloe Vera Gel
obulin	2.7-3.0 gm% (2.2)	3.0	hi	
G Ratio	2:1	1.6/1	Lo	
otein Electrophoresis	TOTAL PROTEIN (7.4)	7.80		
Albumin	3.3-5.0 gm% (5.2)	4.33	Lo	
Globulin	2.7-3.0 gm% (2.2)	3.47	hi	
A/G Ratio	2:1	1.25	Lo	
Alpha 1	0.2-0.4 gm% (0.30)	0.29		
Alpha 2	0.6-1.0 gm% (0.65)	1.01	hi	
Beta	0.6-1.2 gm% (0.95)	1.20	hi	
Gamma	0.7-1.3 gm% (1.15)	0.96	Lo	
tal Lipid	400-1000 mg%	598		
herogenic Index	See Chart 71	48	-213	
Sf 0-12	356	296		
Sf 12-400	252	104	Lo	
RE STS	Non-Reactive	NR		

Wm. A. Ellis, D.O.
2202 Rosedale Ln.
Arlington, Texas 76011
817-649-0036

SPECIMEN REQUIRED:
25 ml blood (12 ml serum)
2 blood slides for differential prepared from fresh blood
1 tube EDTA whole blood

Figure 9: Blood chemistry analysis of a 42 year old man

COMPREHENSIVE PROFILE

Patient: **Female Age: 36** Date

EXAMINATION 1/26/83	NORMAL RANGE	DATE	DATE	REMARKS
Complete Blood Count	Sed Rate 0-15	8		
Leukocytes (WBC)	5,000-10,000	6200		
Erythrocytes (RBC)	M-4.5-6.0M, F-4.0-5.5M	4.53 mil		
Hemoglobin (HGB)	M-14-18, F-12-16 gm%	15.8	[illegible]	RF#2 Reg
Hematocrit (HCT)	M-40-54, F-37-47%	45		
Eosinophils	1-3%	5	[illegible]	OMR Reg.
Basophils	0-1%	0		
Monocytes	2-8%	0	[illegible]	Standard
Lymphocytes	20-40%	30		Thymus 1pc
Segs	50-70%	59		SymF 1pc
Bands	2-6	6	[illegible]	Thyrotophin 1pc
RBC Morphology		N		OrgI [illegible]
Platelet Appearance		Ad		AFFB 1-3 oz [illegible]
Calcium	8.5-10.5% } 2.5:1 3.2/1	9.7	[illegible]	1 month.
Phosphorus, inorganic	2.5-4.5 mg%	3.0	[illegible]	
Glucose	70-125 mg%	100		
BUN	10-26 mg%	6	[illegible]	
Uric Acid	M-3.9-9.0 F-2.2-7.7 mg%	3.8		Enzymes
Cholesterol	~~140-330~~ mg% 120-210	185		Adult 2 QID
Bilirubin, total	0.2-1.2 mg%	0.3		[illegible]
Alkaline phosphatase	30-115 mU/ml	44		
LDH	60-200 mU/ml 230	161		
SGOT 24 (0-45)	0-41 units	24		Bodies
Sodium	135-145 mEq/L } 28:1 36/1	144		Facti - 2 - 30 oz
Potassium	3.5-5.0 mEq/L	4.0		[illegible]
Chloride	96-108 mEq/L	107		[illegible]
CO_2	24-30 mEq/L	24	[illegible]	[illegible]
Creatinine	0.7-1.5 mg%	1.0		[illegible]
Iron	40-150 units	42		Cu 1pc
Triglycerides	30-150 mcg%	55		[illegible] 1pc
T_4 (T_4X.65=P.B.I.)	3.2-8.8 mcg%	3.9	[illegible]	[illegible] 1pc
Inorganic Iodine	0-3 mcg%			Fe 1pc
Protein, total	6.0-8.0 gm% (7.4)	7.20	[illegible]	SE 1 QID
Albumin	3.5-5.0 gm% (5.2)	4.40	[illegible]	
Globulin	2.7-3.0 gm% (2.2)	2.82	[illegible]	
A/G Ratio	2:1	1.57/1	[illegible]	
Protein Electrophoresis	Total Protein (7.4)	7.20	[illegible]	Aloe Vera Gel
Albumin	3.3-5.0 gm% (5.2)	4.18	[illegible]	
Globulin	2.7-3.0 gm% (2.2)	3.02	[illegible]	200 mgC QID
A/G Ratio	2:1	1.38	[illegible]	
Alpha 1	0.2-0.4 gm% (0.30)	0.23	[illegible]	
Alpha 2	0.6-1.0 gm% (0.65)	0.79	[illegible]	
Beta	0.6-1.2 gm% (0.95)	0.79	[illegible]	
Gamma	0.7-1.3 gm% (1.15)	1.21	[illegible]	
Total Lipid	400-1000 mg%	520		
Atherogenic Index	See Chart 48	37	-11	
Sf 0-12	308	283		
Sf 12-400	147	47	[illegible]	
~~VDRL~~ STS	Non-Reactive	NR		[illegible]

Yellow Clear 1.005 6.0 Neg

Wm. A. Ellis, D.O.
2202 Rosedale Ln.
Arlington, Texas 76011
817-649-0036

SPECIMEN REQUIRED:
25 ml blood (12 ml serum)
2 blood slides for differential prepared from fresh blood
1 tube EDTA whole blood

Figure 10: Blood chemistry analysis of a 36 year old woman

Ni & Al irritations
arthritis Poor Circ – nerv.
COMPREHENSIVE PROFILE
Hypo Thyroid.
nervous.
Short Longevity
Hypoglycemia
Demineralization

mild hypo chr anemia
Poor antibody Prod
allergies
Poor Circ – nerv.
Gout – arthritis.
Pre hypoglycemia
D.D.S.K.B.
Kidney Inf

Patient Male Age: 33 .... Date ....

EXAMINATION 2/7/83	NORMAL RANGE	DATE	DATE	REMARKS
Complete Blood Count				
Leukocytes (WBC)	5,000-10,000	6000		
Erythrocytes (RBC)	M-4.5-6.0M, F-4.0-5.5M	4920000		
Hemoglobin (HGB)	M-14-18, F-12-16 gm%	14.5	LO	RF #2 Reg
Hematocrit (HCT)	M-40-54, F-37-47%	46.3	LO	
Eosinophils	1-3%	6	HI	OM12 Reg
Basophils	0-1%	2	HI	
Monocytes	2-8%	1	LO	Standard
Lymphocytes	20-40%	49	HI	Sym M 1pc
Segs	50-70%	38	LO	Calcanode 1+
Bands	2-6	4		Renafood 1pc
RBC Morphology		N		Vit E 1pc
Platelet Appearance		Ad.		Cal L 30 drops
Calcium	8.5-10.5% 2.5:1 2.46/1	9.6	LO	Antronex 1pc
Phosphorus, inorganic	2.5-4.5 mg%	3.9		
Glucose	70-125 mg%	73		Enzyme
BUN	10-26 mg%	14		added 2 QID
Uric Acid	M-3.9-9.0 F-2.2-7.7 mg%	6.4	HI	
Cholesterol	~~140-334~~ mg% 120-290	214		
Bilirubin, total	0.2-1.2 mg%	0.7		
Alkaline phosphatase	30-115 mU/ml	66		Beatus
LDH	60-~~200~~ mU/ml 230	175		Forte 2-3 oz
SGOT 26 (0-45)	0-41 units	21		Int 2-20+pc
Sodium	135-145 mEq/L 28:1 35/1	140		Hydrac 2pc
Potassium	3.5-5.0 mEq/L	4.0		[illegible]
Chloride	96-108 mEq/L	103		Meth 2 QID
CO_2	24-32 mEq/L	27		[illegible] 1pc
Creatinine	0.7-1.5 mg%	1.2		Thymus 1pc
Iron	40-150 units	143		K 3y 1pc
Triglycerides	30-190 mcg%	53		Cu 3y 1pc
T_4 (T_4X.65=P.B.I.)	3.2-8.8 mcg%	6.0		Fe 3y 1pc
Inorganic Iodine	0-3 mcg%	—		Al 3y 1pc
Protein, total	6.0-8.0 gm% (7.4)	7.40		
Albumin	3.5-5.0 gm% (5.2)	4.60	LO	
Globulin	2.7-3.0 gm% (2.2)	2.80	HI	
A/G Ratio	2:1	1.64/1	LO	
Protein Electrophoresis	Total Protein (7.4)	7.40		Aloe Vera Gel
Albumin	3.3-5.0 gm% (5.2)	4.41	LO	Na
Globulin	2.7-3.0 gm% (2.2)	2.99	HI	2000 mg C QID
A/G Ratio	2:1	1.48	LO	
Alpha 1	0.2-0.4 gm% (0.30)	0.24	LO	
Alpha 2	0.6-1.0 gm% (0.65)	0.78	HI	
Beta	0.6-1.2 gm% (0.95)	1.03	HI	
Gamma	0.7-1.3 gm% (1.15)	0.93	LO	[illegible] Na K.
Total Lipid	400-1000 mg%	543		
Atherogenic Index	See Chart 64	40	-2.4	off Microwave.
Sf 0-12	332	341	HI	
Sf 12-400	223	36	LO	
~~VDRL~~ STS	Non-Reactive	NR		

Yellow Hazy 1+ Glucose neg. 1034 7.0
Few Sq Ep.
Heavy mucous
Few Bact
Unidentified material

Wm. A. Ellis, D.O.
2202 Rosedale Ln.
Arlington, Texas 76011
817-649-0036

SPECIMEN REQUIRED:
25 ml blood (12 ml serum)
2 blood slides for differential
prepared from fresh blood
1 tube EDTA whole blood

Figure 11: Blood chemistry analysis of a 33 year old man

COMPREHENSIVE PROFILE

Patient **Female Age: 6** .... Date ....

EXAMINATION	NORMAL RANGE	DATE	DATE	REMARKS
Complete Blood Count		34		
Leukocytes (WBC)	5,000-10,000	9200		
Erythrocytes (RBC)	M-4.5-6.0M, F-4.0-5.5M	5540000		
Hemoglobin (HGB)	M-14-18, F-12-16 gm%	14.1		
Hematocrit (HCT)	M-40-54, F-37-47%	41.8		
Eosinophils	1-3%	3		
Basophils	0-1%	0		
Monocytes	2-8%			
Lymphocytes	20-40%			
Segs	50-70%	46		
Bands	2-6	10		
RBC Morphology				
Platelet Appearance				
Calcium	8.5-10.5%	9.8		
Phosphorus, inorganic	2.5-4.5 mg%	4.4		
Glucose	70-125 mg%	67		
BUN	10-26 mg%	10		
Uric Acid	M-3.9-9.0 F-2.2-7.7 mg%	4.6		
Cholesterol	140-335 mg%	188		
Bilirubin, total	0.2-1.2 mg%	0.4		
Alkaline phosphatase	30-115 mU/ml	280		
LDH	60-200 mU/ml	301		
SGOT	0-41 units	28		
Sodium	136-145 mEq/L	140		
Potassium	3.5-5.0 mEq/L	3.9		
Chloride	96-106 mEq/L	105		
CO_2	24-30 mEq/L	24		
Creatinine	0.7-1.5 mg%	0.5		
Iron	40-150 units	52		
Triglycerides	30-175 mcg%	106		
T_4 (T_4X.65=P.B.I.)	3.2-8.8 mcg%	10.6		
Inorganic Iodine	0-3 mcg%			
Protein, total	6.0-8.0 gm% (7.4)	8.2		
Albumin	3.5-5.0 gm% (5.2)	4.1		
Globulin	2.7-3.0 gm% (2.2)	4.1		
A/G Ratio	2:1	1.0/1		
Protein Electrophoresis	Total Protein (7.4)	8.2		
Albumin	3.3-5.0 gm% (5.2)	4.1		
Globulin	2.7-3.0 gm% (2.2)	4.1		
A/G Ratio	2:1	1.0/1		
Alpha 1	0.2-0.4 gm% (0.30)	0.4		
Alpha 2	0.6-1.0 gm% (0.65)	1.1		
Beta	0.6-1.2 gm% (0.95)	1.1		
Gamma	0.7-1.3 gm% (1.15)	1.6		
Total Lipid	400-1000 mg%	575		
Atherogenic Index	See Chart	36		
Sf 0-12		290		
Sf 12-400		39		
VDRL	Non-Reactive			

Wm. A. Ellis, D.O.
2202 Rosedale Ln.
Arlington, Texas 76011
817-649-0036

SPECIMEN REQUIRED:
25 ml blood (12 ml serum)
2 blood slides for differential prepared from fresh blood
1 tube EDTA whole blood

Figure 12: Blood chemistry analysis of a 6 year old girl

COMPREHENSIVE PROFILE

Patient Male Age: 7 .... Date ....

EXAMINATION 7-15/83

EXAMINATION	NORMAL RANGE	DATE	DATE	REMARKS
Complete Blood Count	Sed Rate 0-7	44		
Leukocytes (WBC)	5,000-10,000	11,700		
Erythrocytes (RBC)	M-4.5-6.0M, F-4.0-5.5M	5,020,000		
Hemoglobin (HGB)	M-14-18, F-12-16 gm%	11.6		RF#2 1 93
Hematocrit (HCT)	M-40-54, F-37-47%	35.4		
Eosinophils	1-3%	0		
Basophils	0-1%	1		
Monocytes	2-8%	9		
Lymphocytes	20-40%	89		
Segs	50-70%	0		
Bands	2-6	0		
RBC Morphology				
Platelet Appearance				
Calcium	8.5-10.5%	8.6		
Phosphorus, inorganic	2.5-4.5 mg%	3.8		
Glucose	70-125 mg%	93		
BUN	10-25 mg%	24		
Uric Acid	M-3.9-9.0 F-2.2-7.7 mg%	5.3		
Cholesterol	~~140-33~~ mg% 120-270	163		
Bilirubin, total	0.2-1.2 mg%	0.3		
Alkaline phosphatase	30-115 mU/ml	149		
LDH	60-200 mU/ml 230	257		
SGOT	0-41 units	34		
Sodium	136-145 mEq/L	131		
Potassium	3.5-5.0 mEq/L	2.17		
Chloride	96-106 mEq/L	97		
CO_2	24-30 mEq/L	20		
Creatinine	0.7-1.5 mg%	1.1		
Iron	40-150 units	50		
Triglycerides	30-195 mcg%	222		
T_4 (T_4X.65=P.B.I.)	3.2-8.8 mcg%	7.7		Aloe Vera Gel
Inorganic Iodine	0-3 mcg%			
Protein, total	6.0-8.0 gm% (7.4)	8.90		
Albumin	3.5-5.0 gm% (5.2)	3.40		
Globulin	2.7-3.0 gm% (2.2)	5.50		
A/G Ratio	2:1	0.61		
Protein Electrophoresis	TOTAL PROTEIN (7.4)	8.90		
Albumin	3.3-5.0 gm% (5.2)	3.40		
Globulin	2.7-3.0 gm% (2.2)	5.50		
A/G Ratio	2:1	0.61		
Alpha 1	0.2-0.4 gm% (0.30)	0.40		
Alpha 2	0.6-1.0 gm% (0.65)	1.20		
Beta	0.6-1.2 gm% (0.95)	0.80		
Gamma	0.7-1.3 gm% (1.15)	3.20		
Total Lipid	400-1000 mg%	561		
Atherogenic Index	See Chart (20) 66	42	-1.8	
Sf 0-12	(10) 291	232		
Sf 12-400	(10) 131	108		
VDRL	Non-Reactive	NR		

Yellow Hazy 1.014 6.0 Neg

Wm. A. Ellis, D.O.
2202 Rosedale Ln.
Arlington, Texas 76011
817-649-0036

SPECIMEN REQUIRED:
25 ml blood (12 ml serum)
2 blood slides for differential
prepared from fresh blood
1 tube EDTA whole blood

Figure 13: Blood chemistry analysis of a 7 year old boy

COMPREHENSIVE PROFILE

Patient Female Age: 37 Date

EXAMINATION 3/7/04	NORMAL RANGE	DATE	DATE	REMARKS
Complete Blood Count		2		
Leukocytes (WBC)	5,000-10,000	6000		
Erythrocytes (RBC)	M-4.5-6.0M, F-4.0-5.5M	4.46		
Hemoglobin (HGB)	M-14-18, F-12-16 gm%	13.3		
Hematocrit (HCT)	M-40-54, F-37-47%	43.4		
Eosinophils	1-3%	0		
Basophils	0-1%	0		
Monocytes	2-8%	2		
Lymphocytes	20-40%	26		
Segs	50-70%	70		
Bands	2-6	0		
RBC Morphology		N		
Platelet Appearance		ad.		
Calcium	8.5-10.5%	9.4		
Phosphorus, inorganic	2.5-4.5 mg%	3.6		
Glucose	70-125 mg%	96		
BUN	10-26 mg%	11		
Uric Acid	M-3.9-9.0 F-2.2-7.7 mg%	5.3		
Cholesterol	140-335 mg%	149		
Bilirubin, total	0.2-1.2 mg%	0.6		
Alkaline phosphatase	30-115 mU/ml	54		
LDH	60-200 mU/ml	106		
SGOT	0-41 units	13		
Sodium	136-145 mEq/L	141		
Potassium	3.5-5.0 mEq/L	3.9		
Chloride	96-106 mEq/L	102		
CO_2	24-30 mEq/L	27		
Creatinine	0.7-1.5 mg%	0.7		
Iron	40-190 units	132		
Triglycerides	30-175 mcg%	40		
T_4 (T_4X.65=P.B.I.)	3.2-8.8 mcg%	6.6		
Inorganic Iodine	0-3 mcg%			
Protein, total	6.0-8.0 gm% (7.4)	6.2		
Albumin	3.5-5.0 gm% (5.2)	4.1		
Globulin	2.7-3.0 gm% (2.2)	2.1		
A/G Ratio	2:1	2/1		
Protein Electrophoresis	TOTAL PROTEIN (7.4)	6.7		
Albumin	3.3-5.0 gm% (5.2)	4.1		
Globulin	2.7-3.0 gm% (2.2)	2.6		
A/G Ratio	2:1	1.5		
Alpha 1	0.2-0.4 gm% (0.30)	0.2		
Alpha 2	0.6-1.0 gm% (0.65)	0.8		
Beta	0.6-1.2 gm% (0.95)	0.8		
Gamma	0.7-1.3 gm% (1.15)	0.8		
Total Lipid	400-1000 mg%	425		
Atherogenic Index	See Chart	22		
Sf 0-12		220		
Sf 12-400		3		
VDRL	Non-Reactive	NR		

Wm. A. Ellis, D.O.
2202 Rosedale Ln.
Arlington, Texas 76011
817-649-0036

SPECIMEN REQUIRED:
25 ml blood (12 ml serum)
2 blood slides for differential
prepared from fresh blood
1 tube EDTA whole blood

Figure 14: Blood chemistry analysis of a 37 year old woman (daughter of Figure 15)

COMPREHENSIVE PROFILE

Patient Female Age: 65 .... Date ....

EXAMINATION	NORMAL RANGE	DATE	DATE	REMARKS
Complete Blood Count	Sed Rate 0-20	2		
Leukocytes (WBC)	5,000-10,000	6300		
Erythrocytes (RBC)	M-4.5-6.0M, F-4.0-5.5M	4.84		
Hemoglobin (HGB)	M-14-18, F-12-16 gm%	14.1		
Hematocrit (HCT)	M-40-54, F-37-47%	45		
Eosinophils	1-3%	4		
Basophils	0-1%	0		
Monocytes	2-8%	2		
Lymphocytes	20-40%	36		
Segs	50-70%	58		
Bands	2-6	0		
RBC Morphology				
Platelet Appearance				
Calcium	8.5-10.5%	10.0		
Phosphorus, inorganic	2.5-4.5 mg%	3.2		
Glucose	70-125 mg%	99		
BUN	10-25 mg%	14		
Uric Acid	M-3.9-9.0 F-2.2-7.7 mg%	5.5		
Cholesterol	140-330 mg%	231		
Bilirubin, total	0.2-1.2 mg%	1.6		
Alkaline phosphatase	30-115 mU/ml	95		
LDH	60-200 mU/ml	157		
SGOT	0-41 units	17		
Sodium	136-145 mEq/L	143		
Potassium	3.5-5.0 mEq/L	4.3		
Chloride	96-106 mEq/L	106		
CO_2	24-30 mEq/L	27		
Creatinine	0.7-1.5 mg%	0.7		
Iron	40-150 units	128		
Triglycerides	30-175 mcg%	59		
T_4 (T_4X.65=P.B.I.)	3.2-8.8 mcg%	3.6		
Inorganic Iodine	0-3 mcg%			
Protein, total	6.0-8.0 gm% (7.4)	6.7		
Albumin	3.5-5.0 gm% (5.2)	4.2		
Globulin	2.7-3.0 gm% (2.2)	2.5		
A/G Ratio	2:1	1.7		
Protein Electrophoresis	TOTAL PROTEIN (7.4)	6.9		
Albumin	3.3-5.0 gm% (5.2)	4.2		
Globulin	2.7-3.0 gm% (2.2)	2.7		
A/G Ratio	2:1	1.5		
Alpha 1	0.2-0.4 gm% (0.30)	0.2		
Alpha 2	0.6-1.0 gm% (0.65)	0.8		
Beta	0.6-1.2 gm% (0.95)	0.8		
Gamma	0.7-1.3 gm% (1.15)	0.9		
Total Lipid	400-1000 mg%	560		
Atherogenic Index	See Chart	42		
Sf 0-12		376		
Sf 12-400		23		
VDRL	Non-Reactive	NR		

Wm. A. Ellis, D.O.
2202 Rosedale Ln.
Arlington, Texas 76011
817-649-0036

SPECIMEN REQUIRED:
25 ml blood (12 ml serum)
2 blood slides for differential prepared from fresh blood
1 tube EDTA whole blood

Figure 15: Blood chemistry analysis of a 65 year old woman (mother of Figure 14)

COMPREHENSIVE PROFILE

Patient Male Age: 23 .... Date ....

EXAMINATION	NORMAL RANGE	DATE	DATE	REMARKS
Complete Blood Count		3		
Leukocytes (WBC)	5,000-10,000	5100		
Erythrocytes (RBC)	M-4.5-6.0M, F-4.0-5.5M	6.2100		
Hemoglobin (HGB)	M-14-18, F-12-16 gm%	20		
Hematocrit (HCT)	M-40-54, F-37-47%	53.9		
Eosinophils	1-3%	0		
Basophils	0-1%	0		
Monocytes	2-8%	0		
Lymphocytes	20-40%	23		
Segs	50-70%	76		
Bands	2-6	1		
RBC Morphology				
Platelet Appearance				
Calcium	8.5-10.5%	10.5		
Phosphorus, inorganic	2.5-4.5 mg%	3.3		
Glucose	70-125 mg%	65		
BUN	10-25 mg%	18		
Uric Acid	M-3.9-9.0 F-2.2-7.7 mg%	6.8		
Cholesterol	140-335 mg%	185		
Bilirubin, total	0.2-1.2 mg%	1.8		
Alkaline phosphatase	30-115 mU/ml	153		
LDH	60-200 mU/ml	175		
SGOT	0-41 units	47		
Sodium	136-145 mEq/L	143		
Potassium	3.5-5.0 mEq/L	4.3		
Chloride	96-106 mEq/L	105		
CO_2	24-30 mEq/L	24		
Creatinine	0.7-1.5 mg%	1.2		
Iron	40-150 units	236		
Triglycerides	30-176 mcg%	58		
T_4 (T_4X.65=P.B.I.)	3.2-8.8 mcg%	6.7		
Inorganic Iodine	0-3 mcg%			
Protein, total	6.0-8.0 gm% (7.4)	7.8		
Albumin	3.5-5.0 gm% (5.2)	4.8		
Globulin	2.7-3.0 gm% (2.2)	3.0		
A/G Ratio	2:1	1.6		
Protein Electrophoresis	TOTAL PROTEIN (7.4)	7.8		
Albumin	3.3-5.0 gm% (5.2)	4.8		
Globulin	2.7-3.0 gm% (2.2)	3.0		
A/G Ratio	2:1	1.6/1		
Alpha 1	0.2-0.4 gm% (0.30)	0.3		
Alpha 2	0.6-1.0 gm% (0.65)	0.7		
Beta	0.6-1.2 gm% (0.95)	0.9		
Gamma	0.7-1.3 gm% (1.15)	1.1		
Total Lipid	400-1000 mg%	416		
Atherogenic Index	See Chart	30	-3.0	
Sf 0-12		289		
Sf 12-400		8		
VDRL	Non-Reactive	NR		

Wm. A. Ellis, D.O.
2202 Rosedale Ln.
Arlington, Texas 76011
817-649-0036

SPECIMEN REQUIRED:
25 ml blood (12 ml serum)
2 blood slides for differential prepared from fresh blood
1 tube EDTA whole blood

Figure 16: Blood chemistry analysis of a 23 year old man (son of Figure 17)

COMPREHENSIVE PROFILE

Patient Male Age: 56 .... Date ....

EXAMINATION 6/23/84	NORMAL RANGE	DATE	DATE	REMARKS
Complete Blood Count		9		
Leukocytes (WBC)	5,000-10,000	6200		
Erythrocytes (RBC)	M-4.5-6.0M, F-4.0-5.5M	5.32		RF #2 [illegible]
Hemoglobin (HGB)	M-14-18, F-12-16 gm%	15.9		
Hematocrit (HCT)	M-40-54, F-37-47%	46.2		Standard
Eosinophils	1-5%	2		
Basophils	0-1%	0		
Monocytes	2-9%	2		
Lymphocytes	20-40%	38		
Segs	50-70%	58		
Bands	2-6	0		
RBC Morphology		N		
Platelet Appearance		ad.		
Calcium	8.5-10.5%	9.5		
Phosphorus, inorganic	2.5-4.5 mg%	3.2		
Glucose	70-125 mg%	313		
BUN	10-26 mg%	21		
Uric Acid	M-3.9-9.0 F-2.2-7.7 mg%	6.9		
Cholesterol	140-330 mg%	214		
Bilirubin, total	0.2-1.2 mg%	0.1		
Alkaline phosphatase	30-115 mU/ml	156		
LDH	60-200 mU/ml	185		
SGOT	0-41 units	30		
Sodium	136-145 mEq/L	141		
Potassium	3.5-5.0 mEq/L	4.2		
Chloride	96-106 mEq/L	104		
CO_2	24-32 mEq/L	32		
Creatinine	0.7-1.5 mg%	1.3		
Iron	40-150 units	197		
Triglycerides	30-190 mcg%	122		
T_4 (T_4X.65=P.B.I.)	3.2-8.8 mcg%	5.0		
Inorganic Iodine	0-3 mcg%			
Protein, total	6.0-8.0 gm%	5.7		
Albumin	3.5-5.0 gm%	3.7		
Globulin	2.7-3.0 gm%	2.0		
A/G Ratio	2:1	1.85		
Protein Electrophoresis		5.8		
Albumin	3.3-5.0 gm%	3.2		
Globulin	2.7-3.0 gm%	2.6		
A/G Ratio	2:1	1.3		
Alpha 1	0.2-0.4 gm%	0.2		
Alpha 2	0.6-1.0 gm%	0.7		
Beta	0.6-1.2 gm%	0.9		
Gamma	0.7-1.3 gm%	0.8		
Total Lipid	400-1000 mg%	557		
Atherogenic Index	See Chart	42		
Sf 0-12		339		
Sf 12-400		43		
VDRL	Non-Reactive	NR		

Wm. A. Ellis, D.O.
2202 Rosedale Ln.
Arlington, Texas 76011
817-649-0036

SPECIMEN REQUIRED:
25 ml blood (12 ml serum)
2 blood slides for differential
prepared from fresh blood
1 tube EDTA whole blood

Figure 17: Blood chemistry analysis of a 56 year old man (father of Figure 16)

COMPREHENSIVE PROFILE

Patient Male Age: 49 Date

4/19/83

EXAMINATION	NORMAL RANGE	DATE	DATE	REMARKS
Complete Blood Count				
Leukocytes (WBC)	5,000-10,000	5300		
Erythrocytes (RBC)	M-4.5-6.0M, F-4.0-5.5M	4390000		
Hemoglobin (HGB)	M-14-18, F-12-16 gm%	14.6		
Hematocrit (HCT)	M-40-54, F-37-47%	43.1		
Eosinophils	1-3%	3		
Basophils	0-1%	0		
Monocytes	2-8%	1		
Lymphocytes	20-40%	33		
Segs	50-70%	60		
Bands	2-6	3		
RBC Morphology				
Platelet Appearance				
Calcium	8.5-10.5%	9.2		
Phosphorus, inorganic	2.5-4.5 mg%	3.4		
Glucose	70-125 mg%	98		
BUN	10-25 mg%	12		
Uric Acid	M-3.9-9.0 F-2.2-7.7 mg%	6.1		
Cholesterol	140-335 mg% 120-270	190		
Bilirubin, total	0.2-1.2 mg%	0.5		
Alkaline phosphatase	30-115 mU/ml	108		
LDH	60-200 mU/ml 230	147		
SGOT 20 (0-45)	0-41 units	16		
Sodium	135-148 mEq/L	147		
Potassium	3.5-5.0 mEq/L	3.9		
Chloride	96-108 mEq/L	109		
CO_2	24-30 mEq/L	26		
Creatinine	0.7-1.5 mg%	1.0		
Iron	40-150 units	79		
Triglycerides	30-170 mcg%	89		
T_4 (T_4X.65=P.B.I.)	3.2-8.8 mcg%	4.2		
Inorganic Iodine	0-3 mcg%			
Protein, total	6.0-8.0 gm% (7.4)	6.40		Aloe Vera Gel
Albumin	3.5-5.0 gm% (5.2)	4.20		
Globulin	2.7-3.0 gm% (2.2)	2.20		
A/G Ratio	2:1	1.9/1		
Protein Electrophoresis	TOTAL PROTEIN (7.4)	6.40		
Albumin	3.3-5.0 gm% (5.2)	3.75		
Globulin	2.7-3.0 gm% (2.2)	2.65		
A/G Ratio	2:1	1.41		
Alpha 1	0.2-0.4 gm% (0.30)	0.26		
Alpha 2	0.6-1.0 gm% (0.65)	0.68		
Beta	0.6-1.2 gm% (0.95)	0.88		
Gamma	0.7-1.3 gm% (1.15)	0.83		
Total Lipid	400-1000 mg%	486		
Atherogenic Index	See Chart 74	32	-4.2	
Sf 0-12	365	298		
Sf 12-400	259	12		
VDRL STS	Non-Reactive	NR		

Yellow Cloudy 1.033

Wm. A. Ellis, D.O.
2202 Rosedale Ln.
Arlington, Texas 76011
817-649-0036

SPECIMEN REQUIRED:
25 ml blood (12 ml serum)
2 blood slides for differential prepared from fresh blood
1 tube EDTA whole blood

Figure 18: Blood chemistry analysis of a 49 year old man

COMPREHENSIVE PROFILE

Patient Female Age: 52 .... Date ....

EXAMINATION 5/11/83

EXAMINATION	NORMAL RANGE	DATE	DATE	REMARKS
Complete Blood Count				
Leukocytes (WBC)	5,000-10,000	6600		
Erythrocytes (RBC)	M-4.5-6.0M, F-4.0-5.5M	4,800,000		
Hemoglobin (HGB)	M-14-18, F-12-16 gm%	15.1		
Hematocrit (HCT)	M-40-54, F-37-47%	43.9		
Eosinophils	1-3%	1		
Basophils	0-1%	0		
Monocytes	2-8%	1		
Lymphocytes	20-40%	34		
Segs	50-70%	64		
Bands	2-6	0		
RBC Morphology		N		
Platelet Appearance		ad		
Calcium	8.5-10.5%	10.0		
Phosphorus, inorganic	2.5-4.5 mg%	2.5		
Glucose	70-125 mg%	100		
BUN	10-25 mg%	9		
Uric Acid	M-3.9-9.0 F-2.2-7.7 mg%	7.8		
Cholesterol	~~140-335~~ mg% 120-270	232		
Bilirubin, total	0.2-1.2 mg%	0.5		
Alkaline phosphatase	30-115 mU/ml	70		
LDH	60-~~200~~ mU/ml 230	139		
SGOT	0-41 units	33		
Sodium	135-148 mEq/L	144		
Potassium	3.5-5.0 mEq/L	4.6		
Chloride	96-108 mEq/L	102		
CO_2	24-32 mEq/L	26		
Creatinine	0.7-1.5 mg%	0.7		
Iron	40-150 units	152		
Triglycerides	30-175 mcg%	120		
T_4 ($T_4X.65$=P.B.I.)	3.2-8.8 mcg%	8.5		
Inorganic Iodine	0-3 mcg%			
Protein, total	6.0-8.0 gm% (7.4)	7.00		
Albumin	3.5-5.0 gm% (5.2)	4.00		
Globulin	2.7-3.0 gm% (2.2)	3.00		
A/G Ratio	2:1	1.33/1		
Protein Electrophoresis	Total Protein (7.4)	7.00		
Albumin	3.3-5.0 gm% (5.2)	3.57		
Globulin	2.7-3.0 gm% (2.2)	3.43		
A/G Ratio	2:1	1.04		
Alpha 1	0.2-0.4 gm% (0.30)	0.41		
Alpha 2	0.6-1.0 gm% (0.65)	0.77		
Beta	0.6-1.2 gm% (0.95)	1.13		
Gamma	0.7-1.3 gm% (1.15)	1.13		
Total Lipid	400-1000 mg%	635		
Atherogenic Index	See Chart 63	54	-0.9	
Sf 0-12	358	367		
Sf 12-400	224	97		
VDRL	STS Non-Reactive	NR		

Wm. A. Ellis, D.O.
2202 Rosedale Ln.
Arlington, Texas 76011
817-649-0036

SPECIMEN REQUIRED:
25 ml blood (12 ml serum)
2 blood slides for differential
prepared from fresh blood
1 tube EDTA whole blood

Figure 19: Blood chemistry analysis of a 52 year old woman

Detoxification

See Detoxification on page 99.

CBC

See Complete Blood Count (CBC) on page 203.

Atherogenic Index

See Atherogenic Index on page 248.

Urinalysis

See Urinalysis on page 333.

Hair Mineral Analysis

See Hair Mineral Analysis on page 337.

Diet Journal/Diary

No diseases can be corrected unless the individual's diet is resolved. When we do our analysis, we need an accurate picture of a patient's diet. We usually tell the patient something like the following.

We want an accurate picture of your diet – everything you put in your mouth and the time that you put it in. The reason is that, if you don't blend food properly, you are not going to digest it properly. Proteins will putrefy, and then you're on your way to disease.

A journal page can be fancy, such as a Daytimer, or appointment book, or it can be drawn on a piece of paper. It needs spaces large enough to list everything eaten in each day for one week, as shown in Figure .

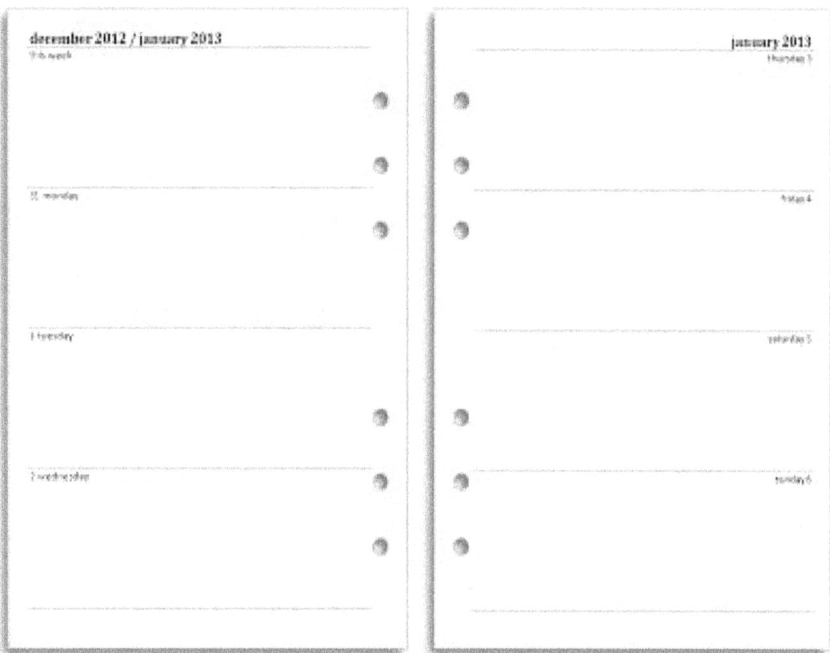

Figure 20: A Daytimer-type journal/diary

The journal can also be a simple notebook with pages divided into segments representing each meal and snack within 24-hour periods. It is also a good idea to write down what digestive, vitamin, and mineral supplements are taken with and between meals. Be honest and complete. You do not have to record the number of calories and percentage of fats for this analysis.

11 Complete Blood Count (CBC)

The complete blood count, or CBC, is an analysis of formed cells in the blood. This group of tests determines the number of circulating red and white blood cells and their subcategories (indices), and platelets. The red cells, or erythrocytes, are characterized by their size and shape, and by their potential to carry oxygen to the tissues. Platelets are characterized by their potential to repair damage to vessel walls. The white cells, or leukocytes, fight infection and specific diseases may be indicated by the relative concentrations of their various morphological subtypes.

From this information, it is possible to detect diseases, such as anemia, infection, and leukemia, to name a few. Abnormal increases or decreases in cell counts indicate medical conditions that need further evaluation. In some instances, the number of a helpful reference is listed in parentheses, referring to the list of references at the end of the chapter. **Do not make a diagnosis of disease based solely on information contained in this chapter.** Check the references listed under Suggested References on page 229 and others for additional conditions, medications, supplements, or chemical exposures that may alter test results.

Red Blood Cell Count (RBCs, Erythrocytes)

The RBC count is the number of erythrocytes present in a microliter sample of whole blood. The cells are formed in the bone marrow, where the nucleated cell becomes a non-nucleated erythroblast. RBCs are destroyed in the spleen and other reticuloendothelial tissues; they have an average life span of 120 days+. Because a normal individual's blood volume is approximately five liters, and his optimum concentration of RBC is five million per microliter of blood, his body must produce over two million RBC per second to maintain this concentration of RBCs in the blood (11).

The primary function of the erythrocyte is to carry oxygen to the tissues and carbon dioxide away from the tissues to the lungs for expulsion. Within normal limits, the RBC count rises during excitement or fear and lowers after drinking water. RBC production is regulated by overabundance and by anemia or hypoxia.

The value of the RBC count lies in its use in calculation of the indices MCV, MCHC, and MCH, which allow for a more accurate description of the anemias. A normal RBC count is associated with numerous diseases that can be described properly only after consideration of the differential count and the morphology of and inclusions within the red cells themselves.

RBC Count Within the Normal Range

A normal RBC count has little pathological significance in itself, but it can be associated with various disease conditions, depending upon deviations of other test values from normal. Some examples are given below (1). It should be understood that these possibilities are not diagnostic; further study is needed to define the specific disorders.

RBC Count Within the Normal Range	
Body System	**Possible Condition**
Circulatory/Blood/Lymph	(See RBC Morphology on page 207.) Hypochromic, microcytic anemia (if the hematocrit and hemoglobin are depressed, with concomitant depression of the MCV and MCH) Acute leukemia (if many blast forms are present) Compensated, acquired hemolytic anemia (if there is spherocytosis, polychromatophilia, and erythrocyte agglutination) Thalassemia major or minor (if there is hypochromia with target cells) Macroglobulinemia (if there is rouleaux formation) Consumption coagulopathy (if the platelet count is depressed with schistocytes and Burr cells present) Infectious mononucleosis (if atypical lymphocytes are present) Agranulocytosis (if the seg count is depressed and the lymphocyte count is elevated) Mechanical hemolysis (if schistocytes and Burr cells are present)
Systemic	Lead poisoning (if basophils are stippled) Vitamin B12 and/or folic acid deficiency (if there is microcytosis with hypersegmented neutrophils) Severe infection (if the seg count is elevated with many band forms and toxic granulations) Allergic reaction (if the eosinophil count is elevated)

RBC Count Above the Normal Range

An elevation of the RBC count above normal is termed polycythemia. This exists strictly when the RBC count exceeds six million cells per microliter of blood and when the the hemoglobin concentration exceeds 17.5 g, with a hematocrit greater than 52%. This is seen in conditions associated with a lack of oxygen to the tissues. Some common symptoms include headache, dizziness, visual disturbances, dyspnea, lassitude, paresthesias, rubor of the skin, and gout (5).

Erythemia (Polycythemia vera) is associated with hyperplasia of bone marrow and an enlarged spleen. Secondary polycythemia results from some other identifiable physiologic or pathologic stimulus (1). The distinctions are shown below.

Primary - Polycythemia vera; there is a postulated relationship to chronic myelocytic leukemia and myelofibrosis. This is seen in oxygen unsaturation caused by cardiovascular disease, extreme obesity, chronic methemoglobinemia (erythrocytosis), and in persons who live at high altitudes.

Secondary - polycthemia resulting from some other identifiable stimulus. Causes may be:

- Compensatory polycythemia from life at high altitudes (hemoglobin elevated)
- Chemical agents coal tar derivatives, cobalt, manganese, mercury, arsenic, digitalis, caffeine, nicotine, testosterone
- Neoplasms (especially of the liver), kidney, uterus
- Hemoconcentration secondary to dehydration

Relative - pseudopolycytemia; this is an acquired condition in which the RBC count may be in the normal range, but the plasma portion of the blood is inadequate. This condition is more common in males with blood pressure problems.

RBC Count Above the Normal Range	
Body System	**Possible Condition (Some Repeated from Above)**
Digestive	Neoplasm of the liver
Circulatory/Blood/Lymph	Primary polycythemia vera Possible relationship to chronic myelocytic leukemia and myelofibrosis (5) Oxygen unsaturation caused by cardiovascular disease, extreme obesity, chronic methemoglobinemia (erythrocytosis), and in persons who live at high altitudes Secondary from some other identifiable stimulus Compensatory polycythemia from living at high altitudes (hemoglobin elevated) Hemoconcentration secondary to dehydration Relative (pseudopolycythemia)
Urinary	Neoplasm of the kidney
Reproductive	Neoplasm of the uterus
Systemic	Common symptoms include headache, dizziness, visual disturbances, dyspnea, lassitude, paresthesias, rubor of the skin, and gout (5). Chemical agents coal tar derivatives, cobalt, manganese, mercury, arsenic, digitalis, caffeine, nicotine, testosterone

RBC Count Below the Normal Range

An RBC count below the normal range indicates the possibility of anemia – a deficiency of the total hemoglobin/red cell mass (1). In all cases, the oxygen-carrying capacity of the blood is reduced. The causes of anemias are many and varied, so the indices must be known to define the cause. Some examples are listed below.

RBC Count Below the Normal Range	
Body System	**Possible Condition**
Digestive	Pernicious anemia due to achlorhydria, which prevents absorption of iron from the digestive tract (see Albumin/ Globulin Ratio (A/G) on page 240) Protein deficiency (see Albumin/Globulin Ratio (A/G) on page 240 and Protein (Total) on page 286) Vitamin B12 and/or folic acid deficiency Ascorbic acid deficiency (prevents absorption of iron from the digestive tract) Deficiency of iron, copper, and/or cobalt, leading to a decrease in RBC production (check these metals by hair mineral assay). In iron deficiency anemia, there is evidence of hypochromia and microcytes; RBC count is low or normal, MCV and MCHC are both depressed.
Circulatory/Blood/Lymph	Bone marrow failure due to chemicals, ionizing radiation, and antineoplastic agents Destruction of RBC resulting from congenital abnormalities in enzyme action as in Thalassemia and sickle cell disease Loss of blood (normochromic, normocytic anemia; the indices are usually normal) Macrocytic anemia (MCV and MCHC are elevated; the cells are larger and contain more hemoglobin than normal, with possible vitamin B12 and folic acid deficiency) Possible aplastic anemia (MCV elevated, hemoglobin is usually normal) Decreased production of RBC is characterized, in these cases, by poikilocytosis, low hemoglobin, possible leukopenia, and thrombocytopenia.
Endocrine	Possible hypothyroidism (MCV elevated, hemoglobin is usually normal; see T4 (Thyroxine) on page 295)

RBC Morphology

The presence of many suspected pathologic conditions may be indicated by the observation of red blood cells under the microscope. Some of these characteristics and related disorders are listed below.

RBC Morphology	
Appearance	**Definition / Possible Conditions**
Anisocytosis	Excessive inequality in the size of RBCs in the total population
Distortion of Shape	Severely distorted red cells, such as Burry Helmet, Acanthoid, and Triangle forms seen in peripheral blood smears. These may be seen in association with acquired hemolytic disorders in which mechanical damage has been caused to the cells, and in some patients with a defibrination syndrome. Other possibilities are: Following insertions of prosthetic heart valves During severe rheumatic valvular disease Hemolytic anemia (associated with uremia) Thrombocytopenia purpura Gastric carcinoma Peptic ulcer with bleeding Microangiopathic hemolytic anemia Cirrhosis of the liver with hemolytic anemia, associated with thrombocytopenia (see Platelets (Thrombocytes) on page 225 and Reticulocytosis, below). Hereditary acanthocytosis (the RBC appears to be covered with thornlike projections) Hereditary pyruvate kinase deficiency Hereditary hexokinase deficiency Following snakebite

Chromicity	Color or density of color of the cell. Color variations are: Achromatic - a colorless cell from which the hemoglobin has been lost Basophilic - the cytoplasm of the RBC stains blue, indicating the presence of basophilic material Hyperchromic - too red; the RBC contains too much hemoglobin Hypochromic - too light; the cell contains an insufficient amount of hemoglobin. The MCHC is usually depressed, and this characteristic is usually accompanied by microcytosis, poikilocytosis, and a low serum iron, achlorhydria is a common finding (see Albumin/Globulin Ratio (A/G) on page 240 and Protein (Total) on page 286), and chronic alimentary tract disorders may be evident (hookworm, diarrhea, etc.). Some other causes are deficiencies of iron (especially if milk is included in the diet), copper, cobalt, vitamin B12, and folic acid. A hair mineral assay may be helpful. Hypochromicity is seen in sickle cell anemia, Thalassemia, hemoglobinopathy C and F, and in vitamin C deficiency. Orthochromatic - the cell stains pink with acid stains only Polychromatic - the cell does not stain uniformly
Erythroblasts Present	See Reticulocytosis, below.
Inclusions Present	Presence of characteristics or elements that are not common to a normal cell, such as: Basophilic stippling - possible heavy metal poisoning (usually lead) Cabot's rings - possible hemolytic or pernicious anemia Heinz-Ehrlich bodies - possible congenital glucose-6-phosphate dehydrogenase deficiency, or drug-induced hemolytic anemia Howell-Jolly bodies - after splenectomy, in hemolytic anemia, pernicious anemia, Thalassemia, some leukemias Pappenheimer bodies - possible defect in incorporating iron into hemoglobin (see Copper on page 359). This is seen in pyridoxine (vitamin B6)-involved anemia, lead poisoning, Thalassemia, and in diGuglielmo's disease. Plasmodium organism - probable malaria

Macrocytes Present	The RBCs are too large. This is indicated by a rise in the MCV, and is commonly associated with: Anemias of pregnancy Anemias of infancy Megaloblastic anemia Sprue Infestation with fish tapeworm Stomach carcinoma Administration of antimetabolite therapy Orotic aciduria Hypothyroidism Chronic liver disease diGuelielmo's disease
Osmotic Fragility	Increased - The cells are very fragile and break open when suspended in a standard salt solution. This is seen in: Some hemolytic anemias After thermal injury (burns) Some neoplasms During pregnancy Some infections Cirrhosis of the liver Decreased - the cells are stronger than normal. This is seen in: Jaundice Liver disease Post splenectomy Nutritional megaloblastic anemia Iron deficiency anemia Thalassemia Sickle cell anemia
Poikilocytosis	The RBCs are irregularly-colored (see Chromicity, above).
Reticulocytosis	The presence of too many immature RBCs (erythroblasts) in the population. Their numbers are increased following blood loss; however, their numbers may increase three- to sixfold following effective therapy for anemia. Decreases from the optimal range are seen in autoimmune hemolytic diseases, during a regenerative crisis, and with decreased erythropoiesis.

Rouleaux Formation	The red cells arrange themselves in a row similar to a row of coins. This condition is commonly seen in: Cryoglobulinemia Macroglobulinemia Multiple myeloma

Hemoglobin (Hgb)

The amount of hemoglobin in a sample of blood is expressed as the number of grams in 10 milliliters (one deciliter) of hemolyzed blood. The normal value for men is above 15, and for women, above 14.5; these are very specific normals. Hemoglobin is the oxygen carrying red pigment of the RBC. It acts like a magnet to carry oxygen to and carbon dioxide away from the tissues. Each red cell is capable of carrying an incredible one billion oxygen molecules (7)! The heme portion, the actual oxygen carrier, is synthesized from glycine, an amino acid, and succinyl CoA. When old red cells are destroyed in the spleen and in other reticuloendothelial tissues, the globin (protein) portion is split off, and the heme is converted to biliverdin and bilirubin. The iron is then returned to the liver for reuse and storage. In the average (70 Kg) individual, there exists about 900 gm of hemoglobin; 0.3 gm of this are synthesized and destroyed every hour (4). Hemoglobin levels can be normal in certain anemias, so it is important to compute and consider the indices, MCV, MCH, and MCHC.

Hemoglobin Within the Normal Range

A normal hemoglobin content may be associated with the following conditions. In these instances, the hemoglobin is usually low normal, the hematocrit is low normal, and the RBC count is within the normal range.

Hemoglobin Within the Normal Range	
Body System	**Possible Condition**
Circulatory/Blood/Lymph	Hypochromic microcytic anemia Iron deficiency anemia Thalassemia major and minor Sickle cell anemia Hemoglobin c disease

Hemoglobin Above the Normal Range

Pathologic increases in the hemoglobin concentration are associated with the following conditions.

Hemoglobin Above the Normal Range	
Body System	**Possible Condition**
Digestive	Intestinal obstruction (the hematocrit is also elevated) Dehydration resulting from diarrhea
Circulatory/Blood/Lymph	Sickle cell anemia Thalassemia Hemoglobin c disease Sickle cell hemoglobin C disease Acquired (autoimmune) hemolytic anemia Polycythemia vera (erythemia) Compensatory polycythemia resulting from living at high altitude Microcytic anemia
Systemic	Dehydration resulting from burns

Hemoglobin Below the Normal Range

A pathologically low hemoglobin level is associated with possible anemia. If the low level is accompanied by an increase in both the MCV and MCHC, a finding of macrocytic anemia is evident. This type of anemia includes the pernicious variety, resulting from a vitamin B12 and folic acid deficiency. Also commonly observed are macrocytosis and hypersegmented neutrophils.

One limitation of considering only the hemoglobin level by itself is that a low hemoglobin level can be associated with a possible normochromic normocytic anemia. There are not many cases in the literature dealing with a low hemoglobin level; this indicates dependence upon other factors, probably the RBC, MCV, and MCHC, to properly characterize anemias.

Hematocrit (Hct)

The hematocrit is the percentage of packed RBCs in a centrifuged sample of whole blood in cubic centimeters per 100 cc. The normal mean for males is 50%, and for females, 45%. It is useful when compared to the level of RBCs in determining the size of the individual red cells (check the MCV). If the number of red cells is constant from one sample to the next, the MCV will change in direct proportion to the hematocrit. Sometimes, the RBC count is normal, but the hematocrit is elevated or depressed; this indicates an abnormality in the size of the red cell (see RBC Morphology on page 207), or it could, in the case of an elevated hematocrit, indicate a state of dehydration.

Hematocrit Within the Normal Range

The hematocrit can fall within the normal range, and, in the absence of other abnormal tests, no further significance is assigned to it. However, the hematocrit can be normal with an elevated or depressed RBC or hemoglobin, altering the MCV and the MCHC, respectively, and a possible pathological condition may be present.

Hematocrit Above the Normal Range

A hematocrit value above the normal range is indicative of abnormally large red cells if the RBC count is within normal limits. If the RBC count is likewise elevated, polycythemia is implied. Calculation of the MCV is also necessary. An elevated hematocrit may be associated with the following.

Hematocrit Above the Normal Range	
Body System	**Possible Condition**
Digestive	Intestinal obstruction (the hemoglobin is also elevated) causes dehydration
Circulatory/Blood/Lymph	Polycythemia (the RBC is also elevated) Decreased blood volume due to dehydration
Endocrine	Addison's disease (chronic adrenal insufficiency) causes dehydration

Hematocrit Below the Normal Range

A reduction in the hematocrit value implies reduced numbers or red cells. If this is indeed true (after considering the MCV and RBC), an anemia is possible. A greater than 10% decrease could also indicate acute pancreatitis.

Sedimentation Rate (Erythrocyte Sed Rate, ESR)

The ESR is defined as the rate (distance vs. time) with which RBCs settle in an uncoagulated blood specimen in one hour. It is a rather nonspecific test, an abnormal value having no organ or disease specificity. A normal value does give some reassurance that significant disease is not present; an abnormal value signifies that further testing should be considered.

The basis for the ESR test is simple. In most diseases, the albumin component of the blood is depleted to some degree. Since albumin is the primary osmotic regulator of blood thickness, the less albumin, the thinner is the blood. As this thickness, or viscosity, of the blood drops, there is less physical resistance to the erythrocytes settling out of the serum due to gravity; they therefore fall faster, as indicated by a higher ESR. The ESR is very useful in following the progress of a diagnosed disease. As the ESR rises, the disease is more severe; as it decreases, the prognosis is more favorable.

ESR Within the Normal Range

There are some disease conditions in which the ESR remains normal, such as the following.

ESR Within the Normal Range	
Body System	**Possible Condition**
Skeletal	Hypertropic arthritis
Digestive	Early acute appendicitis Uncomplicated cholelithiasis Simple peptic ulcer Cirrhosis of the liver
Circulatory/Blood/Lymph	Essential hypertension
Urinary	Hydronephrosis Kidney stones
Endocrine	Diabetes mellitus
Systemic	In various tissues, there may be benign tumors, uncomplicated fibroid cysts. Head colds Asthma Hay fever Functional nervous diseases

ESR Above the Normal Range

A high ESR indicates that any of several disease conditions and/or pregnancy may be present. Further testing is necessary to determine the specific disease. Some possibilities are listed as follows.

ESR Above the Normal Range	
Body System	**Possible Condition**
Skeletal	Rheumatoid or pyogenic arthritis
Digestive	Acute hepatitis
Circulatory/Blood/Lymph	Myocardial infarction Macroglobulinemia Hypoalbuminemia Hemorrhage
Urinary	Nephrosis
Endocrine	Hypothyroidism Hyperthyroidism

Reproductive	Inflammatory pelvic disease Pregnancy (three months to term)
Systemic	In various tissues, there may be necrosis. Tuberculosis Arsenic or lead poisoning Dextran or polyvinyl compounds Rheumatic fever

ESR Below the Normal Range

A low ESR carries no particular significance, except that the lower it is, the more normal it is.

White Blood Cell Count (Leucocytes, WBCs)

The WBC count is the number of leucocytes present in a microliter sample of whole blood. This value varies normally with age, exercise, time of collection with respect to a meal or hot bath, altitude, and the state of hydration of the specimen. A normal value may be meaningless unless the entire hematologic profile is considered. For example, the WBC can be normal even in severe sepsis, but the seg count is usually highly elevated. Conversely, if the differential count (measures the percentage of each type of WBC) and blood smear appear to be normal, a small elevation or depression of the WBC count outside of the normal range may be considered insignificant (1). WBCs are of two types, agranular (lymphocytes and monocytes) and granular (basophils, neutrophils, and eosinophils).

WBC Count Within the Normal Range

As mentioned above, the WBC count can be normal in severe sepsis, but there is usually some alteration in the differential count.

WBC Count Above the Normal Range

A WBC count above the normal range is termed "leucocytosis." The normal range is 5-10,000. This varies normally with age, exercise, relationship to a meal, hot bath, high altitude, and dehydration. A mild to moderate leucocytosis is characterized by a WBC count of 11-17,000 (1). A rise of the WBC count indicates the severity of infection. However, severe sepsis can occur in elderly persons who show only a modest elevation. An elevation may be associated with exposure to mercury, lead, carbon monoxide, and coal tar products. Also, a rise may be seen in allergies. Leucocytosis is commonly associated with the following.

WBC Count Above the Normal Range	
Body System	**Possible Condition**
Digestive	Ulcer Cholecystitis Appendicitis During normal digestion
Circulatory/Blood/Lymph	Acute hemorrhage RBC hemolysis Myeloproliferative disease (basophils are also elevated) Hemopoeitic system disease Coronary occlusion
Urinary	Pyelitis Pyelonephritis
Endocrine	Diabetes mellitus (and acidosis)
Reproductive	Menstruation Obstetrical labor Salpingitis Eclampsia Pregnancy
Systemic	Necrosis In generalized infections (septicemia, pyemia, gangrene, polio, Herpes Zoster, acute rheumatic fever, smallpox, chicken pox, scarlet fever) Localized infections (pyogenic abcesses, carbuncles) Metabolic intoxications (uremia, acidosis) Various physiologic manifestations, (Stress, pain, dehydration, exposure to extreme sunlight, after strenuous exercise, living at high altitude) Tumors Rapidly growing carcinoma Burns Use of various drugs and poisons (vaccines, mercury or lead intoxication, carbon monoxide, camphor, coal tar products, epinephrine, and spider venom)
Miscellaneous	Tonsillitis Mastoiditis Otitis media Pneumonia

WBC Count Below the Normal Range

A WBC count below the normal range is termed "leucopenia." This is commonly seen in overwhelming infections, but a differential count is necessary to more clearly define the disease. Leucopenia may be mild (3,000-5,000), moderate (1,500-3,000), or severe (less than 1,500) (1). Some conditions associated with leucopenia are as follows.

WBC Count Below the Normal Range	
Body System	**Possible Condition**
Skeletal	Systemic Lupus erythematosis Rheumatoid arthritis
Circulatory/Blood/Lymph	Pernicious anemia Aplastic anemia Hypersplenism Primary or secondary splenic neutropenia (seg count is depressed) Drug-induced neutropenia (seg count is depressed) Drugor immunosuppressant-induced leucocyte fragility Leucocyte fragility of lymphocytic leukemia or multiple myeloma
Urinary	
Endocrine	Acromegaly (eosinophil count is also depressed) Excess ACTH, cortisone, or epinephrine
Reproductive	During intermenstrual period (eosinophils are depressed)
Systemic	Infections (acute, chronic, pyogenic) Starvation (seg count is also depressed) Possible acute viral infection (seg count is also depressed) Acute alcohol ingestion (seg count is also depressed) Acute or chronic stress (eosinophils are also depressed) Rickettsial infections Protozoal infections Non-specific protein therapy Cachexia Radiation (X-ray, radium, cobalt) Use of certain drugs and poisons (sulfa, barbiturates)
Miscellaneous	Diurnal variations

Eosinophils (Eos)

Eosinophils are members of one class of the polymorphonuclear leucocytes (granulocytes) that are distinguished by the presence of a bilobed nucleus, as seen through its affinity for eosin, a bright red, acid dye (12). The count is expressed as the percentage of the WBC population that are eosinophils; the normal range is 1-3%.

Eosinophils have an important role in detoxification, because they phagocytize antigen/antibody complexes, disintegrating and removing protein debris from the blood and lymphatic fluid. In patients with allergy diseases, the eosinophil count is often elevated (1), so the eosinophil count is commonly used to monitor the presence of parasites (worms, fungi, certain bacteria) that produce great amounts of antigenic material.

Eosinophil Count Within the Normal Range

There is no particular significance to a normal eosinophil count. The assumption is that there are no allergic manifestations. The count fluctuates during the day in a normal individual (1).

Eosinophil Count Above the Normal Range

An elevation in the eosinophil count above the normal range is termed "eosinophilic leucocytosis." The most frequently encountered pattern is a rise to 10-20%. However, values from 5-90% have been observed (1). Such a high value is commonly elevated in cutaneous and respiratory allergic diseases. Other possible conditions are listed below.

Eosinophil Count Above the Normal Range	
Body System	**Possible Condition**
Skeletal	Bone tumor
Digestive	Colitis Gastroenteritis
Circulatory/Blood/Lymph	Erythema multiforme Polyarteritis nodosa Eosinophilic leukemia (eosinophil count rises to 80-90%) Myelogenous leukemia Pernicious anemia Polycythemia vera Urticaria Basophilic leukemia Chronic hemolytic anemia
Reproductive	Ovarian tumor

Systemic	Psoriasis (responds well to Borage oil applied topically) Cutaneous allergies Drug therapy Parasitic infestation with tissue invasion (trichinosis) Poisoning (phosphorus, copper sulfate, camphor) Neoplasms Specific infections (tuberculosis, brucellosis, chicken pox, smallpox, chronic infection of bony sinuses Administration of non-specific proteins
Miscellaneous	Hay fever Pollenosis Asthma Diseases of unknown etiology

Eosinophil Count Below the Normal Range

A depressed eosinophil count has been shown in marked intoxication and in acute infections (6). Mild to moderate decreases are associated with acute and chronic stress, administration of ACTH, cortisone, or epinephrine, during the intermenstrual period, and in acromegaly. Depressions are also observed in severe infections that reappear upon recovery, in shock, in Cushing's disease, and after major surgical operations.

Eosinophil Count Below the Normal Range	
Body System	**Possible Condition**
Circulatory/Blood/Lymph	With very low value, leucopenia Basophils - 0-1% bring an anticoagulant known as heparin to prevent the clotting of blood in inflamed tissue.
Endocrine	Cushing's disease Acromegaly
Reproductive	Intermenstrual period
Systemic	Acute infections Severe infections that reappear upon recovery Intoxication Acute and chronic stress Shock
Miscellaneous	After major surgery After injections of ACTH or epinephrine

Basophils (Baso)

Basophils are one class of polymorphonuclear leucocytes or granulocytes. They possess a large, lobed nucleus and take on a purplish blue color when subjected to Wright's stain (12). The basophil count is expressed as a percentage of the leucocytes (WBC count) that exist as basophils. Although their role is uncertain (1), these cells have been shown to contain heparin, an anticoagulant that prevents the clotting of blood in inflamed tissues.

Basophil Count Within the Normal Range

No particular significance is assigned.

Basophil Count Above the Normal Range

An elevated basophil count is termed basophilia. It is associated with the following conditions.

Basophil Count Above the Normal Range	
Body System	**Possible Condition**
Circulatory/Blood/Lymph	Chronic myelogenous leukemia (an elevated WBC count with basophilia is uncommon, and suggests myeloproliferative disease) Polycythemia Myeloid metaplasia Hodgkin's disease Postsplenectomy Chronic hemolytic anemia (in some patients; basophilic stippling is often observed in severe anemias)
Urinary	Nephrosis
Endocrine	Myxedema
Systemic	Injection of nonspecific foreign protein Lead or mercury poisoning (causes stippling)
Miscellaneous	Chicken pox Smallpox Chronic sinusitis Chronic malaria (causes stippling)

Basophil Count Below the Normal Range

A rapid fall in the basophil count may indicate an anaphylactic reaction (1). Other conditions associated with a low basophil count are listed below.

Basophil Count Below the Normal Range	
Body System	**Possible Condition**
Endocrine	Hyperthyroidism
Reproductive	Normal pregnancy
Systemic	Postirradiation After chemotherapy After administration of glucocorticoids During the acute phase of infection

Monocytes (Mono)

Monocytes are agranular leucocytes. Their numbers are expressed as a percentage of the total leucocyte count. The normal range for monocytes is 2-8%. These cells lack granules in their cytoplasm, are relatively large, and possess a large, horseshoe-shaped nucleus. The cytoplasm stains grayish-blue with Wright's stain (12). Monocytes are made in the bone marrow.

Their levels can mirror the acuteness of infections; however, a value of 9 or more indicates an acute infection, while the infection becomes clinical at a value of 4. Monocytes do not migrate into inflammatory exudates as rapidly as neutrophils, but they do phagocytize and digest bacteria and protozoa. Monocytes are more commonly seen in chronic inflammatory disorders (1),

Monocyte Count Within the Normal Range

There is no pathological significance associated with a normal monocyte count.

Monocyte Count Above the Normal Range

When the level of monocytes rises above normal, the condition is called monocytosis. Although elevations usually are associated with chronic inflammatory disease (1), a value of 9% or greater indicates the presence of acute infection; the lowering of the value reflects a lessening of the acute condition. Some diseases associated with monocytosis are listed below (2). These disorders can show a count to as high as 10%.

Monocyte Count Above the Normal Range	
Body System	**Possible Condition**
Skeletal	Rheumatoid arthritis
Digestive	Gaucher's disease lipid storage malfunction Chronic ulcerative colitis Chronic regional enteritis
Circulatory/Blood/Lymph	Myelocytic leukemia Various other leukemias Myeloproliferative disorders (plasia, polycythemia vera) Hodgkin's disease Other malignant lymphomas
Systemic	Lupus erythematosis Recovery from agranulocytosis Subsidence of acute infection Protozoal infection (malaria, kala-azar, trypanosomiasis) Rickettsial infection (Rocky Mountain spotted fever, typhus) Bacterial infection (subacute bacterial endocarditis, tuberculosis, brucellosis) Sarcoidosis

Monocyte Count Below the Normal Range

There is no pathological significance assigned to a monocyte count below the normal range.

Lymphocytes (Lymph)

Another class of agranular leucocytes (WBC) is lymphocytes. The amount of lymphocytes in a sample of whole blood is expressed as a percentage of the total numbers of leucocytes, the normal range being 20-40%. Lymphocytes are of two varieties: the longer-lived T cells (formed in the thymus), and the shorter-lived B cells (formed in the lymph nodes and in the bone marrow). These are further categorized into large (predominant in infants and young persons) and small (predominant in adults). The small lymphocytes are capable of producing antigen-specific antibodies. The level of lymphocytes reflects the body's ability to fight infection.

Lymphocyte Count Within the Normal Range

A normal lymphocyte count implies that, in the absence of other indicators of disease, the body is prepared to fight infection.

Lymphocyte Count Above the Normal Range

A value above 40% shows a lack of ingredients within the body to form a good quality antibody to fight infections or inflammations. Usually, the segs are also below 50%, but not always.

Lymphocyte Count Above the Normal Range	
Body System	**Possible Condition**
Circulatory/Blood/Lymph	Blood diseases, such as lymphocytic leukemia
Systemic	Metabolic diseases, such as rickets, malnutrition During convalescence from infection Acute infections, such as infectious mononucleosis, acute infectious lymphocytosis Chronic infections, such as tuberculosis, congenital syphilis If the lymphocytes are Increased with a normal leucocyte count, consider pernicious anemia or acute infections, such as typhoid fever, influenza, brucellosis, infectious hepatitis German measles, and mumps.
Miscellaneous	Normal increase in infants and children

Lymphocyte Count Below the Normal Range

Decreases in the percentage of circulating lymphocytes are associated with the following conditions. If the lymphocyte count is low and the segmented neutrophil count is high, it may signify that the body has the materials necessary to fight infection but is not able to do it.

Lymphocyte Count Below the Normal Range	
Body System	**Possible Condition**
Skeletal	Rheumatoid arthritis
Digestive	Portal cirrhosis

Circulatory/Blood/Lymph	Diseases of hemopoietic system, such as agranulocytosis, aplastic anemia, leukemia, chronic hypochromic anemias Leukopenia Myelocytic leukemia (with increases in myelocytes the immature granulocytes) Neutrophilic leucocytosis (6) Aplastic anemia Agranulocytosis Aleukemic leukemia Chronic hypochromic anemia
Systemic	Overwhelming infections, such as brucellosis, paratyphoid, and pyogenic abcesses Protozoal infestations Nonspecific protein therapy Debilitated states Postirradiation Certain medicines (sulfonamides, barbiturates, benzol, arsenic, quinine, and nitrogen mustards) Certain acute and chronic infections (typhoid, paratyphoid fever, brucellosis overwhelming pyogenic diseases) Viral diseases, such as measles, rubella, smallpox (up to the 4th day only) Drugs and poisons, such as sulfonamides, barbiturates, benzol, arsenic, quinine, nitrogen mustard Radiation, such as X-ray, radium, and cobalt
Miscellaneous	Portal cirrhosis Non-specific protein therapy

Neutrophils (SEG, Poly, PMN)

Neutrophils are also known as polymorphonuclear or PMN cells. However they are commonly called segs. The seg count is expressed as a percentage of the total leucocyte (WBC) count in the sample, and it is the most numerous of all of the WBCs. The nucleus of this type of granulocyte has three to five lobes (hence, segmented), and the fine granules of the cytoplasm stain with neutral dyes. With Wright's stain, these granules appear light purple (12). These neutrophils are produced in the bone marrow in response to infectious organisms (see Bands (Immature SEG, Poly, PMN) on page 225). Their chief role is the phagocytosis of foreign materials (1). These cells, like the other leucocytes, produce powerful digestive enzymes that can act within the cell to dissolve phagocytosed substances or outside the cell to act on surrounding materials.

SEG Count Within the Normal Range

A normal seg count implies that, in the absence of other indicators of disease, the body is prepared to fight infection.

SEG Count Above the Normal Range

An elevated seg count is commonly seen in association with two conditions. One is myelocytic leukemia, but only if mature and immature forms of the other granulocytes are also present. Another is a post-irradiation syndrome, after a dose of less the 300 roentgens; the seg count elevates with the appearance of irradiation sickness (2).

Elevations may imply that the body is manufacturing a poor quality antibody. When the seg count is above 70, it means that the body is unable to produce a good quality antibody although the ingredients are present within the body. When the lymphocytes are above 40, it means that the body does not have the ingredients to build a good quality antibody. There is usually some other reason for it, such as cadmium or lead poisoning, which is found commonly in those who smoke, although that's not the most detrimental part of smoking.

SEG Count Below the Normal Range

A seg count depressed below the normal range is termed "neutropenia." This condition has no symptoms in itself, but it is secondary to a myriad of different disorders. Agranulocytosis, the absence of 98-100% of all nucleated leucocytes in the blood, does have symptoms of extreme weakness, high fever, and oral ulcerations. This condition is usually attributed to exposure to some toxic agent, many of which are listed below (2). Granulocytopenia is seen in infectious mononucleosis, but in this case, the lymphocytes are usually elevated with no sign of agranulocytosis. A depressed seg count implies an inability on the part of the cells to obtain the materials necessary to build a quality antibody.

Toxic Agents That Can Produce Agranulocytosis	
Susceptibility	**Agent**
Anyone/Normal Individual	Nitrogen mustards Methotrexate Mercaptopurine Vinblastine Daunomycin Benzene Radium X-ray irradiation

Sensitive Individual	Aminopyrine (interferes with production in bone marrow) Dipyron Phenylbutazone Phenothiazines Propylthiouracil Diphenylhydantoin Trimethadione Chloramphenicol Sulfonamides Antihistamines Indandiones (pesticide anticoagulant) Gold compounds Arsenicals
Related Disorder	Granulocytopenia (seen in the first week of infectious mononucleosis and primary splenic neutropenia with splenomegaly)

Bands (Immature SEG, Poly, PMN)

Bands are leucocytes that are destined to become mature segmented neutrophils (segs, or polys).

Band Count Within the Normal Range

No significance is assigned to a normal band count.

Band Count Above the Normal Range

The band count increases during acute infections.

Band Count Below the Normal Range

No significance is assigned to a band count below the normal range.

Platelets (Thrombocytes)

The blood platelets, or thrombocytes, function in blood clotting and clot retraction. During this process, called coagulation, the platelet disintegrates and liberates a clot forming substance, cephalin. Also, by adhering to small leaks or tears in the capillary wall, platelets can patch these openings and help close injured vessels (12). Their numbers are usually expressed in thousands per a given volume of whole blood, with a normal range of 150,000 to 450,000 platelets per microliter (cubic millimeter).

Platelet Count Within the Normal Range

In the absence of other indicators of disease, a normal platelet count means that the body can optimally perform the task of blood clotting and vascular repair.

Platelet Count Above the Normal Range

A high platelet count, or "thrombocytosis", may be associated with the following conditions.

Platelet Count Above the Normal Range	
Body System	**Possible Condition**
Circulatory/Blood/Lymph	Polycythemia vera Acute hemorrhage Hemolytic anemias Chronic myelogenous anemia
Systemic	After severe exercise Cachexia Malnutrition Living at high altitudes During suppurative processes Acute rheumatic fever Following surgery, especially after surgery involving the neck of the femur During asphyxia Infections such as suppurative processes, acute rheumatic fever

Platelet Count Below the Normal Range

A depression of the platelet count below the normal range is termed "thrombocytopenia." This is associated with the following conditions.

Platelet Count Below the Normal Range	
Body System	**Possible Condition**
Circulatory/Blood/Lymph	Prothrombocytopenia, idiopathic thrombocytopenia purpura, symptomatic thrombocytopenia purpura Acute and chronic leukemias Hypochromic anemia Aplastic anemia Pernicious anemia Myelothesia
Reproductive	After the first day of the menstrual cycle
Systemic	During certain infections After exposure to certain chemical and physical agents

MCH

The MCH is the **mean corpuscular hemoglobin**, and it reflects the amount of hemoglobin in an RBC. It is calculated by dividing the hemoglobin value by the RBC count. The normal range is typically 27-33 pg/cell.

MCH Within the Normal Range

A normal MCH suggests that the RBC carries a normal amount of hemoglobin. Although MCH can be used to determine if an anemia is hypo-, normo-, or hyperchromic, the MCV must be considered, because the MCH can decrease or increase in parallel with the MCV. The MCHC is believed to be a better parameter than MCH to determine hypochromasia.

MCH Above the Normal Range

A high MCH may indicate macrocytic anemias. The MCH can be falsely elevated by hyperlipidemia resulting in plasma turbidity, spuriously increasing hemoglobin.

MCH Below the Normal Range

A low MCH may indicate hypochromic and microcytic anemias.

MCHC

The MCHC is the **mean corpuscular hemoglobin concentration**, and it reflects the amount of hemoglobin in a volume of packed RBCs, indicating the amount of hemoglobin relative to the size of the red cell. It is calculated by dividing the hemoglobin value by the hematocrit. MCHC correlates the hemoglobin content with the volume of the cell. The normal range is typically 32-36 g/dL,

MCHC Within the Normal Range

A normal MCHC suggests that the RBC carries a normal amount of hemoglobin. However, in megaloblastic anemia caused by vitamin B12 or folic acid deficiency, the MCHC remains normal, but the MCV is increased, and there is anisocytosis.

MCHC Above the Normal Range

A high MCHC may indicate an autoimmune hemolytic anemia (Thalassemia), be the result of severe burns, or be associated with a rare disorder called hereditary spherocytosis.The MCHC can be falsely increased in autoagglutination and hyperlipidemia caused by a spuriously low hematocrit and a spuriously high hemoglobin.

MCHC Below the Normal Range

A low MCHC can indicate iron-deficiency anemia, possibly caused by insufficient iron intake or inability to absorb it or to use it to make hemoglobin. Another cause is blood loss over time.

MCV

The MCV is the **mean corpuscular volume**, or **mean cell volume**, and it reflects the average volume of an RBC, indicating the size of the cell. It is calculated by multiplying the volume of the blood sample by the hematocrit and dividing that product by the number of RBCs in that volume. The normal reference range is typically 80-94 fL (femtoliters = 10^{-15} liters).

MCV Within the Normal Range

A normal MCV value suggests that the RBCs are of normal size. However it is possible to have a normocytic anemia from the loss of blood; check for a low RBC value.

MCV Above the Normal Range

A high MCV is termed macrocytic, or pernicious, anemia, and the value can reach 150 fL. An elevated MCV is also associated with alcoholism, vitamin B12 and/or folic acid deficiency, and liver disease.

MCV Below the Normal Range

A low MCV (60-70 fL) is termed microcytic anemia and is associated with iron deficiency (inadequate, malabsorption, or blood loss), Thalassemia, sideroblastic anemia, or chronic disease.

VDRL

The VDRL (Venereal Disease Research Laboratory) slide flocculation test indicates the presence (positive) or absence (negative) of syphilis in the blood. Ordinarily, the test result should be negative, receiving an NR, or non-reactive, designation. A positive reaction may be given a 1-4 designation, or a weakly reactive, or reactive designation. If the patient's sample gets a positive reaction, call the laboratory immediately and request another test be done on the same sample, because this particular test shows many false positives. It is only reliable in 80% of the cases; in other words, it is 20% inaccurate.

Suggested References

1. Tilkian, S. M., and Conover, M. H., *Clinical Implications of Laboratory Tests*, The C. V. Mosby Company, St. Louis, 1975.(1)

2. Wallach, J., *Interpretation of Diagnostic Tests*: A Handbook Synopsis of Laboratory Medicine, 3rd edition, Little, Brown and Company, Boston, 1978.(2)

3. Harper, H. A., *Review of Physiological Chemistry*, 14th edition, Lange Medical Publications, Los Altos, California, 1973.(3)

4. Garong, W. F., *Review of Medical Physiology*, 5th edition, Lange Medical Publications, Los Altos, California, 1971.(4)

5. Holvey, D. N., ed., *The Merck Manual of Diagnosis and Therapy, 12th edition*, Merck, Sharp, and Dohme Research Laboratories, Rahway, New Jersey, 1972.(5)

6. Medical Services Company of Arizona, *Quick Reference Laboratory Manual*, 2nd edition, Medical Services Company of Arizona, Phoenix, 1977.(6)

7. Asimov, I., *The Bloodstream*, Collier Books, London, 1961.(7)

8. Garb, S., *Laboratory Tests in Common Use, 5th edition*, Springer Publishing Company, Inc., New York, 1971.(8)

9. Widmann, F. K., *Goodale's Clinical Interpretation of Laboratory Tests, 7th edition*, F. A. Davis Company, Philadelphia, 1973.(9)

10. Benson, E. S., and Strandjord, P. E., eds., *Multiple Laboratory Screening*, Academic Press, New York, 1969.(10)

11. Thomas, C. L., ed., *Taber's Cyclopedic Medical Dictionary*, 14th edition, F. A. Davis Company, Philadelphia, 1981.(11)

12. Steen, E. B., and Montagu, A., *Anatomy and Physiology, Vol. 1*, Barnes and Noble, New York, 1959.(12)

13. Schutte, K. H. and Myers, J. A., *Metabolic Aspects of Health: Nutritional Elements in Health and Disease*, Discovery Press, Kentfield, California, 1979.(13)

12 Correlated CBC Patterns

Correlation of complete blood count resulting value patterns can help to narrow the focus of a diagnosis. They are included as a learning experience to show possibilities other than what may be commonly found in laboratory manuals.

Test Pattern vs. Possible Condition

Test patterns are listed in the left column, with possible associated conditions listed in the right column. In this section, **N** = a value within the normal range; **<** = a value below the normal range; and **>** = a value above the normal range.

To make it easier to compare actual combinations of test results with the indicated pattern or patterns, arrange values (usually only those that deviate from laboratory normals) in ascending alphabetical order of the name of the test.

Bands (Immature Forms of SEG)

BANDS>	Acute infection
BANDS> RBC=N SEGS> + toxic granulations	Possible severe infection

Basophils (Baso)

BASO (stippled)	Lead or mercury poisoning, severe anemia, check MCV and MCHC for confirmation
BASO (stippled) ESR>	Possible arsenic or lead poisoning
BASO<	Possible anaphylaxis (if the fall is rapid)
BASO>	A process involving heparin release is occurring.
BASO> EOS> WBC<	Infestation with worms, parasites, or microorganisms

Eosinophils (Eos)

EOS<	Stress, administration of adrenal hormones, shock, after major surgery
EOS< WBC<	Stress; ACTH, cortisone, or epinephrine administration; acromegaly, diurnal variation; intermenstrual period
EOS>	Allergy, infestation by parasites; also eosinophilic granulomatosis or leukemia (if EOS are highly elevated)
EOS> HCT> LYMPH> WBC<	Addison's disease (NA/K < 28, GLU < 50 mg, BUN > 20 mg/dl, CO_2 (28 meq/dl)
EOS> RBC=N	Allergic reaction

Erythrocyte Sedimentation Rate (SED Rate)

ESR>	Possible hypothyroidism or hyperthyroidism, arsenic or lead poisoning (if there is other corroborating evidence, as in a hair mineral analysis), indicative of an infectious process that is depleting the serum of protein components
ESR> LDH> SGOT> SGPT>	Myocardial infarction, hepatitis

Hematocrit (Hct)

HCT< (more than 10% low)	Anemia or pancreatitis
HCT< HGB< RBC=N	Hypochromic, microcytic anemia, iron deficiency, (Thalassemia, sickle cell anemia, hemoglobin C disease
HCT=LN HGB=LN RBC=N	Hypochromic microcytic anemia (check MCV, MCHC for confirmation)
HCT>	Dehydration
HCT> HGB>	Intestinal obstruction
HCT> RBC>	Possible polycythemia

Lymphocytes (Lymph)

LYMPH<	The body has the materials needed to fight infection, but such antibodies are not being produced (check A/G, CA, NA/K, MCV, MCHC, and TP for deviations from normal).
LYMPH> (> 40%)	Probable infection, specific antibodies are required in a relatively short period of time in response to some type of invasive organism. The ingredients for making these antibodies are probably lacking.
LYMPH> RBC=N SEGS<	Agranulocytosis, poor antibody formation
LYMPH> WBC=N	Pernicious anemia, typhoid fever, influenza, undulant fever, infectious hepatitis, German measles, mumps. The ingredients needed to build a healthy immune system are probably lacking.

Mean Cell Hemoglobin Concentration (MCHC)

MCHC< MCV< RBC=N or <	Hypochromic, microcytic anemia due to iron deficiency (check the levels of cobalt, copper, and iron in a hair mineral analysis)
MCHC< RBC=N + hypochromia and target cells	Thalassemia
MCHC=N MCV=N RBC< + loss of blood	Normochromic, normocytic anemia
MCHC< MCV> RBC<	Macrocytic anemia, possible vitamin 812 and folic acid deficiency (check A/G ratio to determine if hypochlorhydria is involved)

Mean Cell Volume (MCV)

MCV> RBC=N + macrocytosis and hypersegmented neutrophils	Vitamin B12 and folic acid deficiency

Monocytes (Mono)

MONO>	Chronic inflammatory disorder (> 4 clinical disease; > 9 acute infection is evident)

Platelets (Plat)

PLAT>	Lack of vascular leak repairing capability, lack of T factors, found in sesame oil
PLAT>	Possible hypoxia, bone surgery, hemopoeitic disorder (check MCHC, MCV)

Red Blood Cells (RBC, Erythrocytes)

RBC<	Probable oxygen unsaturation
RBC=N + atypical lymphocytes	Possible infectious mononucleosis
RBC=N + basophilic stippling	Possible lead poisoning (check the level of lead in a hair mineral analysis)
RBC=N + hypochromia with target cells	Thalassemia major or minor
RBC=N + macrocytosis, hypersegmented neutrophils	Vitamin B12 and folic acid deficiency
RBC=N + many blast forms	Possible acute leukemia
RBC=N + parasites in cells	Possible malaria
RBC=N + polychromatophilia, spherocytosis	Hereditary spherocytosis
RBC=N + rouleaux formation	Multiple myeloma or macroglobulinemia
RBC=N + schistocytes and burr cells	Possible mechanical hemolysis of the cells during or after collection of the specimen
RBC=N + spherocytosis, polychromatophilia, RBC agglutination	Possible compensated, acquired hemolytic anemia
RBC=N PLAT< + schistocytes and burr cells coagulopathy	Possible consumption coagulopathy
RBC>	Possible polycythemia

Segmented Neutrophils (Segs, Polys, PMN)

SEGS<	Possible drug or chemical poisoning
SEGS< WBC<	Acute viral infection, splenic neutropenia, drug-induced neutropenia, acute alcohol ingestion. Even though the ingredients to build a healthy immune system may be present, the body is unable to do so; check the levels of minerals in the hair.

SEGS>	Large numbers of phagocytic cells are needed. If the value exceeds 70%, a good quality antibody cannot be synthesized, even though the patient may contain sufficient ingredients (as evidenced by albumin, A/G ratio, and total protein).

White Blood Cells (Leucocytes)

WBC=N	Severe sepsis is still a possibility
WBC>	Presence of an acute or long-standing chronic infection

13 Blood Chemistry

This section describes important elements found in the liquid portion of the blood — the blood chemistry of the serum. The lists of disease conditions under each test are not exhaustive, but they may point to problems with particular body systems. **Do not make a diagnosis of disease based solely on information contained in this chapter.** Check the references listed under Suggested References on page 302 and others for additional conditions, medications, supplements, or chemical exposures that may alter test results.

Functions of Blood

What does the circulating blood do for us? The body's weight is about 8% blood. Males have about 5.5 liters, and females have about 4.5 liters, these differences due mostly to body size. The pH of the blood is between 7.35 and 7.45, making it slightly alkaline. Blood is about five times as viscous as water, giving it just the right amount of resistance to be pumped efficiently by the heart. Arterial blood is much redder than that in the veins, because it carries oxygen. An amazing fluid, blood carries out the following functions.

- **Respiration** - The transportation of O_2 coming from the air in the lungs, to get to the tissues and the CO_2 from the tissues to be expelled by the lungs.
- **Nutrition** - The conveyance of food materials, such as glucose, amino acids, and fats from the alimentary canal to the tissues.
- **Excretion** - The removal of waste products and metabolism such as urea, uric acid, creatinine, etc.
- **Maintenance of H_2O Content of Tissues** - A constant interchange of fluid through the vessel walls takes place. This is the lymph; the final stage in the transportation of O_2 and food materials to the tissues and the first stage in the journey of CO_2 and waste products from the tissues are made through the medium of the transudated fluid.
- **Body Temperature Regulation** - The body owes its ability to regulate the temperatures to the water of blood and the tissue fluids.
- **Protection and Regulation** - The blood and lymph contain certain chemical antitoxins and antibodies that are the basis of the body's defense against injurious

agents of various kinds. The circulating fluid also brings the endocrine principles from the ductless glands into direct contact with the cells of the tissue.

Acid Phosphatase

This enzyme is present in the capsule of the prostate, and the basis of the laboratory test is to detect amounts in excess of those that are normally present in the blood. A slight elevation is observed in benign hypertrophic prostatitis (BHP) and after especially vigorous massage of the gland. This enzyme is occasionally elevated in nephritis, hepatitis, Paget's disease, and hyperparathyroidism; and elevations are seen in about 67% of patients with prostatic carcinoma. However, multiple myeloma and Gaucher's disease (abnormal accumulations of cerebrosides in reticuloendotheilal tissue) also may manifest elevations in acid phosphatase, as does metastatic carcinoma invading the bone from the breast, the thyroid, or the colon. It can rise as high as 30 units. Because this enzyme is present in platelets and erythrocytes, care must be taken to collect and separate the specimen properly to minimize contamination of the serum by the particulate component (5).

The reason that we want to know the acid phosphatase level is that we talk so much about cancer of the prostate, and neither this nor the alkaline phosphatase test will definitely show you cancer of the prostate. The acid phosphatase is much more accurate in the diagnosis of the cancer of the prostate than the alkaline, but why should we run an alkaline phosphatase on women? They don't have a prostate. It is because we want to make sure we know what that liver is doing and whether or not there may be a malignancy in either sex.

Albumin

Albumin is the raw material needed to rebuild every cell, enzyme, and hormone in the body. Of the serum proteins, albumin is normally the most abundant; it is synthesized in the liver and has a molecular weight of about 69,000. It serves to mediate osmotic balance, to buffer the blood, to act as the protein reserve mentioned above, and to act as a transporter of substances that would otherwise be insoluble in the blood (drugs, for example) (3).

In diseases, the albumin component is commonly depressed, this substance being used to manufacture elements involved with healing and the immune response. Further, protein inavailability or leakage through capillary walls may result in diminished albumin concentration. In this case, the globulin component may be called upon to maintain osmotic pressure. This is a task for which globulin is poorly suited, primarily because of the larger size of the molecules, and some edema may ensue. Shifts in the sodium/potassium relationship may follow.

Albumin Within the Normal Range

Normal albumin levels imply that disease is absent. However, a normal level may be associated with the following conditions. For our purposes, we do not accept just any value within the usual laboratory range of 4.5-5.5 gm%. We believe that the best value is 5.2 gm%, which ensures a sufficient reservoir of albumin for protein synthesis.

Albumin Within the Normal Range	
Body System	**Possible Condition**
Digestive	Obstructive jaundice (the bilirubin will probably exceed 1.5 mg/dL)
Circulatory/Blood/Lymph	Hemolytic anemia/iron-deficiency anemia Agammaglobulinemia
Urinary	Acute glomerulonephritis (BUN and creatinine are both elevated; the BUN/creatinine ratio is greater than 10)
Systemic	A1 antitrypsin deficiency

Albumin Above the Normal Range

High albumin levels are referred to as hyperalbuminemia. This is a very rare condition that is not seen except in cases of dehydration where the globulin rises as well. Various medications may elevate the albumin value; some of these are steroids, digitalis, epinephrine, insulin, oral contraceptives, and thyroid hormones.

Albumin Level Below the Normal Range

Hypoalbuminemia is the condition in which serum albumin levels fall below normal. The normal pregnant value is lower (46.6% of the total protein, as opposed to the usual adult normal of 64.2%). A low albumin level is very characteristic of chronic liver disease. This depression also occurs in many other conditions, as listed below.

Albumin Level Below the Normal Range	
Body System	**Possible Condition**
Skeletal	Rheumatoid arthritis
Digestive	Alcoholic hepatitis (globulin increases) Various liver diseases, such as cirrhosis, cystic fibrosis of the liver, pyogenic liver abcess (globulin increases) Protein losing enteropathy (total protein and globulin are both lowered)
Circulatory/Blood/Lymph	Analbuminemia IgA, IgG myeloma Waldenstrom's macroglobulinemia Heavy chain disease (marked depression of albumin) Chronic constrictive pericarditis Hypoanabolic hypoalbuminemia (albumin falls below 0.3 mg/dL)
Urinary	Nephrotic syndrome Chronic renal insufficiency (total protein is also depressed)
Endocrine	Cystic fibrosis of the pancreas
Reproductive	Pregnancy; the normal value is lower
Systemic	Amyloidosis Inflammations Systemic Lupus erythematosis Chicken pox Hypervitaminosis A Leprosy Rickettsial disease Sarcoidosis Trichinosis Use of estrogen and oral contraceptives

Albumin/Globulin Ratio (A/G)

The acceptable range for the albumin/globulin (A/G) ratio is 1.5-2.5, with the ideal being 2.0. A drop to 1.7 indicates a need for a digestive supplement of hydrochloric acid – the condition called hypochlorhydria. Complete achlorhydria, the absence of hydrochloric acid secretions in the stomach, is signaled by a drop in the ratio to a value of 1.1 or less. In many disease conditions, the A/G ratio is lowered or even reversed. I have done more than 25,000 patient's blood chemistries. Out of these, I have found only five that had an adequate level of protein in their bodies, according to my adjusted working normal maximum values of total protein 7, albumin 5.2, and globulin 2.2, with a better than two to one ratio. Five out of 25,000 people! Now you know why I say that we don't find healthy people anymore.

Albumin/Globulin Ratio Within the Normal Range

See the information concerning normal levels for albumin and globulin, above.

For our treatment, we do not accept just any value within the usual laboratory range of 1.5-3.5. We believe that the best value is 2.0. This indicates a sufficient reservoir of albumin for protein synthesis and a sufficiently low globulin level to suggest the absence of disease.

Albumin/Globulin Ratio Above the Normal Range

A rise in the A/G ratio is not commonly observed; hence no significance has been assigned to an elevation in this value.

Albumin/Globulin Ratio Below the Normal Range

A depression of the A/G ratio is common in infectious disease and malnutrition. Some examples of such conditions follow.

Albumin/Globulin Ratio Below the Normal Range	
Body System	**Possible Condition**
Skeletal	Rheumatoid arthritis
Digestive	Cirrhosis of the liver
Circulatory/Blood/Lymph	Heavy chain disease Macroglobulinemia (total protein is elevated) Chronic constrictive pericarditis (total protein is usually normal)
Urinary	Nephrotic syndrome (total protein is decreased, albumin is approximately 2.5 g)
Endocrine	Cystic fibrosis of the pancreas
Reproductive	Normal pregnancy (A/G ratio is always decreased in the last two trimesters)
Systemic	Amyloidosis Chickenpox Possible hypervitaminosis A Kwashiorkor Leprosy Marasmus Use of certain medications (see those for depressed albumin level)

Alkaline Phosphatase (Alk Phos, AP)

Alkaline phosphatase is an enzyme that mediates the formation of bone tissue. When the osteoblasts are depositing bone matrix, they secrete large amounts of this enzyme. The other main source of alkaline phosphatase is the liver. Therefore, elevations should direct attention to these two tissues, and the value for alkaline phosphatase should correlate well with other findings, such as jaundice, injury to bone, elevated SGOT, etc. (1). Heat inactivation is commonly used to differentiate bone alkaline phosphatase from that of the liver.

Alkaline Phosphatase Level Within the Normal Range

A normal alkaline phosphatase value suggests that there exists a satisfactory balance between bone formation and destruction. Growing children will exhibit as much as a threefold higher normal level as an adult, so laboratory normals must take this factor into consideration.

Alkaline Phosphatase Level Above the Normal Range

A high alkaline phosphatase level is called hyperphosphatasemia. This usually results from increased deposition of calcium in bone. Associated conditions are listed below (2). An extreme elevation is considered to be five times the normal mean (1).

Alkaline Phosphatase Level Above the Normal Range	
Body System	**Possible Condition**
Skeletal	Osteitis fibrosa cystica Paget's disease (extreme elevation with no liver disease) Healing of fractures Osteoblastic bone tumors (osteosarcoma shows extreme elevation with no liver disease) Osteogenesis imperfecta Familial osteoectasia Osteomalacia (alkaline phosphatase is not elevated in osteoporosis) Rickets Polyostotic fibrous dysplasia Metastatic carcinomas of bones resulting in osteoblastic changes
Digestive	Liver disease with any obstruction of the biliary system. An extreme elevation with abnormal levels of bilirubin, SGOT, and SGPT indicates early stages of obstructive jaundice at the major ducts – gallstone or tumor of the head of the pancreas. Also, there is the possibility of widespread metastasis (1). Cholangiolar obstruction in hepatitis or cirrhosis (moderate or slight elevation in alkaline phosphatase with abnormal bilirubin, SGOT, and SGPT) Alimentary hyperglycemia
Circulatory/Blood/Lymph	Myelogenous leukemia Myocardial or pulmonary infarction (seen in some patients during the organization phase)
Urinary	Renal rickets (associated with fistulas of the biliary system)
Endocrine	Hyperparathyroidism (moderate or slight elevation with no liver disease and usually accompanied by hypercalcemia) Marked hyperthyroidism
Reproductive	Late pregnancy Prostatic cancer (possible elevation of acid phosphatase)

Systemic	Administration of ergosterol Adverse reaction to a therapeutic drug (The alkaline phosphatase may be the first indication that the drug should be discontinued.) Hyperphosphatasia Primary hypophosphatemia (depressed serum phosphates) Following intravenous injection of albumin Following repeated insertions of syringe needle in an attempt to puncture the vein Advanced tuberculosis

Alkaline Phosphatase Level Below the Normal Range

A low alkaline phosphatase level is termed hypophosphatemia. It is associated with the conditions listed below. A chronically low value should suggest the possibility of rare disorders such as hypophosphatasia, achondroplasia, cretinism, and a possible vitamin C deficiency (1). This is where we like to do our checking before a woman becomes pregnant, to make sure that we have all of these things working right; just like when we talk about zinc and hair analysis. Usually, by the time a woman knows she's pregnant, she doesn't have enough zinc in her body; her baby, in all probability will have a hair lip and a cleft palate.

Alkaline Phosphatase Level Below the Normal Range	
Body System	**Possible Condition**
Digestive	(Burnett's) milk-alkali syndrome Excessive intake of vitamin D Scurvy (see note above) Celiac disease Malnutrition
Circulatory/Blood/Lymph	Pernicious anemia
Urinary	Chronic nephritis Renal dwarfism (in the absence of rickets)
Endocrine	Hypothyroidism Cretinism
Systemic	Hypophosphatasia Collection of the specimen in EDTA, fluoride, or oxalate anticoagulant (2)

Alpha Globulins

The globulins are manufactured by cells of the reticuloendothelial system. The alpha globulins are related to tissue destruction. An increase, particularly in the alpha globulins, glycoproteins and mucoproteins, is a common feature of febrile diseases. In many cases, there is an inverse relationship between albumin (falls) and alpha globulins (rises), such as that observed in pneumonia, acute rheumatic fever, and typhus. The abnormal constituent of the blood, CRP, or C-reactive protein – diagnostic for inflammation – moves in the electrophoretic group with alpha globulins (3).

Alpha-1 Globulin Level Within the Normal Range

The alpha-1 globulin level may be normal in the following situations.

Alpha-1 Globulin Level Within the Normal Range	
Body System	**Possible Condition**
Digestive	Laennec's cirrhosis (hobnail liver)
Circulatory/Blood/Lymph	Hypogammaglobulinemia Analbuminemia (the alpha-2 fraction rises)
Urinary	Chronic glomerulonephritis (the alpha-2 fraction rises)

Alpha-1 Globulin Level Above the Normal Range

The alpha-1 globulin level may be elevated in the following situations.

Alpha-1 Globulin Level Above the Normal Range	
Body System	**Possible Condition**
Digestive	Various gastrointestinal diseases Peptic ulcer Ulcerative colitis Protein-losing enteropathy
Circulatory/Blood/Lymph	Hodgkin's disease
Systemic	Stress Metastatic carcinomatosis

Alpha-1 Globulin Level Below the Normal Range

A fall in the alpha-1 globulin fraction to less than 0.25 gm% suggests that the cells producing the globulin are not being given enough raw materials in the form of amino acids. The cells will eventually break down if the deficiency is not corrected. Amino acids and/or pancreatic enzymes may be necessary. Low values for this component are observed in acute viral hepatitis.

Alpha-2 Globulin Level Within the Normal Range

A normal value for this fraction may be observed in hypogammaglobulinemia, in Laennec's cirrhosis, and in hyperthyroidism.

Alpha-2 Globulin Level Above the Normal Range

Elevation of the alpha-2 fraction to a value above 0.65 gm% indicates a catabolic state in which protein is being pulled out of cellular structures. It also indicates a hormone imbalance in that optimal levels of male or female hormones are necessary to place protein in the tissues. Some diseases associated with this elevation are as follows.

Alpha-2 Globulin Level Above the Normal Range	
Body System	**Possible Condition**
Skeletal	Rheumatoid arthritis
Digestive	Various gastrointestinal diseases Peptic ulcer Ulcerative colitis Protein losing enteropathy
Circulatory/Blood/Lymph	Hodgkin's disease Analbuminemia
Urinary	Nephrosis Chronic glomerulonephritis
Endocrine	Diabetes mellitus
Systemic	Stress Systemic Lupus erythematosis Metastatic carcinomatosis Various infections (meningitis, pneumonia, osteomyelitis)

Alpha-2 Globulin Level Below the Normal Range

A depression of the alpha-2 globulin fraction to a value of less than 0.60 gm% suggests an insufficiency of raw materials being supplied to the synthesizing cells. This could imply a hormone imbalance. Acute viral hepatitis is often associated with such a low value for this fraction.

Beta Globulins

The beta globulins are proteins that are characteristic of bone and joint material. This fraction is highly influenced by the amount of lipids in the blood because many of the lipoproteins migrate electrophoretically together with the beta globulins. Changes in the levels of the beta globulin component of the lipoproteins account for the positive thymol turbidity test that is shown to be of value in diagnosis of hepatitis and cirrhosis. Certain arthritic syndromes may be predicted on the basis of alterations in the beta fraction (3) with respect to alterations in serum uric acid, calcium, phosphorus, and alpha-2 globulin values.

Beta Globulin Level Within the Normal Range

The beta globulin fraction is usually normal in the following disorders.

Beta Globulin Level Within the Normal Range	
Body System	**Possible Condition**
Digestive	Laennec's cirrhosis
Circulatory/Blood/Lymph	Hypogammaglobulinemia Essential hypertension Congestive heart failure
Urinary	Chronic glomerulonephritis
Endocrine	Hyperthyroidism
Systemic	Acute rheumatic fever

Beta Globulin Level Above the Normal Range

An elevation above 0.96 gm% of beta globulins is indicative of an arthritic condition; a catabolic state exists with protein being pulled out of existing cell structures. If the uric acid level and the calcium/phosphorus ratio are also elevated, one may assume that an arthritic syndrome is present. If the uric acid exceeds 6.0 mg for males and 5.0 mg for females, gout, gouty arthritis, or rheumatoid arthritis may be indicated. If the alpha-2 fraction exceeds 1.0 gm% as well, rheumatoid arthritis is definite. The beta globulin fraction may also be elevated in a condition called analbuminemia.

Beta Globulin Level Below the Normal Range

A depression in the level of beta globulins below 0.89 gm% indicates that the cells that synthesize bone and joint protein are not getting enough raw materials. If the situation is not corrected, some type of arthritic disease will probably develop. Further, beta globulins may be depressed in the following.

Beta Globulin Level Below the Normal Range	
Body System	**Possible Condition**
Digestive	Ulcerative colitis
Circulatory/Blood/Lymph	Lymphatic leukemia Lymphoma Myelogenous leukemia Monocytic leukemia
Urinary	Nephrosis
Systemic	Metastatic carcinomatosis

Atherogenic Index

The atherogenic index is an estimation of the risk of a person of a certain age having a heart attack due to arteriosclerosis. It is based on levels of various classes of serum lipoproteins that are classified according to their density, as measured in an ultracentrifugal field. The basics are:

- Triglycerides are transported in the blood bound to very low density beta lipoproteins (VLDL, beta).
- Cholesterol is bound to low density beta lipoproteins (LDL, beta).
- Phospholipids are bound to alpha lipoproteins (HDL, LDL2).
- Free fatty acids are bound to albumin.
- Globular proteins, the alpha and beta globulins, are termed alpha and beta lipoproteins when complexed to their respective carrier lipids.
- Lipoprotein complexes are least dense (LDL) when they contain more lipid and less protein.
- Lipoprotein complexes are more dense (tending to become HDL) when they contain less lipid and more protein.

The alpha lipoproteins comprise the HDL and LDL2 classes, and these fall into the Sf 0-12 range. The beta lipoproteins comprise the LDL1 and VLDL classes and fall within the Sf 12-400 range. **The HDL fraction is thought to be the major transport vehicle for cholesterol between the peripheral tissues and the liver. Therefore, high HDL levels probably indicate promotion of more efficient removal of cholesterol from the blood and a lesser risk of cholesterol deposition.**

Although there seems to be no relationship between HDL-cholesterol and age, studies conducted at the University of Illinois show a definite relationship between alpha lipoproteins and age. Thus the Atherogenic Index is calculated from the Sf 0-12 and the Sf 12-400 values. It is known that, as the protein, cholesterol, cholesterol ester, and phospholipid content decreases, the triglyceride content increases progressively.

Sf 0-12

The Sf **0-12, are the lipids complexed to the alpha globulins, including the phospholipids.** These are glycerol attached to two fatty acids, typically palmitic, stearic, and oleic acids, along with a third component such as phosphate, inositol, choline (to form lecithin), ethanolamine (to form cephalin), or serine. These substances are derived from the dietary intake of fats, oils, and greases; these are split apart by pancreatic lipases to form glycerol, fatty acids, monoglycerides, and diglycerides. Phospholipids can be absorbed directly into the mucosa of the digestive tract and pass, via the lymphatic system, to the liver.

This group of lipids is commonly controlled by limiting the proportion of fats in the diet to 300 calories, which translates to approximate 15% of the daily intake. Further, the dietary fat should consist primarily of unsaturated vegetable fats. Saturated, solid fats should be avoided. See Food and Diet, Fats on page 72.

Sf 12-400

The Sf **12-400 are the lipids complexed to beta globulins, including the triglycerides and cholesterol.** Only about 30% of the body's total cholesterol component is provided by the diet; the rest arises from acetyl coenzyme A, which is synthesized mainly from carbohydrate, either directly via oxidation of pyruvate or indirectly from stored fats that originally came from the ingestion of carbohydrates. Therefore, cholesterol in the blood is primarily determined by the amount of dietary carbohydrates. In the normal condition, hepatic triglycerides are also derived from carbohydrates.

This group of lipids is commonly controlled by limiting dietary carbohydrates. Carbohydrates should be complex, such as found in raw vegetables. Sugars, breads, and processed foods should be avoided. See Food and Diet on page 59, Editor: At the end of Dr. Ellis' career, he became aware of research involving tests for food, preservative, and coloring intolerances (not allergies) being carried out in San Antonio, Texas and Miami, Florida. He was hopeful that he would be able to incorporate such testing into his comprehensive plan, but the field was not commercialized by the time Dr. Ellis began his struggle with a terminal illness. Subsequent to Dr. Ellis' passing, researchers developed what is called the ALCAT test and made it available to the public. Current information about this service is found at https://cellsciencesystems.com/patients/alcat-test/. A book about food intolerance and weight control is Your Hidden Food Allergies Are Making You Fat by Roger Deutsch and Rudy Rivera M.D., July 23, 2002, available from Amazon.com. For a list of undesirable food additives, visit the MPH website at http://mphprogramslist.com/50-jawdroppingly-toxic-food-additives-to-avoid/. on page 60.

Calculating the Atherogenic Index

Although laboratories providing blood chemistry testing usually provide the atherogenic index value when requested, it is valuable to know how it is calculated, as shown below. See the normal values in Figure 21.

$$AI = \frac{\text{Standard Sf 0-12} + (\text{Standard Sf 12-400} \times 1.75)}{10}$$

Figure 21: Atherogenic Index normal values

	Male			Female		
Age	AI	Sf 0-12	Sf 12-400	AI	Sf 0-12	Sf 12-4
10		291	131		279	117
11		287	131		277	115
12		284	131		276	113
13		280	131		274	111
14		277	131		273	109
15		273	131		271	107
16		270	131		270	105
17		274	131		271	105
18		278	137		272	105
19		282	143		274	105
20	60	286	149	45	275	106
21	60	290	155	45	277	106
22	60	294	161	45	279	106
23	60	298	167	45	280	106
24	60	300	173	45	282	106
25	60	302	178	45	284	107
26	60	305	183	45	286	110
27	60	309	189	45	288	114
28	60	313	195	45	290	117
29	60	317	201	45	292	121
30	61	321	207	45	294	125
31	62	324	212	46	296	128
32	63	328	217	46	298	132
33	64	332	223	47	290	135
34	65	336	229	47	302	139
35	66	340	236	48	304	143
36	67	342	238	48	308	147
37	68	344	240	49	312	151
38	69	347	243	49	316	155
39	70	349	245	50	320	159
40	70	352	248	51	325	164
41	70	354	250	52	329	168
42	71	356	252	53	333	172
43	71	359	255	54	337	177
44	72	361	257	55	341	181
45	72	364	260	56	346	187
46	72	364	259	57	347	192
47	73	364	259	59	351	202
48	73	364	259	60	352	208
49	74	365	259	60	352	208
50	74	365	258	61	354	213
51	74	365	258	62	356	218
52	74	366	258	63	358	224
53	74	366	257	64	360	229
54	74	366	257	65	362	235
55	74	367	257	66	363	240
56	74	366	254	67	363	245
57	74	365	241	68	364	250
58	74	364	240	69	365	260
59	75	363	245	70	366	270
60	74	363	242	71	367	280
61	74	361	240	73	368	290
62	74	360	239	74	369	300
63	74	360	239	76	369	300
64	73	360	239	79	369	300
65	73	360	239	79	369	300
70	72	360	239	86	369	300

Bilirubin (Total) (Bili)

Bilirubin is formed mostly in the reticuloendothelial tissues of the spleen, from the destruction of erythrocytes and the reclamation of hemoglobin. It is the predominant pigment that gives bile the characteristic golden yellow color. The normal range is 0.3 to 1.9 mg/dL. Because bilirubin is a waste product of hemoglobin metabolism, it must be excreted, and the bilirubin level reflects the efficiency of the excretory function of the liver or the degree of hemolysis occurring. If the bilirubin is elevated, the bile is too thick and needs to be thinned. Never give a B complex when the bile Is thick.

The test for bilirubin is a colorimetric determination, the reagent (Ehrlich)/sample mixture's color being compared to a standard. Therefore, any foods or drugs that give the serum a yellow or orange color may alter the true reading. Likewise, drugs that temporarily modify liver function may cause an elevated bilirubin reading through real, not spurious changes, in the liver, without reflecting liver disease! A complete list of these drugs may be found in (8). One important consideration is that the thicker the bile, the more restricted the flow. This is also seen in elevations of the BUN; as the BUN is elevated, the thicker the bile (see BUN Level Above the Normal Range, below).

Bilirubin Level Within the Normal Range

A normal bilirubin value suggests a normal excretory function of the liver and a normal degree of hemolysis (1). However, one may want to further consider the relative concentrations of indirect and direct bilirubin.

Bilirubin Level Above the Normal Range

This condition is termed hyperbilirubinemia; it is most often associated with liver disease, but other conditions are included below. By definition, a greatly elevated serum bilirubin level is equal to or greater than 12 gm% (1).

Bilirubin Level Above the Normal Range	
Body System	**Possible Condition**
Digestive	Liver disease due to any number of causes (hepatitis, obstructions, infections, poisonings, intoxications, tumors) (see Liver Pathology and Related Bilirubin Type, below) A 48-hour fast produces a mean increase of 240 in the bilirubin of normal individuals and only a 194 mean increase in individuals with liver dysfunction (2). Fatty liver Ulcerative colitis Gilbert's disease (impaired uptake of bilirubin by the liver) Jaundice (By definition, jaundice occurs when the total serum bilirubin level reaches 1.5 mg; it becomes clinically apparent at 3.0 mg.) Cholecystitis (If this is suspected, there is a 75% chance of elevation of the SGOT.)
Circulatory/Blood/Lymph	Hematologic diseases Sickle cell disease
Endocrine	Various disorders
Systemic	Collagen diseases Mucopolysaccharidosis Glycogen storage disease Wilson's disease Use of marijuana Use of certain medicines (aimaline, antimalarials, salicylates, cholinergics, coumarin, ethoxazene, morphine, oral contraceptives, penicillin, phenylbutozone, primaquine, procainamide, quinidine, quinine, radiographic agents, rifampin, streptomycin, sulfa drugs, tetracycline, thiazides)

Liver Pathology and Related Bilirubin Type

There is a host of specific conditions that bring about liver pathology; they are too numerous to mention here. However, to better diagnose these conditions, a distinction must be made between prehepatic and posthepatic bilirubin. Prehepatic bilirubin exists in the free, or unconjugated form in the serum. It has not yet passed through the liver. It is measured as indirect bilirubin. Posthepatic bilirubin is conjugated to glucuronic acid as it passes through the liver cells. It is measured as direct bilirubin. Accurate diagnosis is based on relative elevations of these two classes in addition to the total bilirubin. Elevations of these are seen in the following disorders.

Liver Pathology and Related Bilirubin Type	
Type	**Possible Condition**
Indirect (Prehepatic)	Anemias Polycythemia Internal hemorrhage Malaria Septicemia Streptococcal or staphylococcal infections During fasting
Direct (Posthepatic)	Extrahepatic obstruction of the biliary system (if the direct bilirubin is greater than 30 of the total bilirubin) (5). Tumors of the bile duct Hepatitis Infections Toxic conditions Carbon tetrachloride poisoning After X-rays Acute yellow atrophy of the liver

Bilirubin Level Below the Normal Range

A low bilirubin level carries no significance until it reaches 0.1 mg. At this concentration, it is suggested that aplastic anemia is a possibility. Also possible are secondary anemias especially those brought about by toxic agents of carcinoma and chronic nephritis. Certain drugs may also depress the bilirubin level, such as barbiturates, corticosteroids, phenobarbital, sulfonamides, and thioridazine. If the BUN is high with a low bilirubin – the other test that indicates a thick bile – never give a B complex.

Blood Urea Nitrogen (BUN)

The BUN is an indicator of kidney function. Urea is a waste product of the digestion and metabolism of protein in the tissues. Ammonia formed by the delamination of amino acids in the liver is converted to urea in the urea cycle for excretion from the body. Normal human adult blood should contain 10-25 mg of urea nitrogen per 100 ml of blood, or mg/dL. This test must be done on a fasting blood.

BUN Level Within the Normal Range

A normal BUN indicates normal glomerular function. Small deviations within the normal range indicate the efficiency of liver function and protein metabolism. A low BUN within normal limits can occur if the liver is inefficiently converting amino acids to urea and if the diet is low in proteins and high in carbohydrates. Since proteins contribute to enzyme, hormone, structural, and oxygen-carrying components of the body, it is wise to consider the values for total protein, albumin, and globulin along with the BUN.

BUN Level Above the Normal Range

The most common cause of an elevated BUN is impaired kidney function. A moderate elevation suggests that protein intake is too great or that excessive protein catabolism, such as seen in disease, is occurring. One interesting aspect of an elevated BUN is lowered efficiency of protein metabolism, less-than-optimal liver function, and a concomitant thickening of the bile. The BUN begins to rise when the glomerular filtration rate falls below 50 ml/min, the normal rate for the average-sized man is approximately 125 ml/min (1). Kidney disease is likely to develop if the physiology is not modified, and one should check for infection. If the BUN is high with a low bilirubin – the other test that indicates a thick bile – never give a B complex. Some disease conditions related to an elevated BUN are as follows.

BUN Level Above the Normal Range	
Body System	**Possible Condition**
Digestive	Liver disease Hemorrhage into the gastrointestinal tract (protein catabolism through digestion of the serum proteins and the cellular mass)
Circulatory/Blood/Lymph	Congestive heart failure Acute myocardial infarction (Both of the conditions listed exhibit reduced blood flow to the kidneys, and, in the case of myocardial infarction, protein catabolism is operating.)
Urinary	Impaired kidney function: Serious renal impairment (BUN = 50-150 mg) Conclusive evidence of severely impaired kidney function (150-250 mg/dL) Check the following: Renal infarction (LDH and SGOT may both be elevated) Acute glomerulonephritis (creatinine is elevated; BUN/creatinine is 10 or greater)
Endocrine	Hyperparathyroidism (calcium level is usually normal) Addison's disease (glucose may be depressed; potassium may be elevated, and sodium may be abnormally high or low)

Systemic	Salt and water depletion Shock Stress Sepsis Fever Use of thiazide diuretics (uric acid is usually elevated; calcium and glucose may be elevated; phosphorus may be depressed)

BUN Level Below the Normal Range

A BUN below the normal range indicates the presence of liver and/or kidney disease. A low and sometimes pathologically low value can occur in any of the conditions listed below. A BUN less than 10 mg, in the 6-8 mg range suggests overhydration, with a concomitant edema and a feeling of fullness. Check the total protein to see if it is depressed. There is a possibility of liver or kidney disease, involving infection, protein non-utilization, malabsorption, adrenal malfunction, etc. The flow of bile is not as good as desired.

A BUN in the 8-10 mg range suggests impaired absorption and/or a low protein/high carbohydrate diet; increased protein utilization may be indicated by an abnormal albumen level and sedimentation rate. Check for other signs of disease, pregnancy, or an increased rate of growth.

BUN Level Below the Normal Range	
Body System	**Possible Condition**
Digestive	Liver damage from many causes (drugs, poisons, hepatitis) Impaired absorption
Urinary	Nephrotic syndrome
Systemic	Increased protein catabolism (pregnancy, infancy, acromegaly) Intravenous feeding

Calcium (Ca)

Calcium is absorbed into the body from the upper part of the small intestine, the jejunum. The efficiency of absorption depends on the degree of acidity of the intestinal contents and on the amount of phosphorus and magnesium present (these tend to block the absorption of calcium). The body contains about 1,100 gm of calcium, most of which is found in the skeleton; the plasma contains 10 mg per 100 milliliters of fluid. This total plasma calcium is either bound to proteins, bound to organic or inorganic compounds, or is free and ionizable. It is the free form, only 2% of the total body complement, that is available to coagulate blood, regulate smooth and cardiac muscle contraction, and to regulate nerve function (1). Calcium levels in the plasma are raised by parathormone (increases urinary phosphate excretion) and lowered by thyrocalcitonin. A normal interaction of these regulatory factors maintains the plasma calcium level within 5% of normal levels. Of course, calcium is stored in the bones and eliminated from the body in the urine and feces.

Calcium Level Within the Normal Range

We use specific normals of 10 mg/dL for calcium and 4 mg/dL for phosphorus; we want a 2.5/1 ratio. A normal calcium level is not necessarily reflective of optimal calcium metabolism. Therefore, the normal serum calcium level must be assessed in the light of other test values. For example, if a normal calcium level is accompanied by an abnormal phosphorus level, disease may still be present (see Calcium/Phosphorus Ratio). If one multiplies the calcium value by the phosphorus value, 50 is normal for children; if the resultant value is less than 30, rickets may be a possibility. Secondly, a normal calcium level with an elevated BUN suggests hyperparathyroidism.

Additionally, since free calcium ions are not measured directly, one must consider serum protein levels in estimating the level of ionizable calcium. For instance, a normal calcium level with a marked decrease in the serum albumin concentration is still indicative of abnormal hypercalcemia. The reason for this is that 50% of serum calcium is protein-bound; the calcium level should be depressed in the presence of hypoproteinemia (actually hypoalbuminemia)!

Calcium Level Above the Normal Range

Elevation of the serum calcium level above the normal range is termed hypercalcemia; this condition is characterized by a calcium level well above 10.5 and is associated with the following:

Calcium Level Above the Normal Range	
Body System	**Possible Condition**
Skeletal	Metastatic carcinoma of bone (elevation seen in 10% of patients) Acute osteoporosis Paget's disease (calcium and alkaline phosphatase are both elevated) Osteomalacia
Digestive	Consumption of alcohol Consumption of large amounts of fruit juices (most of these contain acids that are metabolized to alkaline products *)
Circulatory/Blood/Lymph	Hematologic malignancies (myeloma, lymphoma, leukemia) Polycythemia vera Multiple myeloma (calcium and gamma globulin are both elevated) Conditions that cause excess CO_2 tension in the blood, emphysema and cardiac decompensation

Urinary	Chronic nephritis with uremia During hemodialysis Acute renal failure (diuretic phase)
Endocrine	Hyperparathyroidism - both primary (due to hyperplasia or adenoma of the gland) and secondary. The common pattern in hyperparathyroidism is an elevated calcium level and depressed phosphorus level. Hyperthyroidism (seen in only some patients) Cushing's syndrome Addison's disease Myxedema (hypofunction of the thyroid) Basophilic adenoma of the pituitary gland
Reproductive	Following ovarectomy
Systemic	Milk-alkali (Burnett's) syndrome (the calcium, CO_2, and pH of the blood all rise) Excessive dosage of vitamin D Idiopathic hypercalcemia of infants Infantile hypophosphatasia Berylliosis Sarcoidosis (calcium and gamma globulin are both elevated) Laboratory artifacts (venous stasis during collection of the specimen, use of cork stoppers on the test tubes) Use of certain drugs and medications (anabolic steroids, calcium-containing antacids, estrogens, hydralazine, oral contraceptives, secretin, thiazide diuretics)
Miscellaneous	* Any condition that causes the CO_2 level to rise (possible alkalosis) will probably cause the calcium level to rise also. This is because calcium cannot be used by the tissues in a relatively alkaline environment. The pattern for metabolic alkalosis is an elevated calcium, normal or elevated CO_2, and an elevated blood pH.

Calcium Level Below the Normal Range

A calcium level that is depressed below the normal range is termed hypocalcemia. However, as in the cases of normal and elevated levels of serum calcium, the protein picture must be considered before proper interpretation of calcium levels can be accomplished. The method of choice is protein electrophoresis (1). If the albumin is greatly depressed, a lowered calcium may not reflect true hypocalcemia; the best procedure is to check the ratio of calcium to albumin. If this is normal, hypocalcemia may be ruled out; the condition is pseudohypocalcemia. Only after the determination is made that true hypocalcemia exists can the following conditions be possible (2).

Calcium Level Below the Normal Range	
Body System	**Possible Condition**
Skeletal	Osteomalacia Rickets
Digestive	Obstructive jaundice Malabsorption of calcium and vitamin D Sprue Celiac disease
Urinary	Nephrotic syndrome Chronic renal disease with uremia and phosphate retention
Endocrine	Hypoparathyroidism (both surgical and idiopathic) Cystic fibrosis of the pancreas Acute pancreatitis with extensive fat necrosis
Reproductive	Late pregnancy
Systemic	Cachexia Any condition that results in a depressed serum protein or albumin (see the introductory statement under Calcium, above), e.g., malignancy, leishmaniasis, starvation, etc. Insufficient calcium, phosphorus, and/or vitamin D intake Manic depressive psychoses Hypomagnesia Respiratory alkalosis with hyperventilation (The common pattern for hypocalcemia with respiratory alkalosis is depressed calcium, normal albumin, depressed CO_2, and a normal or elevated blood pH.) Laboratory artifact (If the cells are allowed to stand in the serum or plasma too long before separation, calcium can adsorb to the surface of the red cells, and a false depression of the serum calcium level will result.) Use of certain drugs and medications (corticosteroids, mercurial diuretics, gastrin, Insulin, excessive use of laxatives, mestranol, oral contraceptives, chronic use of phenytoin sodium, and sulfates)

Calcium/Phosphorus Ratio (Ca/P)

Calcium and phosphorus combine to form carbonate apatite, the main constituent of bones and teeth. Ratios are more important than the actual amounts that we find. Calcium is absorbed from the upper parts of the small intestine. The amount of absorption depends on the acidity of the intestinal contents and the amount of phosphate present. Calcium salts are soluble in acids.

Phosphorus should not be taken when taking calcium. Calcium should be taken in the morning on an empty stomach; the phosphorous supplement should be taken half way between breakfast and lunch and lunch and supper; and the magnesium supplement should be taken at night. Also, do not mix magnesium with calcium or it will also block absorption. The same precaution applies to taking manganese with calcium.

Calcium/Phosphorus Ratio Within the Normal Range

The ideal value for this ratio is 2.5. Generally, those foods that cause the calcium level to rise will, at the same time, cause the phosphorus to go down. This is a characteristic of refined foods, a diet rich in proteins, fats, and unrefined carbohydrates will tend to stabilize the calcium and phosphorus levels in a more desirable ratio.

Calcium/Phosphorus Ratio Above the Normal Range

When the calcium level rises and the phosphorus level drops, free calcium is available for combination and precipitation. The kidneys will attempt to excrete the excess, but while the free calcium is in the body, it can form dental or vascular plaques, as well as stones and calcifications within various organs and joints. The higher the ratio, the greater the potential for an arthritic syndrome. A high ratio may indicate hyperparathyroidism, the disease of stones, bones, and groans in the absence of renal dysfunction (the BUN and creatinine values are normal).

Calcium/Phosphorus Ratio Below the Normal Range

In the absence of renal dysfunction, a low calcium/phosphorus ratio suggests hypoparathyroidism. The typical pattern is a depressed calcium and an elevated phosphorus, with normal values for BUN and creatinine. If the ratio is low enough, muscle aches and pains as well as periodontal disease may be experienced.

Carbon Dioxide (CO_2)

The test for plasma CO_2-combining power measures the total carbonic acid and bicarbonate. It is a rather indirect indicator of acid/base abnormalities. Determination of the blood pH is desirable, but this test is not practical in ordinary laboratory circumstances, therefore CO_2 levels are used to determine acidic or alkaline tendencies. Carbon dioxide neutralizes metabolically-produced acids, such as lactic acid and hydrochloric acid. The pH of the blood rarely becomes relatively acidic in disease, but it can reach as low as 6.8 in diabetic coma.

Measuring the pH of a patient's circulating blood in vitro would be very useful. For many years, we have been trying to interest some company in making a low-priced pH meter with a sensing needle that could be inserted into a vein or an artery to measure the pH. The test must be done in three seconds, because whenever air hits the sample, the blood immediately coagulates and turns black, and the pH changes. So you can't get an accurate reading from the outside. In the mid-1950s, Beckman made such a machine, but the price to me was $1,100. For me to sterilize equipment, get it ready, and do the test to find out what their acid-alkaline balance was in the bloodstream would cost me $25 per test. This meant that I would have to charge patients $50 each to perform a three-second test while they were watching me? No way!

What we are left with is using the CO_2 as an indicator of pH. But it has little to do with the pH of the blood. We know in supplementation therapy that certain minerals leave alkaline residues, other minerals leave acid residues. And some researchers say that blood pH ranges from 7.34 to 7.44. If it rises to 7.45, one could die of alkalosis; if it drops to 7.33, one could die of acidosis. The pH varies little, but we would like to know this.

Carbon Dioxide Level Within the Normal Range

A normal CO_2 level with an increased blood pH indicates metabolic alkalosis (2).

Carbon Dioxide Level Above the Normal Range

A high serum CO_2 level is termed hypercapnia, and this is commonly equated with alkalosis. However, if the blood pH is decreased, respiratory acidosis is suggested; if the pH is normal, respiratory acidosis with compensated metabolic alkalosis is implied. If the pH is elevated, metabolic alkalosis is indicated (2). Generally, an elevated CO_2 level is associated with any state in which oxygen is limited to the tissues (hypoxemia, hypoxia, anoxia). Some specific examples of disorders are given below.

Carbon Dioxide Level Above the Normal Range	
Body System	**Possible Condition**
Skeletal	Any skeletal abnormality with limits (flat chest, injury to the rib cage or ribs after trauma, etc.)
Digestive	Ingestion of citric acid (found in most soft drinks and citrus juices)
Circulatory/Blood/Lymph	Congenital heart disease Cardiac shunts Pulmonary hemangioma
Endocrine	Severe hypothyroidism

Systemic	Any condition that limits the amount of lung area available for diffusion of gasses (lymphangitic carcinomatosis, pulmonary adenomatosis, Hamman-Rich syndrome, pulmonary hemosiderosis, lung collapse, loss of lung tissue due to injury of surgery, emphysema, etc.) Any condition that limits respiration (seizures, polio, tetanus, use of depressive drugs, injury to the head, stroke, massive obesity, reaction to pain, etc.) Severe electrolyte disturbances Acute intermittent porphyria Exposure to carbon monoxide or smoke After anaesthesia After near drowning Sarcoidosis Berylliosis Administration of calcium or sodium bicarbonate Living at high altitudes or high temperatures After hot baths During hysteria Concomitant with a loss of potassium After prolonged exposure to radium and/or X-rays After exposure to ultraviolet light Use of certain drugs and medications (aldosterone, bicarbonates, ethacrynic acid, hydroxycortisone, chronic abuse of laxatives, metolazone, prednisone, thiazides, tromethamine, and viomycin)

Carbon Dioxide Level Below the Normal Range

Hypocapnia is the term for low serum CO_2. It is usually associated with acidosis, and it is commonly brought about by mechanisms causing hyperventilation. Such mechanisms produce acids faster than they can be neutralized by CO_2. Just as the alternative condition, hypercapnia, hypocapnia is not related to the pH of the blood. If the blood pH is decreased; metabolic acidosis with respiratory alkalosis is suggested, if the blood pH is normal, respiratory alkalosis with compensated metabolic acidosis is implied. If the blood pH is elevated, respiratory alkalosis is indicated (2). Some conditions associated with hypocapnia are listed below.

Carbon Dioxide Level Below the Normal Range	
Body System	**Possible Condition**
Digestive	Liver failure
Circulatory/Blood/Lymph	Severe anemia Congestive heart failure
Urinary	Kidney disease Prolonged obstruction of the urinary tract
Endocrine	Diabetes mellitus
Reproductive	Toxemia of pregnancy Hypertrophy of the prostate Fibroid tumor of the uterus
Systemic	Pneumonia Asthma Emphysema Terminal tuberculosis Lesion of the central nervous system Living at high altitudes Psychogenic (fear) Use of a mechanical breathing device Deep breathing in excess Infection (usually gram negative sepsis) Excessive use of ammonium or calcium chlorides Use of certain drugs and medicines (acetazolamide, salicylates, dimercaprol, dimethadione, methicillin, morphine, nitrofurantoin, opium, phenformin, tetracycline, and triamterene)

Chloride (Cl)

Chlorides are mainly extracellular. It is an anion (bears a negative charge) present in large quantities in the serum and which exerts a significant influence on the acid/base and osmotic balances. The normal adult value for chloride is 97-107 mEq/liter. The RBC contains only half as much chloride as the plasma. Chlorides are excreted mainly in the urine and, to some extent, in the feces.

Chloride Level Within the Normal Range

A normal chloride level indicates potential optimal conditions; however, one must assess its level with respect to the levels of sodium and potassium. Chlorides can be absolutely normal in starvation and malabsorption, while a loss of potassium is experienced!

Sometimes, the chloride level can be normal in chronic renal failure, even though sodium and potassium levels are both depressed. However, it is more usual to observe alterations in the chloride level in association with pathologic conditions.

Chloride Level Above the Normal Range

Elevated chlorides in the blood is termed hyperchloremia, which is an electrolyte imbalance. The kidneys control the levels of chloride, so a disturbance in the level often involves the kidneys. Elevated chlorides are associated with the following disorders.

Chloride Level Above the Normal Range	
Body System	**Possible Condition**
Urinary	Renal tubular acidosis (usually associated with decreased CO_2, sodium, and potassium) Acute renal failure Obstruction in any location of the urinary tract Acute glomerulonephritis without excessive loss of fluids Chronic glomerulonephritis with a low protein intake and a high salt intake Essential hypertension with chronic nephritis and increased intake of chlorides by mouth or through intravenous administration
Endocrine	Diabetes insipidus
Systemic	Dehydration Administration of ammonium chloride Use of certain drugs and medicines (aspirin, prolonged therapy with chlorothiazide, corticosteroids, guanethidine, marijuana, and phenylbutazone)

Chloride Level Below the Normal Range

Hypochloremia is the condition of low serum chlorides. It is often associated with hypokalemia (decreased potassium) and alkalosis (elevated CO_2) (1). Low serum chlorides are observed in the following instances.

Chloride Level Below the Normal Range	
Body System	**Possible Condition**
Digestive	Diarrhea Starvation Fistulas Post-gastrointestinal surgery Vomiting Pyloric obstruction
Circulatory/Blood/Lymph	Congestive heart failure Rheumatic fever
Urinary	Chronic renal failure (chlorides may, however, be normal) Nephrosis Nephritis
Endocrine	Primary aldosteronism Adrenocortical insufficiency Diabetes mellitus Addison's disease
Systemic	Emphysema Pneumonia Excessive sweating Bromine intoxication Infectious diseases, rheumatic fever, pulmonary tuberculosis After major operations, especially gastrointestinal Use of diuretics (If potassium is to be replaced, it should be accompanied by chloride in a 1:1 ratio; thereby lessening the possibility of hypochloremia and hypochloremic alkalosis (1).) Use of certain drugs and medicines (aldosterone, bicarbonates, corticosteroids, corticotropin, cortisone, chronic abuse of laxatives, and prednisone)

Cholesterol (Serum Cholesterol)

Cholesterol exists in the body in a free form and in an esterified form (combined with a fatty acid). For those whose age is below 40 years, the ideal normal is 140-270; for those above 40 years, the ideal normal is 150-330. When women enter their menstrual cycle, their cholesterol levels rise. Therefore, it is important to know at what time in their menstrual cycle this blood has been drawn.

Dietary cholesterol is esterified in the lining of the intestine and is absorbed into the lymphatic system. Sources of preexisting cholesterol are the so-called fatty foods that contribute only 15% of the cholesterol that appears in the serum. Consequently, too much importance has been assigned to limiting cholesterol-containing foods in the diet. The greater part (85%) of serum cholesterol is derived chemically from acetate, an end product of carbohydrate metabolism! Therefore, when confronted with deviations in the cholesterol level from normal, one must attend to the comsumption of starches, sugars, and dairy products to pinpoint the cause.

Cholesterol is used by the liver to form cholic acid which, in turn, is converted into bile salts for fat digestion. A steroid alcohol, cholesterol is involved in maintaining the integrity of blood cells, cellular membranes, and nervous tissues, as well as in the transport of fat soluble vitamins. Much cholesterol is used to protect the skin from water soluble substances (1), and upon exposure to the sun, cholecalciferol forms vitamin D.

The importance of cholesterol is emphasized when one considers that some 50 steroids have been isolated from the adrenal cortex, including glucocorticoids, mineralocorticoids, androgen, and estrogen. Cholesterol serves as a precursor to these steroids, which are converted to hormones by the adrenal gland and gonads.

The serum cholesterol level is regulated by assimilative and hormonal factors. When the circulating cholesterol level is high, synthesis of cholesterol from acetate is inhibited; estrogen and thyroid hormones effect a decrease in the serum level also. Other, pathologic conditions cause irregularities in the cholesterol level, and these are discussed below.

Unfortunately, normal cholesterol values show populational variation as well as age-dependent differences. This accounts for the often seen wide laboratory normal ranges. Therefore, one usually depends on the levels and types of other blood lipids to predict the risk factor for coronary artery disease, even though hypercholesterolemia is one of the closely associated characteristics (see Atherogenic Index, above).

Cholesterol Level Within the Normal Range

A normal serum cholesterol level implies that dietary habits and supplementation schedules are adequate to maintain potentially optimal levels of this raw material for its role in metabolism. However, one must consider other factors such as the CBC and the indices, MCH, MCHC, and MCV; as well as the serum bilirubin and iron levels to monitor the status of the hemopoeitic system. Likewise, one must check adrenal and gonadal functioning (serum sodium, serum potassium, and the protein electrophoretic spectrum) to see if the cholesterol is being properly converted into hormones.

Cholesterol Level Above the Normal Range

Elevation of the serum cholesterol level above the normal range is termed hypercholesterolemia. By definition, a marked hypercholesterolemia is reached when the cholesterol level exceeds 400 mg/dL (1).

Sugar appears to be the most instrumental in maintaining elevated cholesterol levels. The use of alcohol, caffeine, and tobacco also contribute to such an elevation, because, in the case of alcohol, it is metabolized via the same pathway as are sugars; and in the case of tobacco, the tobacco industry uses sugar in the processing of their products. A diet that contains a daily allowance of at least two eggs and a quarter pound of butter tends to optimize cholesterol, bringing the level down.

When dietary control is not completely successful, one should check for chromium and magnesium deficiencies (1). When thyroid activity goes down, the cholesterol level rises. If the thyroid is back up again, the cholesterol level goes down. Dr. Broda Barnes believes that it is impossible to have a heart attack unless the thyroid is in a hypothyroid condition.

Psoriasis is nothing more than cholesterol coming out of the pores of your skin. So your treatment at all times, is to lower cholesterol and you'll find it's what we are doing today with emulsions of RNA-DNA, hydrochloric acid, and pancreatic enzymes. We are clearing up most of these conditions in 6-8 weeks.

High cholesterol levels are often associated with the following conditions.

Cholesterol Level Above the Normal Range	
Body System	**Possible Condition**
Skeletal	Hypertropic arthritis
Digestive	Biliary obstruction Cholangiolytic cirrhosis Celiac disease
Circulatory/Blood/Lymph	Amyloidosis Periarteritis Sudden, severe hemorrhage Atherosclerosis
Urinary	Chronic glomerulonephritis
Endocrine	Pancreatitis Total pancreatectomy Diabetes mellitus Hypothyroidism Amyloid diseases

Systemic	Psoriasis (cholesterol is literally oozing out of the pores of the skin) Cataracts Systemic Lupus erythematosis Ether anesthesia Idiopathic hypercholesterolemia Use of certain drugs and medicines (anabolic steroids, cinchophen, cortisone, epinephrine, heparin, oral contraceptives, phenytoin sodium, Promazine, sulfonamides, thiazides, and thiouracil)

Cholesterol Level Below the Normal Range

A low cholesterol level is termed hypocholesterolemia. By definition, a significant hypocholesterolemia is reached when the cholesterol level drops below 150 mg/dL (1). Runners and joggers exhibit low cholesterol levels. However, these levels are not permanent; they rise within a few days after discontinuance of exercise. Hypocholesterolemia is often associated with the following.

Cholesterol Level Below the Normal Range	
Body System	**Possible Condition**
Digestive	Severe liver damage (due to chemicals, drugs, hepatitis) Malnutrition (resulting from starvation, neoplasms, malabsorption) Intestinal obstructions Acute pancreatitis
Circulatory/Blood/Lymph	Pernicious anemia in relapse Hemolytic anemias Hypochromic anemia Arteriosclerosis Coronary artery thrombosis
Urinary	Diseases of the urinary tract
Endocrine	Administration of cortisone and ACTH Hyperthyroidism Cachexia Arteriosclerosis Infectious diseases, pulmonary tuberculosis
Reproductive	During menstruation After birth

Systemic	Polyneuritis (especially in alcoholism, malnutrition) Hypobeta and alpha-beta lipoproteinemia Tangier's disease (alpha lipoproteinemia) Infections Cachexia Uremia Utilization of certain drugs and medicines (allopurnol, azathioprine, clofibrate, clomiphene, corticotropin, erythromycin, garlic, isoniazid, kanamycin, MAO inhibitors, neomycin, tetracycline, and thiouracil)

Gamma Globulins

The gamma globulin fraction contains the circulating antibodies. These are divided into five groups: IgG (80% of all circulating antibodies), IgA, IgM, IgD, and IgE, in their descending order of concentration in the serum. These are produced by the plasma cells of the reticuloendothelial system, and the level of these molecules depends on the body's exposure to infectious agents, as well as its ability to produce sufficient numbers of these molecules to meet the challenge.

Gamma Globulin Level Within the Normal Range

The gamma globulin level may be normal even in acute cholecystitis, chronic glomerulonephritis, polyarteritis nodosa, and hyperthyroidism.

Gamma Globulin Level Above the Normal Range

Elevation of gamma globulin to a value greater than 1.15 gm% suggests a catabolic condition in which great demands are being made on the synthesizing cells to produce antibody molecules at an accelerated rate. In this case, the cells are always unable to produce enough of these antibodies to fight the infections.

Injection Schedule: If the value reaches 1.5 gm%, injections of gamma globulin and painless liver at a rate of two injections of each per week for five weeks is recommended. Wait four weeks, and if there is no improvement, repeat the injection schedule for another five weeks until there is no longer a letdown. Some diseases associated with elevated gamma globulins are listed below.

Gamma Globulin Level Above the Normal Range	
Body System	**Possible Condition**
Skeletal	Rheumatoid arthritis
Digestive	Laennec's cirrhosis

Circulatory/Blood/Lymph	Macroglobulinemia Myelogenous leukemia Monocytic leukemia Analbuminemia
Systemic	Collagen diseases (lupus) Hypersensitivity (allergies, stings, bites, etc.)

Gamma Globulin Level Below the Normal Range

A depression in the gamma globulin fraction suggests an insufficiency in the raw materials to make antibodies. If the value falls below 0.7 gm%, an injection schedule is indicated (the same as listed under Gamma Globulin Level Above the Normal Range). Decreased levels of gamma globulins are associated with protein losing enteropathy, hypogammaglobulinemia, lymphatic leukemia, lymphoma, and nephrosis.

Glucose

Glucose is also the main building block from which amino acids, purines, and pyrimidines arise through chemical conversions. These substances are further used to make proteins and nucleic acids. Glucose levels rise with the amount of carbohydrate in the diet and tend to normalize and stabilize with the high protein and high fat diet.

We use some normals that are slightly different from the usual laboratory normals. We use a normal range of 70-125 mg per 100 ml of blood, which includes most age groups. Below 50 years, the best normal is 70-115 mg /100; above 50 years, it is 85-125 mg /100.

When sugars and starches (complex carbohydrates) are ingested, they are digested by various enzymes to form glucose or fructose. They are acted upon first by the ptyalin in saliva. Then, they move into the stomach and into the small intestine. Other monosaccharides found in small amounts are levulose and galactose. Ptyalin itself provides minimum digestion, but it starts the process, triggering the stomach to produce hydrochloric acid, which triggers the liver to produce bile and the pancreas to produce more digestive enzymes.

It is important in nutrition that you teach your patients to make sure that all food, when it leaves the mouth is in liquid form. You tell them to chew it that much! I would like to see the old Fleturizing system come back; his method was, Everything you put in your mouth, chew it 50 times. Do you want to have some fun? Go to a dining room and watch people eat! I think I am a fast eater at times, and I go into many restaurants where people come in five to 10 minutes after I start eating my meal, and leave 10 minutes before I do. Most of them will chew each mouthful only four or five times, especially the soft food that ptyalin is supposed to be mixed with.

From the small intestine, these sugars are taken by the portal vein to the liver where fructose is converted to glucose, the main fuel constituent in the body. The glucose level reflects the amount of energy available for the many metabolic reactions inside the body. Other sources of glucose are certain amino acids and lactic acid released by the muscles.

These are changed into glycogen in the liver for storage; later, when needed, glycogen is converted back into glucose, with the assistance of potassium.

Glucose Level Within the Normal Range

A serum glucose within the normal range indicates the possibility for normal sugar-handling capacity of the individual. However, patients who have latent diabetes or a prediabetic tendency will show a normal fasting glucose level, so a normal glucose level does not rule out diabetes (1).

Glucose Level Above the Normal Range

A high glucose level is termed hyperglycemia. This is usually equated with diabetes. However, it may be associated with a variety of disorders as listed below. Some working definitions pertaining to hyperglycemia are as follows: a mild hyperglycemia is usually considered to be 120-130 mg, a moderate hyperglycemia is 300-500 mg, and a marked hyperglycemia is represented by values above 500 mg (1).

The glucose level may be elevated in persons with a good diet if certain minerals are absent or in suboptimal amounts. Among these minerals are chromium, zinc, magnesium, manganese, potassium, and calcium. These levels should be assayed in the hair by a spectrographic hair mineral analysis to get an accurate picture.

Glucose Level Above the Normal Range	
Body System	**Possible Condition**
Digestive	Vomiting
Circulatory/Blood/Lymph	Hemachromatosis
Nervous/Sensory	Some lesions of the central nervous system (subarachnoid hemorrhage, convulsion)
Endocrine	Diabetes mellitus (moderate hyperglycemia is diagnostic) Cushing's syndrome (mild hyperglycemia) Acromegaly Giantism Increased levels of circulating adrenalin (ACTH or adrenalin injection, hyperadrenalism, hyperpituitarism, pheochromocytoma (mild hyperglycemia), acute stress (regardless of the cause – mild hyperyglycemia)) Hyperthyroidism (if the cholesterol level is depressed, mild hyperglycemia) Acute or chromic pancreatitis (mild hyperglycemia) Adenoma of the pancreas (mild hyperglycemia)
Reproductive	Normal pregnancy

Systemic	Wernicke's encephalopathy (a vitamin B1 deficiency) After various muscular exercise After anaesthesia In dehydration In possible chromium and/or zinc deficiency Possible ketoacidosis with uncontrolled diabetes (This is a dangerous situation; the CO_2 is also depressed.) Possible nonketotic and nonacidotic hyperglycemia (The CO_2 is normal; this is also a serious condition, characterized by abnormal carbohydrate metabolism and uncoupling of oxidative phosphorylation. It is commonly associated with vascular disease in the elderly with accompanying dehydration and hypernatremia. Check for elevations in total protein, BUN, and sodium.) Hyponatremia (For an increase in serum glucose of 100 mg, there is usually a decrease in serum sodium of 3 mEq/liter (2).) Medications that may affect a false elevation of serum glucose are: aminosalicilic acid, aspirin, caffeine, chlorpromazine, chlorthalidone, corticosteroids, ephnephrine, estrogens, ethacrynic acid, Furosamide, Hydralazine, Levodopa, Phenylbutazone, Phenytoin, Prednisolone, Reserpine, Secretin, thiazides, and thyroxine.

Glucose Level Below the Normal Range

A low glucose level is termed hypoglycemia. This characteristic is responsible for such a wide variety of symptomatology, that it is only in recent times that physicians have popularly recognized its devastating role! Hypoglycemia is often called the Great Imitator because it manifests so many symptoms.

If a patient comes in to your office, and you try very hard to make a diagnosis, but you still can't figure out what's wrong. Just write down hypoglycemia, and you'll be correct probably 80% of the time. Are you familiar with all of the various symptoms? Here is a list; see how many of these hit home.

Anxiety	Fear	Pallor
Blurred vision	Hallucinations	Palpitation
Cold sweats	Headaches	Phobias
Compulsive eating	Insomnia	Staggering
Confusion	Irritability	Suicidal motivation
Crime spells	Itching	Undue fatigue
Depression	Lack of concentration	Vertigo
Drowsiness	Muscular pain	Weak spells
Exhaustion	Nervousness	Worry
Fatigue on awakening	Night terrors	

In all cases of hypoglycemia, the potassium level must be checked because this mineral is used in the conversion of glycogen to glucose in the liver (see Sussman, et. al., Diabetes 12:38, 1963). Diseases associated with hypoglycemia are listed below.

Glucose Level Below the Normal Range	
Body System	**Possible Condition**
Skeletal	Some cases of arthritis
Digestive	Carcinoma of the stomach Liver disease (hepatitis, cirrhosis, carcinoma, poisoning) Gastroenterostomy
Circulatory/Blood/Lymph	Marked anemia (check MCV, MCHC)
Urinary	Chronic nephritis with renal failure
Endocrine	Pancreatic disorders (tumor or hyperplasia of the Islets of Langerhans, pancreatitis, glucagon deficiency) Carcinoma of the adrenal gland Hypopituitarism Addison's disease (adrenocortical hypofunction) The typical pattern is a < GLU, < NA, > K, > BUN. Hypothyroidism Administration of exogenous insulin Hyperinsulinism
Reproductive	Prematurity Infant of a diabetic mother Normal pregnancy Normal lactation

Systemic	Starvation Severe prolonged muscular exercise Fibrosarcomas Early diabetes mellitus Ketotic hypoglyemia Zetterstrom's syndrome Leucine sensitivity Von Gierke's disease (glycogen storage disease) Galactosemia Maple syrup urine disease Fructose intolerance Malnutrition Starvation Following severe and prolonged muscular exercise The following medications may falsely depress the serum glucose level: dicumarol, erythromycin, ethacrynic acid, guanethidine, insulin, sulfonamides, sulfonylureas, sulfaphenazole.

Iron (Fe)

Both the organic and inorganic forms of iron are absorbed chiefly from the stomach and duodenum. Iron must be in the ferrous (+2 charge) form to be absorbed from the digestive tract, but because most dietary iron is in the ferric state (+3 charge), many reducing substances (electron donors) must be present along with the iron for the iron the be absorbed. Such reducing substances include gastric or supplemental hydrochloric acid, ascorbic acid, and the amino acid, cysteine. Phytates (plant fiber), phosphates. oxalates (found in chocolate, tomatoes, spinach, rhubarb, etc.), and pancreatic secretions inhibit absorption of iron.

After absorption, which is controlled by the level of body stores and the rate of RBC production, iron is transported in the blood attached to a beta-1 globulin (transferrin – a metalloprotein), and it is deposited in the liver, where it is either stored or withdrawn and excreted (4). Iron is found in storage in the spleen and bone marrow, as well as in the liver in a form known as ferritin. Only seven of the 27 mg of iron used each day comes from the diet; the rest is derived from the breakdown of old RBCs (3)! However, since copper is a cofactor essential for the production of heme, the iron containing portion of the hemoglobin molecule, the dietary supply and tissue levels of copper should be known before considering the role of iron in anemia. Dr. John Myers pointed out that iron deficiency anemia is morphologically indistinguishable from copper deficiency anemia (1). Females, incidentally, are not able to absorb iron as efficiently as males.

Iron Level Within The Normal Range

Men: 70-175 mcg/dL or 12.5-31.3 micromoles per liter (mcmol/L)

Women: 50-150 mcg/dL or 8.9-26.8 mcmol/L

Children: 50-120 mcg/dL or 9.0-21.5 mcmol/L

A normal iron level reflects only that in transit between storage and absorption sites to utilization sites. It does not accurately reflect, by itself, the amount of iron actually used in the hemoglobin molecule. Other tests, such as the RBC, HCT, and HGB, and the indices MCV, MCH, and the MCHC are necessary. When considered with these values, as well as with the level of bilirubin, the iron level can be helpful in clarifying the status of the hemopoeitic system. A normal iron level can be observed in patients with biliary obstruction.

Iron Level Above The Normal Range

An elevated level of iron is termed hemochromatosis and is an accumulation of iron in the body. Untreated, the iron level can become dangerously high, leading to liver and heart damage, diabetes, and arthritis. Hemochromatosis can be genetic, but it can also be caused by too many blood transfusions, liver disease, alcoholism, or from taking iron pills unnecessarily. Men are more likely than women to have too much iron, because women flush iron during menstrual cycles and pregnancy.

Because accumulation is slow, symptoms often don't appear until a person is age 40 or older. Early symptoms are somewhat vague, so this condition is sometimes mistaken for another. Some symptoms are fatigue, joint pain, weight loss, and frequent urination. An elevated serum iron level is associated with the following conditions.

Iron Level Above the Normal Range	
Body System	**Possible Condition**
Skeletal	Possible liver and heart damage, diabetes, and arthritis
Digestive	Acute liver damage (the SGOT and SGPT are probably elevated, and the level of iron parallels the extent of liver necrosis), e.g., hepatitis (6)
Circulatory/Blood/Lymph	Hemochromatosis (idiopathic, check for other symptoms Hemosiderosis (via transfusion) Hemolytic anemia (the MCV is 80-95%, and the MCHC drops to 30 (6)) Anemias in which there is decreased RBC formation (the iron is not being used)
Reproductive	Use of birth control pills Progesterone therapy

Iron Level Below The Normal Range

It is important to check the RBC, MCV, and MCHC before attempting to diagnose an anemia as hypochromic; a correct diagnosis of this condition cannot be made on the basis of a low serum iron level alone. Depressed serum iron levels are observed in the following situations.

Iron Level Below the Normal Range	
Body System	**Possible Condition**
Digestive	Achlorhydria Hypochlorhydria Malabsorption Deficient intake of iron Deficient intake of reducing substances and/or consumption of dietary fiber with iron-containing substances
Circulatory/Blood/Lymph	Iron deficiency anemia (the MCV is less than 80, and the MCHC is less than 30) (6) Normochromic anemias of infection and chronic disease (the MCV is 80; 95, and the MCHC is less than 30) (6) Pernicious anemia (the MCV is less than 95, and the MCHC is less than 30) (6)
Urinary	Nephrosis (due to iron-binding protein in the urine; the BUN/creatinine ratio is less than 10) (6)
Systemic	Neoplastic disease (see normochromic anemias, above) Chronic infection (see normochromic anemias, above)

Lactic Dehydrogenase (LDH)

Lactic dehydrogenase is an enzyme that brings about reversible oxidation of lactic acid to pyruvic acid. The normal range differs with the method of testing, but is commonly thought of as 140-330 units/liter. LDH is present in many tissues, the highest concentrations occurring in the heart, liver, kidney, brain, skeletal muscle, and in RBCs. Damage to any of these tissues brings about release of LDH molecules into the bloodstream. An electrophoretic separation and identification of the isoenzymes is necessary to determine the origin of serum LDH. Levels are normally elevated in children and are highly variable in pregnant females.

LDH Level Within the Normal Range

Although the acceptable range of LDH in the bloodstream may seem rather wide, elevations may be in excess of fifteen times the normal mean. Therefore, normal values are indicative of optimal integrity of the tissues that contain this class of enzymes.

LDH Level Above the Normal Range

Elevations of LDH are indicative of damage to the tissues mentioned above. By definition, an extreme elevation means that the LDH is above 1,500 Wroblewski units; a slight elevation implies that the LDH is 500-700 Wroblewski units. A normal elevation (approximately three times that of the adult mean) are seen in healthy children. However, slight elevations that persist should direct attention to many chronic conditions as possibilities; among these are chronic viral hepatitis, malignancies of the various tissues, lung destruction, generalized viral infections, brain damage, and destruction of kidney tissue (1). Suspicion may be cast in the direction of a diet high in carbohydrates. Always look at an elevated SGOT along with the elevated LDH; if both are elevated, there is a strong indication of myocardial infarction. If only one is elevated, myocardial infarction is not probable. Many conditions associated with an elevated LDH are as follows.

LDH Level Above the Normal Range	
Body System	**Possible Condition**
Skeletal	Various muscular diseases (the serum creatinine is probably altered)
Digestive	Hepatitis Poisoning by carbon tetrachloride, chlorpromazine Cirrhosis Biliary obstruction
Circulatory/Blood/Lymph	Acute myocardial infarction (extreme elevations, elevated SGOT and SGPT) Insertion of intracardiac prosthetic valves Untreated acute leukemia Malignant lymphoma Sickle cell anemia Untreated pernicious anemia (probable extreme elevation) Lymphocytic leukemia Acute leukemia Lymphatic leukemia Myelogenous leukemia Hemolysis (various causes)
Urinary	Carcinoma of the kidneys and/or bladder Other kidney diseases (the elevations are not high and not clinically useful)

Systemic	Pulmonary embolus Malignant tumors (a high LDH with a normal SGOT and SGPT indicates the need for further testing) Chromium toxicity (Usually no elevation in SGOT or SGPT; the LDH may be in the high normal category. One should check the level of selenium in a hair mineral analysis; selenium exerts a protective effect against malignancy if the levels are not in the toxic range.) Aluminum toxicity Nickel toxicity Lead toxicity (check the WBC morphology for basophilic stippling) Laboratory artifacts (The technician may have performed a poor venipuncture, or the blood was heated; possibly the clot was not separated from the serum quickly enough.) Muscular exercise Certain medications elevate LDH, such as anaesthetic events, codeine, dicumarol, morphine, and estrogens

LDH Level Below the Normal Range

A depressed LDH usually means that sufficient amounts of this class of enzymes are not being produced; probably, this is a result of some inhibition of protein synthesis. This condition is often seen after X-ray irradiation. Another factor to consider is a mineral inavailability to the tissues. A hair mineral analysis may reveal a deficiency of the minerals that make up of the prosthetic group of enzymes involved in protein synthesis. Total protein, albumin, and globulin values should be checked in the blood. The hair should be assayed for low levels of beneficial minerals as well as for high levels of toxic, inhibitory metals.

Lipids (Total)

Bodily fats or lipids represent a dynamic tissue that is constantly tearing down and rebuilding itself. The reason is that fat is a major energy source for most of the other tissues. In fact, much of the dietary carbohydrate is converted into fat before it is used as energy via the Kreb's cycle.

Fats are essential for other functions, such as the provision of essential fatty acids (polyunsaturated) and fat soluble vitamins and for efficient absorption of other compounds from the gastrointestinal tract. Separation of a plasma sample by electrophoresis shows that it contains triglycerides, phospholipids, cholesterol, cholesterol esters, and free fatty acids. These materials are hydrophobic (water-hating) and are therefore insoluble in the water portion of the blood. They are, by necessity, transported by proteins, that, by virtue of their function, are termed, lipoproteins. The category, Total Lipids, excludes those fatty acids that are esterified to cholesterol.

Total Lipid Level Within the Normal Range

Because the total lipid fraction contains so many components, the fact that the value may be within the normal range is not diagnostic. The acceptable normal range is so wide that a normal value may even hide the presence of some metabolic disorder. It is for this reason that measurements of blood lipids usually take into account the important categories, high density and low density lipoproteins.

Total Lipid Level Above the Normal Range

An elevation of total serum lipids is termed hyperlipemia or hyperlipidemia. This condition can occur normally after meals, during a fast, and in association with an exclusively meat diet. Hence, the necessity for a preparatory fast before the patient is tested. Abnormal elevations of serum lipids are observed in the following conditions.

Total Lipid Level Above the Normal Range	
Body System	**Possible Condition**
Circulatory/Blood/Lymph	Hypertension Pernicious anemia Hypochromic anemia Hemolytic anemia Hemolytic anemia Leukemia
Urinary	Nephrosis
Endocrine	Hypothyroidism Diabetic acidosis
Systemic	Hypernatremia After administration of drugs Ether or chloroform anaesthesia Alcohol ingestion

Total Lipid Level Below the Normal Range

Hypolipidemia, or low serum lipids, is usually associated with hyperthyroidism. Possible conditions are indicated as follows for an elevated T4; these are repeated here to indicate hypothetical situations in which the total lipids may be depressed.

Total Lipids Below Normal Range If T4 Level is Elevated (Hypothetical)	
Body System	**Possible Condition**
Digestive	Certain cases of hepatitis
Endocrine	Thyroiditis Cretinism
Reproductive	Normal pregnancy
Systemic	Following administration of certain drugs, such as estrogens, birth control pills, d-thyroxine, thyroid extract, thyroid-stimulating hormone. After use of certain cough syrups, toothpastes, and antiseptics Overconsumption of fish
Miscellaneous	The specimen over 72 hours old Recent radioactive testing (brain scan)

Phosphorus (PO_4)

About 85% of the body's phosphorus is in bones and teeth, but small amounts exist in tissues throughout the body. Phosphorus is a component of DNA and RNA. Further, it is an essential element in the role of ATP in energy metabolism and in the synthesis of important brain and membrane phospholipids, such as phosphatidylcholine and phosphatidylserine. On a conscious scale, phosphorus helps to reduce muscle pain after a workout. The normal mean for phosphorus is 4 mg/dL, and it is absorbed into the blood from the jejunum. It is excreted into the intestines and reabsorbed into the lower part of the small intestinal tract. It is eliminated mainly in the feces but also in the urine. Phosphorus should not be taken when taking calcium.

Phosphorus Level Within the Normal Range

We strive for a specific normal for both calcium and phosphorus — 10 mg/dL for calcium and 4 mg/dL for phosphorus, with an ideal ratio of 2.5/1.

Phosphorus Level Above the Normal Range

A phosphorus level above the normal range is termed hyperphosphatemia. This condition is observed in the following situations:

Phosphorus Level Above the Normal Range	
Body System	**Possible Condition**
Skeletal	Certain bone diseases, multiple myeloma, during the healing of fractures
Digestive	Yellow atrophy of the liver After a high intestinal obstruction
Circulatory/Blood/Lymph	Myelogenous leukemia
Urinary	Renal diseases
Endocrine	Hypoparathyroidism Addison's disease
Systemic	Hypervitaminosis (excessive vitamin d)

Phosphorus Level Below the Normal Range

A phosphorus level below the normal range is termed hypophosphatemia. **If someone has a low phosphate level, such as 3.0 mg/100 or below, and the calcium is quite normal, one may predict that the person has or will have periodontal disease.** He or she should be examined by a dentist, who should consider altering the diet and possibly supplementing with phosphorus. Another situation in which low phosphorus plays a part is in the development of abnormal calcium deposits, such as spinal or cervical stenosis, which often requires surgical intervention, such as a laminectomy.

Phosphorus Level Below the Normal Range	
Body System	**Possible Condition**
Skeletal	Osteomalacia (adults) or rickets (children) Abnormal deposition of calcium, such as spinal stenosis
Digestive	Deficient absorption from the intestinal tract Probable periodontal disease and caries
Endocrine	Hyperparathyroidism Hyperinsulinism, as in adenomas of the islets of Langerhans or after insulin injection Diabetes mellitus or after ingestion of carbohydrates or intravenous glucose
Reproductive	During normal pregnancy
Systemic	Probable muscle aches and pains

Here is a true story. I consult with 300 doctors around the world. They send me blood chemistry results of their patients, and I analyze them and send back my observations. One recent case involved a doctor's patient; it was a woman with a phosphate level of 2.6. The calcium was about 10.1. So I predicted that she had or was going to have periodontal disease. I recorded my findings on an audio tape and sent it to the doctor, who played the recording for the patient. After she listened to the tape, the doctor asked, Are there any questions? She responded, Well, I question about this periodontal disease. I haven't had an ache or pain in my mouth for a long time. I am not quite sure whether or not I want to believe what Dr. Ellis says in that report. The doctor later told me that, the next day, she called and said, Doctor, I have to see you right away. She arrived at his office and told him that, when her dentist checked her mouth with X-ray, she was shown to have not only one, but two abscessed teeth alongside one another. She added, Well, if he can predict this by the blood that has been taken out three weeks earlier, all of what he says in this report must be true, so I am to do exactly the way he tells it.

Potassium (K)

Potassium is the major cation of the intracellular fluid, or cytoplasm. Potassium is more abundant in cells than is sodium. It helps to regulate osmotic pressure and acid-base balance. It is absorbed from the intestinal tract into the bloodstream, and about 90% is excreted into the urine. Potassium is concentrated in the cells that line the lumen of the blood vessels and inside the nerve cells. **The optimum situation in the body is 28:1 ratio of sodium to potassium (see Sodium/Potassium Ratio (Na/K)); this results in a stable pH, proper osmotic balance, and the proper functioning of smooth and striated muscle tissue.** Potassium plays a major role in the conversion of glycogen to glucose; therefore, hypoglycemic patients' serum potassium level must be monitored during treatment.

Rich dietary sources include avocados, bananas, and parsley. Bananas are rich in potassium, but you must eat them very ripe to benefit from it. Eat a banana when the skin is very thin and almost black. Don't eat it otherwise. Bananas are always picked green; then they are gassed to turn them yellow. If you don't wait long enough for the enzymes that are in the skin to ripen it, all you're getting is the pure starch. Here again, it is starch that forms cholesterol. If you use a ripened banana in baking, you lose all of the nutritive value from heating. Anything over 120° starts to destroy many of the enzymes and also make the minerals insoluble. It is better to eat bananas in their natural state.

Parsley, by the way, is one of the best vegetable sources of minerals. Restaurants use it as garnish on your plate, and almost everybody puts it aside. It is the most important thing they should eat first. You get more out of parsley than from the rest of the food on your plate.

Potassium Level Within the Normal Range

A normal serum potassium level, although indicative of potentially properly functioning mechanisms, is not good evidence of the absence of disease. One must attend to the levels of sodium, chloride, and the sodium/potassium ratio before discounting the possibility of electrolyte imbalances based on the normal potassium level alone. Several conditions are associated with a normal serum potassium level; some of these are listed below (2).

Potassium Level Within the Normal Range	
Body System	**Possible Condition**
Circulatory/Blood/Lymph	Congestive heart failure
Urinary	Chronic renal failure (potassium may be depressed) Nephritis
Endocrine	Diabetes insipidus
Systemic	Excessive sweating Dehydration Salicylate intoxication (potassium may be depressed) Diabetic acidosis (potassium may be increased) Metabolic acidosis or alkalosis *
Miscellaneous	Pulmonary emphysema * If the potassium is normal with a highly elevated CO_2 (greater than 35 mEq/liter), this indicates probable metabolic alkalosis; potassium would tend to migrate into the cell and be excreted in the urine. If the potassium level is normal with a greatly depressed CO_2 (less than 10 mEq/ liter), potassium would leave the cell (1).

Potassium Level Above the Normal Range

A high serum potassium level is termed hyperkalemia or hyperpotassemia. It may result from excessive intake beyond the ability of the kidneys to excrete it. Further, it may be associated with the following conditions.

Potassium Level Above the Normal Range	
Body System	**Possible Condition**
Skeletal	Periodic paralysis (epilepsy)
Circulatory/Blood/Lymph	Any cause of hemolysis of the RBCs
Urinary	Renal failure with oliguria or anuria Nephrosis Obstruction or trauma

Endocrine	Addison's disease (the potassium may rise as high as 6.5) Adrenocortical insufficiency Hypofunction of rennin-angiotensin aldosterone system Administration of an aldosterone antagonist (spironolactone) Pseudohypoaldosteronism
Systemic	Respiratory acidosis or alkalosis (the potassium may rise as high as 5.5) Any process of tissue breakdown Dehydration Diabetic acidosis (the potassium level may be normal) Fasting Hyperchloremic acidosis (check the level of serum chloride) Administration of potassium-retaining drugs (triamterene) Rapid potassium infusion Excessive dietary intake Poor venipuncture technique (hemolysis and lysis of platelets) Incomplete or late separation of clot from serum in a specimen Certain medications can elevate the serum potassium; some are: Amphotericin B, epinephrine, heparin, histamine (IV), marijuana, methicillin, and tetracycline.

Potassium Level Below the Normal Range

This condition is termed hypokalemia or hypopotassemia and is associated with the following disorders (2). If potassium is to be supplemented, it should be accompanied by chloride in a 1:1 ratio, thereby lessening the possibility of hypochloremia and hypochloremic alkalosis (1).

Potassium Level Below the Normal Range	
Body System	**Possible Condition**
Digestive	Vomiting Diarrhea Gastric suctioning Colon cancer Villous adenoma Chronic abuse of laxatives Chronic and severe diarrhea Zollinger-Ellison syndrome (peptic ulceration with pancreatic tumor) Uterosigmoidostomy Malabsorption (serum sodium is also increased) Pyloric obstruction Starvation Duodenal obstruction
Urinary	Salt-losing nephropathy * Renal tubular acidosis ** Chronic pyelonephritis ** Diuresis following relief of urinary tract obstruction ** Chronic renal failure (serum potassium may be normal)
Endocrine	Primary aldosteronism * Pseudoaldosteronism * Cushing's syndrome * Insulin therapy
Systemic	Administration of diuretics (thiazides and mercurials*) (serum chloride may be depressed) Salicylate intoxication Infusion of potassium-deficient fluids Administration of ammonium chloride Administration of Diamox Certain medications may depress the serum potassium; some are: aldosterone, Amphotericin B, bicarbonates, corticosteroids, ethacrynic acid, furosemide, gentamycin, insulin, and estrogens (licorice may effect the same changes).

Miscellaneous	* These are renal and adrenal conditions associated with metabolic alkalosis. ** These are renal conditions associated with metabolic acidosis.

Protein (Total)

The serum total protein complement contains all of those proteins present in plasma except fibrinogen and clotting factors II, V, and VIII. Included are albumin (synthesized in the liver) and globulin (made in reticuloendothelial tissues). Proteins are made from amino acids contained in the amino acid pool, the total body complement of amino acids. This pool is kept replenished from breakdown and assimilation of dietary proteins and from recycling amino acids derived from previously existing proteins that have outlived their usefulness in their original forms. The amino acids are chopped apart enzymatically and put into a different order, thus creating new proteins. Dietary replenishment of the amino acid pool is dependent upon the quality and quantity of the protein being ingested.

Beef serum and lactalbumin seem to be the best sources of protein with respect to their effectiveness in replenishing the albumin portion of the blood (3). Also important is the ability of the digestive tract to assimilate the proteins. This factor is dependent on the sufficiency of hydrochloric acid, pepsin, bile, and pancreatic juices. Endogenous replenishment depends upon the amount and activity of the body's proteolytic enzymes and the energy efficiency of the tissues.

Total Protein Within The Normal Range

In disease processes, the total protein concentration is usually altered in some manner, due to the common depression of albumin and elevation of the globulin portion. However, the condition, polyarteritis nodosa may exhibit a normal total protein, even though the albumin is decreased and the globulins are increased (IgG and IgA).

For our purposes, we do not accept just any value within the usual laboratory range of 6-8 gm%. We believe that the best value is 7.4 gm%, accounted for by an albumin level of 5.2 gm% and a globulin level of 2.2 gm%. These ensure a sufficient reservoir of albumin for protein synthesis and a sufficiently low globulin level to suggest the absence of disease.

Total Protein Above The Normal Range

A rise in total protein is termed hyperproteinemia and generally occurs in any condition associated with a loss of body fluids. One may observe elevations in the following situations.

Protein Level Above the Normal Range	
Body System	**Possible Condition**
Skeletal	Rheumatoid arthritis (the ESR, CRP, IgG, and IgA are increased)
Digestive	Liver disease
Circulatory/Blood/Lymph	Monoclonal gammopathies Malignant lymphoma (increased IgA, decreased albumin) Myxoma of the left atrium of the heart Bacterial endocarditis (increased IgG) Macroglobulinemia (marked increased in IgM)
Endocrine	Cystic fibrosis of the pancreas (increased IgA and IgM, decreased albumin)
Systemic	Skin diseases Systemic Lupus erythematosis Acute rheumatic fever General infections Hypercalcemia (if total protein is increased due to sarcoidosis or multiple myeloma) Granuloma Malnutrition Hypochlorhydria or achlorhydria

Total Protein Below The Normal Range

A low total protein value is termed hypoproteinemia. Generally, it can be said that this condition is brought about by protein inavailability or by a destruction of preexisting proteins. Edema is common due to the decreased osmotic pressure within vessel walls. The various conditions associated with hypoproteinemia are listed below.

Protein Level Below the Normal Range	
Body System	**Possible Condition**
Digestive	Hepatic failure (due to decreased albumin) Protein-losing enteropathy (albumin and globulin are decreased) Cirrhosis of the liver
Circulatory/Blood/Lymph	Heavy chain disease (marked decrease in albumin and IgM) Congestive heart failure (decreased albumin) Agammaglobulinemia
Urinary	Chronic renal insufficiency (decreased albumin) Nephrotic syndrome (the albumin is less than 2.5 mg/dL)
Endocrine	Hyperparathyroidism (an electrophoresis is necessary; the calcium can reach as high as 20 mg/dL)
Systemic	Heavy infestation of hookworms Trichinosis Rickettsial infections Kwashiorkor (lowered albumin) Sprue Prolonged starvation

SGOT (Serum Glutamic Oxaloacetic Transaminase, AST)

The transaminase enzymes, SGOT and SGPT, catalyze the transfer of an amine (NH3) group from one amino acid to a keto acid to form a second, new amino acid. The normal range is 5-40 units/liter. Widely distributed in animals and in the tissues; SGOT (now referred to as Aspartate Aminotransaminase, or AST) is concentrated greatest in the heart muscle, skeletal muscles, brain, liver, kidneys, and RBCs in decreasing order. When this value rises in myocardial infarction, the peak usually occurs within 24 hours. Then it starts to decrease.

The important point to remember is that the enzyme normally exists only within the cell. Therefore, only cellular damage will increase the level of this enzyme in the bloodstream. SGOT and SGPT levels are used generally to determine the extent of heart or liver damage; however, the creatinine phosphokinase (CPK) level should be known to more accurately define the tissues involved.

SGOT Level Within the Normal Range

Normal SGOT levels can often be observed in angina pectoris, coronary insufficiency, pericarditis, and in congestive heart failure without liver damage. Therefore, other indicators such the LDH, CPK, and possibly their isoenzymes may have to be checked in the presence of overt clinical symptoms. Fluctuations in the SGOT level as great as 10 units may occur in a normal individual; values may vary with age and pregnancy.

SGOT Level Above the Normal Range

The level of SGOT in the bloodstream is directly proportional to the number of tissue cells damaged and the amount of time elapsing between the injury and the test. Values usually elevate within eight hours after the injury and peak within two to three days; normal values are usually reached within four to six days (1). Extreme elevations are characterized by values in excess of 100 units/ml; minor elevations involve values between 40 and 100 units/ml. Elevations of SGOT are often associated with the following disorders.

SGOT Level Above the Normal Range	
Body System	**Possible Condition**
Skeletal	Musculoskeletal disease * Muscle injury Intramuscular injection
Digestive	Liver disease Severe fulminating hepatitis (extremely high SGOT) Intestinal injury Postsurgical to GI tract Cirrhosis Cholangiolitic jaundice * Metastatic liver disease *
Circulatory/Blood/Lymph	Acute myocardial infarction (extreme elevations with peak in 24 hours) ** Congestive heart failure * Tachyarrhythmia (in the presence of shock) * Dissecting aneurysm *
Urinary	Renal infarction

Systemic	Pulmonary infarction * Local irradiation injury Myoglobinuria Drugs, aspirin type or opiates (some examples are dicoumerol, papaverine, isoniazid, phenothiazides, erythromycin, Dialose Plus, oral contraceptives, sulfonamides, anabolic/androgenic steroids, phenylbutazone, diphenylhydantoin, halothane, methyldopa, monoamine oxidase inhibitors, indomethacin, pyrazinamide, drugs that induce hypersensitivity and cholestasis) Degenerative central nervous system diseases, multiple sclerosis, cerebral infarction, brain tumors Head injuries
Miscellaneous	Minor elevations of SGOT are commonly observed. ** Sometimes a pseudomyocardial infarction: pattern is observed. It is usually brought about by administration of opiates to patients with no gallbladder or with a diseased biliary tract. Elevations in LDH and SGOT occur, but the elevation in SGOT peaks in five to eight hours; the peak may persist for 24 hours.

SGOT Below the Normal Range

Decreases in SGOT are not usually assigned a pathologic significance. However, depressions are seen in diabetic ketoacidosis, beriberi, severe liver disease, during hemodialysis, and in uremia (check the BUN). Such depressions are described in the literature (2) as being false decreases, because these conditions increase the serum level of lactate-consuming enzymes during the in vitro test.

SGPT (Serum Glutamic Pyruvic Transaminase, ALT)

The transaminase enzymes, SGOT and SGPT, catalyze the transfer of an amine (NH3) group from one amino acid to a keto acid to form a second, new amino acid. The normal range of values for SGPT is 7-56 units/liter. SGPT (now referred to as Alanine Aminotransaminase, or ALT) is an enzyme found primarily in the liver but also to a lesser degree, the heart and other tissues. It is more useful in diagnosing liver function than SGOT levels. However, the creatinine phosphokinase (CPK) level should be known to more accurately define the tissues involved.

The SGOT/SGPT (AST/ALT) ratio may indicate acute and chronic liver injury, fatty liver, or hepatitis C (the ratio is less than or equal to 1). However, an AST/ALT ratio greater than 2 is characteristic of alcoholic hepatitis.

SGPT Level Within the Normal Range

Test results can be normal in people with liver disease. Malignant tumors may show a high LDH with normal SGOT and SGPT; further testing is indicated. Also, chromium toxicity usually shows no elevation in SGOT or SGPT; the LDH may be in the high normal category. One should check the level of selenium in a hair mineral analysis; selenium exerts a protective effect against malignancy if the levels are not in the toxic range.

SGPT Level Above the Normal Range

SGPT (ALT) is an enzyme normally present in liver and heart cells. When the liver or heart is injured, this enzyme is spilled into the bloodstream, raising the enzyme levels in the blood. Some medications can also raise SGPT levels. An elevated SGPT level is associated with the following.

SGPT Level Above the Normal Range	
Body System	**Possible Condition**
Digestive	Hepatitis Liver damage from salicylates, carbon tetrachloride Fatty liver
Circulatory/Blood/Lymph	Myocardial infarction
Endocrine	Pancreatitis
Systemic	Acute infections Alcoholism Some medications such as: acetaminophen, aspirin and ibuprofen; anti-seizure medications and antibiotics; cardiovascular drugs, cholesterol lowering drugs, and antidepressants.

SGPT Below the Normal Range

A low SGPT level can indicate a normal healthy liver, but it may not necessarily be the case. A low-functioning or non-functioning liver, lacking normal levels of SGPT activity, would release diminished amounts of the enzyme into the blood when damaged. People infected with the hepatitis C virus initially show high SGPT levels in their blood, but these levels fall over time. Because the SGPT test measures levels at only one point in time, people with a chronic hepatitis C infection may already have experienced the peak before blood was drawn for the test. Urinary tract infections or malnutrition may also cause low levels.

SGPT Level Below the Normal Range	
Body System	**Possible Condition**
Digestive	Long-term hepatitis infections
Urinary	Some urinary tract infections
Endocrine	Low-functioning liver
Systemic	Malnutrition

Sodium (Na)

Sodium is the major cation of the extracellular fluid. The normal range is 136-145 mEq/liter. It is present at a higher concentration on the inside of blood vessels and on the outside of the nerves. Sodium is concentrated outside cells; potassium is concentrated inside cells (see Sodium/Potassium Ratio (Na/K)); through interaction of these two elements, the body is protected against large swings in blood pH, an excessive loss or retention of fluids, and the malfunction of muscular activity.

Sodium Level Within the Normal Range

A normal sodium level implies a potentially optimal osmotic balance. However, one should not consider sodium alone; he must know the potassium level, the chloride concentration, and the sodium/potassium ratio before discounting the possibility of electrolyte imbalances based on a normal sodium level alone.

Sodium Level Above the Normal Range

Elevation of serum sodium is very rare (1). This condition is termed hypernatremia and usually results from some type of water loss. Hypoproteinemia can also cause an elevated sodium level, so it is wise to check total protein, albumin, and globulin levels. **No patient should ever be put on a salt-free diet unless the physician knows the absolute and relative concentrations of serum sodium and potassium!** Conditions associated with hypernatremia are listed below.

Sodium Level Above the Normal Range	
Body System	**Possible Condition**
Digestive	Vomiting Diarrhea
Circulatory/Blood/Lymph	Congestive heart failure Hyproproteinemia

Urinary	Nephrotic Diabetes insipidus Acute tubular necrosis Urinary tract obstruction Hypercalcemic nephropathy Hypokalemic nephropathy Lower nephron nephrosis Chronic renal failure Renal tubular acidosis
Endocrine	Diabetes insipidus Diabetes mellitus Hypothalamic lesions (check for elevated serum glucose) Cushing's syndrome Administration of ACTH, cortisone Adrenocortical insufficiency
Systemic	Hyperpnea Excessive perspiration Improper administration (iatrogenic) of excess sodium following loss of fluids Administration of ACTH Dehydration Hypoproteinemia Certain medications can effect elevation of serum sodium; some are: salicylates (intoxication), diuretics (thiazides, mercurials), ammonium chloride, Diamox, anabollc steroids, bicarbonate, Clonidine, estrogens, guanethidine, marijuana, methoxyflurane, oral contraceptives, prolactin (1M), and tetracyclines.

Sodium Level Below the Normal Range

Decreased sodium levels, hyponatremia, are common and observed in the following conditions.

Sodium Level Below the Normal Range	
Body System	**Possible Condition**
Digestive	Vomiting Diarrhea Pyloric obstruction Malabsorption Cirrhosis (with ascites) Intestinal fistula

Circulatory/Blood/Lymph	Congestive heart failure
Urinary	Nephrosis Acute renal failure Nephritis Chronic glomerular nephritis with uremia
Endocrine	Adrenocortical insufficiency Inappropriate secretion of ADH Priimary aldosteronism Myxedema Addison's disease (Depressed sodium is accompanied by elevated potassium, elevated BUN, and mild dehydration (see Protein (Total), above).
Systemic	Lobar pneumonia Pulmonary emphysema Excessive perspiration Hyperlipidemia (see Total Lipids) Hyperglycemia (The serum sodium decreases 3 mEq/liter for every increase of serum glucose of 100 mg/100 ml (2).) Diabetic acidosis Metabolic alkalosis with pyloric obstruction Administration of ether anaesthesia Certain medications may depress the serum sodium level; some are: ammonium chloride, cathartics (excessive), chlorpropamide, ethacrynic acid, furosemide, mannitol, metolazone, spironolactone, thiazides, and Triamterene.

Sodium/Potassium Ratio (Na/K)

The ideal ratio between sodium and potassium in the body fluids is 28/1. This represents the ratio of concentrations of the two elements that must be maintained for optimum osmotic balance, stable pH, and proper nerve firing and muscle contraction. Any deviation from this ratio is undesirable, manifesting overt circulatory problems and a sluggish or nervous personality. Edema is a result of sodium/potassium imbalance; so is sluggishness, poor circulation, and nervous hyperirritability. If the ratio rises above 32/1, look for poor circulation and a highly nervous demeanor.

The balance must be kept between sodium and potassium. In the use of any salt or salt-free diet, you must check these two to know whether the body needs them or does not need them. We have seen more people who do not have enough sodium or enough potassium in their bodies, and we have to give supplements of both of them to bring them up to where they belong to get their proper nerve and blood circulation. I often say, "If you put your patient on a salt-free diet without having checked their potassium, you, sir, are a quack; you are not a doctor!"

T4 (Thyroxine)

The T4 test is a test for the presence of thyroxine, a molecule that bears four iodine atoms. Ingested iodine is converted to iodide and absorbed, the thyroid gland taking up iodide via a mechanism called the iodide pump. Within the gland, iodide is oxidized to iodine and bound to the 3-position of the tyrosine molecules, which are attached to the protein, thyroglobulin. Iodination forms 23% mono-iodotyrosine, 33% di-iodotyrosine, 35% thyroxine, and 7% tri-iodotyrosine. About 80 micrograms per day of thyroxine is secreted into the blood where it is bound to plasma proteins. The protein bound iodine (PBI) is contained 95% within the thyroxine molecule. Since 65% of the weight of thyroxine is due to iodine, PBI ranges approximate 65% of the normal range values given for the T4.

T4 Level Within the Normal Range

A normal T4 indicates the possibility of a normally functioning thyroid. However, it is still necessary to know if the level of inorganic iodine is within normal limits (2.0 ideal) before any assumption is made that the thyroid gland is functioning normally. The T4 level may be normal even following the administration of non-thyroidal iodine, radiopaque substances, or mercurial diuretics.

T4 Level Above the Normal Range

An elevated T4 indicates the possibility of the condition called hyperthyroidism. However, true hyperthyroidism displays symptoms such as tachycardia, tremors (especially of the protruding tongue), sweating (especially moist skin on the palms of the hands), weight loss with increased appetite, vertigo, an intense personality, and a frightened appearance. Some conditions associated with an elevated T4 are as follows.

T4 Level Above the Normal Range	
Body System	**Possible Condition**
Digestive	Certain cases of hepatitis
Endocrine	Thyroiditis Cretinism
Reproductive	Normal pregnancy
Systemic	Following administration of certain drugs, such as estrogens, birth control pills, d-thyroxine, thyroid extract, thyroid-stimulating hormone. After use of certain cough syrups, toothpastes, and antiseptics Overconsumption of fish
Miscellaneous	The specimen over 72 hours old Recent radioactive testing (brain scan)

T4 Level Below the Normal Range

A depressed T4 may indicate hypothyroidism. This condition is associated with a host of symptoms such as sensitivity to cold, fatigueability, skin rashes, vague abdominal symptoms, weight gain (especially of the upper body), mental dullness, inability to work under stress, retardation of bone development, enuresis, menstrual disorders, male sterility, coarse hair, thickening brittle nails, lowered body temperature, numbness and tingling sensations, and a slow personality. Diagnosed conditions found in conjunction with hypothyroidism are listed below.

T4 Level Below the Normal Range	
Body System	**Possible Condition**
Urinary	Nephrosis Hypoalbuminuria
Endocrine	Myxedema Cretinism
Systemic	Following administration of certain drugs, such as Dilantin, ACTH, corticosteroids, triiodothyronine, testosterone, mercury compounds. Hypoproteinemia (There may not be enough circulating proteins in the blood. Therefore, the T4 can be low, not because of hypofunction of the thyroid, but because of too little available protein to act as a thyroxine carrier.)

Triglycerides

Triglycerides, or neutral fats, consist of a glycerol molecule connected to three fatty acids. These fatty acids may be saturated (no double bonds) or unsaturated (one or more double bonds) and may be of various length. Short chain fatty acids (less than 10 carbon atoms) are split off from the glycerol portion in the intestine and are absorbed into the portal blood.

Dietary sources high in short chain fatty acids are starches, sugars, and fruits, the cltrus fruits being especially rich. Long chain fatty acids (more than 10 carbon atoms) are reassembled into triglycerides in the intestine, complexed with proteins, cholesterol, and phospholipids to form chylomicrons. These complexes enter the lymphatic ducts and move into the bloodstream. Chylomicrons are about one micron in diameter and are so numerous in the blood after meals, that the plasma takes on a milky appearance. These bodies are cleared from the blood by the clearing factor (a lipase enzyme), and the fats are stored in the body's fat deposits or depots. From these depots, fat is discharged into the blood as free fatty acids (4).

Triglyceride Level Within the Normal Range

A normal triglyceride level may be an indicator of the absence of significant arteriosclerosis, but a more reliable indicator is the atherogenic index, which takes into account the density pattern of the various lipids contained in the blood. A normal value for triglycerides indicates, however, that the patient has probably fasted properly before the test.

Triglyceride Level Above the Normal Range

Elevated triglycerides implies a condition called hyperlipidemia. This usually indicates that there are more sugar and starches in the diet than the body can tolerate. To more accurately assess the significance of such an elevation, an electrophoretic separation of the various classes of lipids should be performed.

Elevation of serum triglycerides may be observed if the patient has not properly fasted before the test or if the diet is high in starchy or sugary foods, citrus fruits being one of the most troublesome. The high fructose diet is especially undesirable, because fructose causes an accumulation of glycerol in the liver, followed by attachment of fatty acids to form triglycerides.

If there is insufficient consumption and assimilation of proteins, these triglycerides cannot be efficiently transported out of the liver. Hence, elevated triglycerides and low serum proteins can effect liver congestion. Use of alcohol and tobacco can bring about chronic elevations of triglycerides; some disorders associated with elevated triglycerides are listed below.

Triglyceride Level Above the Normal Range	
Body System	**Possible Condition**
Digestive	Liver disease Alcoholism (the total bilirubin will probably also be elevated) Obesity Von Gierke's disease Pancreatitis
Circulatory/Blood/Lymph	Hyperlipidemia Atherosclerosis After myocardial infarction (The triglyceride value may not normalize for one year; there are also elevations of LDH, SGOT, and SGPT.)
Urinary	Nephritis Nephrosis
Endocrine	Hypothyroidism Diabetes mellitus
Systemic	Gout Certain medications may raise serum triglycerides; some are: estrogens, birth control pills, and cholestyramine. **Note:** There is a pattern of test values for cholesterol, triglycerides, and the various types of lipoproteins that characterize the different types of hyperlipoproteinemias. For a chart of these patterns, see (2), Table 50, pages 352-353.

Triglyceride Level Below the Normal Range

A depressed triglyceride level does not carry any particular pathologic significance. It may suggest malnutrition or congenital alpha-beta lipoproteinemia, in which the LDL fraction is absent, the HDL fraction is within normal limits, and the values for triglycerides and cholesterol are markedly decreased. Some medications that may depress serum triglycerides are ascorbic acid (vitamin C therapy), asparaginase, Clofibrate, Metformin, and Phenformin.

Uric Acid (UA)

Uric acid is the end product of purine metabolism. Purines are derived from the diet directly from foods high in nucleic acids, and indirectly from the condensation of amino acids. Amino acids are supplied in the diet in the form of proteins, or they can be manufactured from glucose. Therefore, it is easy to see how imbalances and indiscretions in eating habits can raise the uric acid level.

Dietary sources of uric acid itself are pork, red meat, and shellfish; foods that do not contain significant amounts of uric acid, but which cause elevations in the serum uric acid levels are milk, alcohol, and foods rich in nucleic acids, such as yeast and sardines.

Uric acid is cleared from the bloodstream by the kidneys via glomerular filtration and tubular secretion (1). It is stored in the kidneys to be released and destroyed by the liver. The working maximum of the normal range for men is 6 mg% and for women is 5 mg%. Any value above this maximum is indicative of gout.

Uric Acid Level Within the Normal Range

Although a normal uric acid level makes the diagnosis of gout unlikely, it should not be ruled out as a possibility. It should be remembered that uric acid levels show day-to-day and seasonal variations and are much influenced by stress and total fasting (effect elevation) (2).

It is practical to assign a lower working normal maximum value to detect problems before gout becomes clinical. Over the years, it has become useful to assign any value over 5.0 mg for females and 6.0 mg for males as potentially pathological! The patient that shows such values is a prime candidate for gout or gouty arthritis, depending on the relative levels of calcium and phosphorus in the blood (see Calcium/Phosphorus Ratio (Ca/P), above).

Uric Acid Level Above the Normal Range

A uric acid level above accepted laboratory normals is termed hyperuricemia. This condition is usually synonymous with gout and found to be increased in 25% of the relatives of patients with gout. Kidney damage is a common occurrence with gout, but the uric acid level is not a good indicator of the extent of kidney damage; the BUN and creatinine levels are usually elevated, and their values are better indicators.

Certain population groups display higher normal values; these include the Blackfoot and Pima Indians, Filipinos, and the New Zealand Maoris. Further, persons with high blood pressure and arteriosclerosis commonly show elevated uric acid in 80% of those with elevated triglycerides (2).

A high amount of uric acid indicates the inability of the person to produce enough hydrochloric acid. The main foods that he or she should not eat are pork, red meat (muscle meat), shellfish, milk, and alcohol. Excessive elevations of serum uric acid are observed in the following situations.

Uric Acid Level Above the Normal Range	
Body System	**Possible Condition**
Skeletal	Rheumatoid arthritis
Digestive	A high protein, weight reduction diet Ingestion of excess nucleoproteins (sweetbreads, liver, etc.) Liver disease Consumption of caffeine
Circulatory/Blood/Lymph	Leukemia * Multiple myeloma * Hemolytic anemia * Sickle cell anemia * Severe heart failure Remission from pernicious anemia
Urinary	Renal failure Polycystic kidneys Acute and chronic nephritis (especially before a rise in nonprotein nitrogen (NPN), urea, and creatinine) Pyelonephritis Pyelonephrosis Hydronephrosis Reflex anuria
Endocrine	Hypoparathyroidism Primary hyperparathyroidism Hypothyroidism
Reproductive	Eclampsia (monitor progress with successive serum assays) *

Systemic	Psoriasis (A third of all patients exhibit elevated uric acid; see also possible elevation in cholesterol.) Chronic dermatitis Lobar pneumonia Resolving pneumonia * Gout Various disseminated neoplasms * During cancer chemotherapy Alcoholism Von Gierke's disease Lead poisoning (possibly associated with drinking moonshine whiskey) Lesch-Nyhan syndrome Maple syrup urine disease Down's syndrome Calcinosis universalis and circumscripta Sarcoidosis Chronic berylliosis Asymptomatic hyperuricemia Use of certain drugs and medications, such as thiazides, furosemide, nitrogen mustards, vincristine, mercaptopurine, ethacrynic acid, salicylates, acetazolamide, hydralazine, and propylthiouracil.
Miscellaneous	* In these situations, the mechanism is the destruction of nucleoproteins to purines and pyrimidines with subsequent conversion to uric acid.

Uric Acid Level Below the Normal Range

A depression of the uric acid level is termed hypouricemia. It is often observed in conjunction with the following conditions.

Uric Acid Level Below the Normal Range	
Body System	**Possible Condition**
Digestive	Celiac disease (slight decrease)
Circulatory/Blood/Lymph	Pernicious anemia (slight decrease in relapse)
Urinary	Fanconi's syndrome (proximal renal tubular abnormalities) Dalmation dog mutation (defective tubular transport)
Endocrine	Admnistration of ACTH Acromegaly
Systemic	Wilson's disease (copper accumulation in the tissues) Xanthinuria Some neoplasms (carcinomas, Hodgkin's disease) Use of certain agents, such as X-ray contrast medium, glyceryl guaiacolate Use of certain drugs and medications, such as salicylates, probenecid, cortisone, allopurinol, coumarins, chlorpromazine, cinchophen, clofibrate, corticotropin, and phenylbutazone.

Suggested References

1. Tilkian, S. M., and Conover, M. H., *Clinical Implications of Laboratory Tests*, The C. V. Mosby Company, St. Louis, 1975. (1)

2. Wallach, J., *Interpretation of Diagnostic Tests: A Handbook Synopsis of Laboratory Medicine*, 3rd edition, Little, Brown and Company, Boston, 1978. (2)

3. Harper, H. A., *Review of Physiological Chemistry, 14th edition*, Lange Medical Publications, Los Altos, California, 1973. (3)

4. Garong, W. F., *Review of Medical Physiology, 5th edition*, Lange Medical Publications, Los Altos, California, 1971. (4)

5. Holvey, D. N., ed., *The Merck Manual of Diagnosis and Therapy, 12th edition*, Merck, Sharp, and Dohme Research Laboratories, Rahway, New Jersey, 1972. (5)

6. Medical Services Company of Arizona, *Quick Reference Laboratory Manual, 2nd edition*, Medical Services Company of Arizona, Phoenix, 1977. (6)

7. Asimov, I., *The Bloodstream*, Collier Books, London, 1961. (7)

8. Garb, S., *Laboratory Tests in Common Use, 5th edition*, Springer Publishing Company, Inc., New York, 1971. (8)

9. Widmann, F. K., *Goodale's Clinical Interpretation of Laboratory Tests*, 7th edition, F. A. Davis Company, Philadelphia, 1973. (9)

10. Benson, E. S., and Strandjord, P. E., eds., *Multiple Laboratory Screening*, Academic Press, New York, 1969. (10)

11. Thomas, C. L., ed., *Taber's Cyclopedic Medical Dictionary, 14th edition*, F. A. Davis Company, Philadelphia, 1981. (11)

12. Steen, E. B., and Montagu, A., *Anatomy and Physiology, Vol. 1*, Barnes and Noble, New York, 1959. (12)

13. Schutte, K. H. and Myers, J. A., *Metabolic Aspects of Health: Nutritional Elements in Health and Disease*, Discovery Press, Kentfield, California, 1979. (13)

14 Correlated Blood Chemistry Patterns

I have used many laboratories that have provided reliable test results; they generally do a good job. However, the problem with using blood chemistry results is with the person reviewing them. **Inattention to the meaning of slight deviations of patient values from the optimum and, further, a lack of understanding of important correlations among individual tests can result in these reports losing much of their usefulness.**

Usually, a physician will scan a blood panel report and look only for extremely high or low values on individual tests. Occasionally, he will correlate a few values, such as LDH, SGOT, SGPT, and triglycerides, but he usually misses other high or low normal values and important ratios – especially those that have not been calculated for him and, therefore, do not appear on the report. This is unfortunate, because correlation of blood serum chemistry values can reveal tendencies and narrow down the focus of a diagnosis. In short, there is very little about the physiology of the body that cannot be resolved by proper analysis of blood, urine, and hair.

Test Pattern vs. Possible Condition

in the following array of test results, the patterns are listed in the left column, with possible associated conditions listed in the right column. In this section, **N** = a value within the normal range; **<** = a value below the normal range; and **>** = a value above the normal range. A <> entry indicates that a test result is abnormal, being outside of the normal range, under or over.

Editor: Correlations not marked with an asterisk were derived from Dr. Ellis' personal notes. Correlations marked with an asterisk (*) were obtained from Reese, R. L. and Hobbie, R. K., *Computer evaluation of chemistry values: a reporting and diagnostic aid, American Journal of Clinical Pathology,* 57:664-675, 1972. For detail on how the investigators resolved these patterns, see the article.

Dr. Ellis' values are assigned relative strengths, such as a **<** may signify one standard deviation below (low); a **<<** may signify two standard deviations below (very low); and a **<<<** may signify three standard deviations below the normal mean (extremely low). Likewise, a single **>** may signify one standard deviation above (high); a **>>** may signify two standard deviations above (very high); and a **>>>** may signify three standard deviations above the normal mean (extremely high). **Reese and Hobbie define values as low (<) or high (>), but do not attempt any further subdivision.**

To make it easier to compare actual combinations of test results with the indicated pattern or patterns, arrange test result values (usually only those that deviate from laboratory normals) in ascending alphabetical order based on the name of the test. Albumin/Globulin Ratio (A/G)

A/G<	Hypochlorhydria (if < 1.7), achlorhydria (if < 1.1)

Alpha-1-Globulin (A1G)

A1G< (< 0.25 gm)	Protein is not being made available to the cells (may indicate the need for pancreatic enzymes)
A1G>	Protein is being depleted from cellular structures

Alpha-2-Globulin (A2G)

A2G<	Protein is not being made available to the cells (may indicate the need for a hormone-related supplement)
A2G> (> 1.0 gm%) BG> CA/P> UA>	Rheumatoid arthritis
A2G>	Possible hormone imbalance

Albumin (Alb)

ALB<	Chronic liver disease, lack of hydrochloric acid and pepsin
ALB< AP< BILI> BUN< CHOL< GLU< LDH> SGOT> TP>	Acute or chronic viral hepatitis *
ALB< AP< CA< CHOL> TP<	Use of estrogens or oral contraceptives *
ALB< AP> BILI> BUN< CHOL> LDH> SGOT> TP>	Subacute hepatitis or biliary cirrhosis (an elevated SGOT is essential) *
ALB< AP> BILI> BUN< GLU> LDH> P> SGOT> TP<>	Liver disease (fatty degeneration) or cirrhosis (a rise in the bilirubin is essential *)

ALB< AP> BILI> BUN> CHOL> GLU> LDH> SGOT> UA>	Degenerative vascular disease that may be associated with generalized arteriosclerosis, heart failure, hypertension, and obesity *
ALB< AP> BILI> CA> LDH> P> SGOT> TP> UA>	Metastatic tumor in the liver (a rise in the AP is essential) *
ALB< AP> BILI> CA> LDH> P> SGOT> TP> UA> + lipemic serum	Ingestion of alcohol or alcoholic hepatitis (a rise in the SGOT is essential) *
ALB< AP> BILI> CA> LDH> P> SGOT> TP< UA>	Carcinoma *
ALB< AP> BILI> CHOL< LDH> SGOT> TP<	Hepatic or biliary damage due to drugs or cholecystitis *
ALB< AP> BILI> CHOL> LDH> SGOT> TP< + lipemic serum	Obstructive hepatic disease
ALB< AP> BILI> LDH> SGOT> TP>	Collagen disease (especially lupus and lupus hepatitis) *
ALB< AP> BUN< CA< CHOL> GLU> TP< + lipemic serum	Normal in pregnancy *
ALB< AP> BUN> CA< CHOL< GLU> LDH> P> SGOT> TP< UA>	Renal insufficiency (an elevated BUN is essential) *
ALB< AP> BUN> CA< GLU> LDH> TP< SGOT> + lipemic serum	Pancreatitis *
ALB< AP> BUN> CA< GLU> LDH> P> SGOT> TP< UA>	Prerenal azotemia due to cardiac heart failure, shock, etc. (an elevated BUN is essential)
ALB< AP> BUN> CHOL> GLU> LDH> SGOT> UA>	Myocardial infarction (an elevated SGOT is essential) *
ALB< AP> CA< CHOL< GLU> P< TP<	Ulcerative colitis or intestinal obstruction
ALB< AP> CA< CHOL< SGOT> TP<	Regional enteritis *
ALB< AP> CA> CHOL< P<	Hyperthyroidism *
ALB< AP> CA> LDH> P> SGOT> TP< UA>	Bone metastasis *
ALB< AP> CA> P>	Paget's disease *, immobilization due to paraplegia fracture
ALB< AP> CA> TP<	Prolonged immobilization *
ALB< BILI> BUN> P< UA>	Gastrointestinal bleeding *
ALB< BILI> CA<> LDH> TP<> UA>	Leukemia, other myeloproliferative diseases *
ALB< BUN< CA< CHOL< GLU<> P< TP< UA<	Malabsorption or malnutrition *
ALB< BUN< CA< CHOL< P< TP< UA<	Overhydration (excessive fluids) *
ALB< BUN> CHOL> GLU> LDH> SGOT>	Stroke *

ALB< BUN> CHOL> GLU> TP< + lipemic serum	Nephrotic syndrome *
ALB< CA<	Possible pseudohypocalcemia, especially if the percentage of deviation from the ideal mean of each are identical
ALB< CA=N	Possible hypercalcemia (CA should be depressed if ALB is depressed)
ALB< CA> LDH> TP<> UA>	Lymphoma (Hodgkin's disease) *
ALB< GLOB< TP<	Protein losing enteropathy
ALB< GLOB> TP<	Lack of HCl and pepsin
ALB< IgA> IgM> TP>	Cystic fibrosis of the pancreas
ALB< LDH> TP> UA>	Rheumatic fever *
ALB< P< TP<	Peptic ulcer *
ALB<< CA<	False hypocalcemia (pseudohypocalcemia)
ALB=N BILI> (> 1.5 mg/dL)	Obstructive jaundice
ALB=N BUN> B/C> (> 10) CREAT>	Acute glomerulonephritis
ALB=N CA< C02< PH=N or >	Hypocalcemia with respiratory alkalosis
ALB>	Possible dehydration, malignancy
ALB> AP> BILI> BUN> CA> CHOL> GLU> LDH> P> SGOT> TP> UA>	Dehydration of patient or evaporation of the specimen (an elevated TP is essential) *
ALB> AP> BUN> CA> CHOL> GLU> LDH> P< SGOT> TP> UA> + lipemic serum	A non-fasting specimen or hyperlipoproteinemia (lipemic serum is essential) *
ALB> AP> BUN> GLU> P< + lipemic serum	A non-fasting specimen *
ALB> AP> GLU< LDH> P> SGOT> TP>	Serum artifact (The specimen is old, has been overheated, or the serum has remained in contact with the clot for an excessive period of time.) *
ALB> BUN> CHOL> GLU> UA>	Recent ingestion of a high-protein meal (values borderline) *
ALB> CA> TP>	Contamination of test tubes by detergent *
ALB> CA> TP>	Dehydration from enemas for X-ray studies (elevation of all three values are essential) *
ALB> TP>	Administration of BSP dye *

Alkaline Phosphatase (Alk Phos, AP)

AP< BILI> CHOL< LDH> SGOT> UA>	Pernicious or macrocytic anemia (check the MCV and MCHC for confirmation) (an elevated LDH is essential) *
AP< P<	Hypophosphatasia, achondroplasia, cretinism, or vitamin deficiency (hypophosphatasia is very rare)
AP> BILI> CHOL> LDH> SGOT>	Hypersensitivity, cholestatic hepatitis from drugs (a rise in the SGOT is essential)
AP> BILI> CHOL> LDH> SGOT> UA>	Infectious mononucleosis *
AP> BILI> LDH> P> SGOT> UA>	Tissue necrosis, abcess, gangrene, peritonitis *
AP> BILI> LDH> SGOT> UA>	Pulmonary embolism or infarction *
AP> BUN> CA< GLU> TP< UA>	Toxemia of pregnancy *
AP> BUN> CA> P< UA>	Hyperparathyroidism (an elevated CA is essential)
AP> BUN> CA> P<>	Hypervitaminosis D (an elevated CA is essential) *
AP> BUN> CA> P> TP> UA> + lipemic serum	Plasma cell myeloma (an elevated TP is essential) *
AP> BUN> CHOL> GLU> LDH> SGOT> UA> + lipemic serum	Diabetes mellitus *
AP> CA< P<	Osteomalacia, steatorrhea, vitamin D deficiency, rickets *
AP> CA< P>	Pseudohypoparathyroidism *
AP> CA=N or > P<	Rickets or osteomalacia
AP> CA>	Paget's disease, multiple myeloma, osteomalacia, rickets, or hyperparathyroidism, prostatic cancer (see the level of acid phosphatase – a specialized test, not part of a standard battery of tests)
AP> SGOT> SGPT>	Cholangiolytic hepatitis or cirrhosis
AP>> SGOT=N SGPT=N	Paget's disease or osteogenic sarcoma
AP>>> (5X normal mean) BILI> SGOT> SGPT>	Early stages of obstructive jaundice

BUN/Creatinine Ratio (B/C)

B/C< (< 10)	Loss of protein through diet, dialysis, severe diarrhea, or vomiting (hepatic insufficiency is also possible)
B/C< (< 10) FE<	Nephrosis due to an iron-binding protein in the urine
B/C> (> 10)	Impaired kidney function

Beta Globulin (BG)

BG>	Loss of bone and joint protein, arthritis
BG> CA/P> UA> (> 5.0 mg/dL)	Arthritic syndrome (if UA >5.0, arthritis is probable)

Bilirubin (BILI)

BILI<< (< 0.1 mg/dL)	Aplastic anemia (check MCHC, MCV, HGB, FE, and TP) This usually results from toxic agents of carcinoma or chronic nephritis (check B/C ratio and BUN).
BILI> (> 1.5 mg/dL)	Obstructive jaundice, bile is too thick (By definition, jaundice occurs when the BILI level exceeds 1.5 mg/dL.) Never give a B complex when the bile Is thick.
BILI>	May bring about false elevations of ALB CHOL and TP *
BILI> BUN> CHOL> LDH> SGOT> TP> UA> + hemolyzed specimen	Hemolysis due to venipuncture
BILI> FE=N	Possible biliary obstruction
BILI> GLU> SGOT> UA>	Strict diet with rapid weight loss *
BILI>> (> 3.0 mg/dL)	Clinical signs of jaundice appear
BILI>>> (> 12.0 mg/dL) HGB < + reticulocytosis	Massive hemolysis

Blood Urea Nitrogen (BUN)

BUN< (6-8 mg/dL)	Overhydration, check TP to see if it is depressed (possible liver or kidney disease, involving infection, protein non-utilization, malabsorption, adrenal malfunction, etc.)
BUN< (> 8 mg/dL)	Impaired absorption, low protein/high carbohydrate diet, increased protein utilization (check ALB and ESR). Also check for other signs of disease, pregnancy, or an increased rate of growth.
BUN=N CA< CREA=N P>	Hypoparathyroidism
BUN=N CREA=N P=N	Milk-alkali syndrome or sarcoidosis if clinical symptoms are present
BUN>	Lowered efficiency of protein metabolism, thick bile, less-than-optimal liver function. The kidneys are not necessarily diseased, but any elevation of the BUN indicates that the glomerular filtration rate is less than 50 ml/min (the normal rate is 125 ml/min). Kidney disease is likely to develop if the physiology is not modified. The physician is well-advised to check for infection.
BUN> CA< UA>	Excessive transfusions *
BUN> CA> GLU> P< UA>	Use of thiazide diuretics (an elevated UA is essential) *
BUN> CA> P> UA>	Milk-alkali syndrome *
BUN> CA> UA>	Acute renal failure (an elevated BUN is essential) *
BUN> CA> UA>	Certain cases of hypertension *
BUN> CREAT> B/C> (> 10)	Acute glomerulonephritis
BUN> GLU< K> NA<>	Adrenocortical hypofunction (Addison's disease)
BUN> GLU>>> (> 500 mg/dL) NA> TP>	Vascular disease (dehydration and hypernatremia are usually associated with hyperglycemia in the elderly)
BUN> K> NA<	Mild dehydration, possible Addison's disease (check TP>)
BUN> LDH> SGOT>	Renal infarction *
BUN>> (50-150 mg/dL)	Serious renal impairment

BUN>>> (150-250 mg/dL)	Conclusive evidence of severely impaired glomerular function

Calcium (Ca)

When considering the serum calcium level, one must always take into account the albumin (ALB) level. If the CA is high, but if the ALB is also high, this may not indicate hypercalcemia. If the CA is high, accompanied by a normal ALB, hypercalcemia is a distinct possibility. If CA is normal, but the ALB is low, hypercalcemia is also possible.

CA< P<	Use of alkaline antacids *
CA< P>	Hypoparathyroidism * (probable muscular pains with periodontal disease)
CA>	Laboratory artifact (if no other tests are elevated, the screening tests should be performed again)
CA> BUN> GLU>	Cushing's syndrome *
CA> CO_2=N or > pH>	Milk-alkali syndrome, peptic ulcer (suggests ingestion of large quantities of milk and antacids)
CA> GG>	Sarcoidosis, multiple myeloma, malignancy
CA> GG> LDH)	Possible malignancy, selenium poisoning, sarcoidosis, multiple myeloma
CA> GLU<	Adrenal insufficiency *
CA> P<	Hyperparathyroidism, periodontal disease, arthritic syndrome (possibly the result of a diet high in refined foods)
CA> P< TP>	Sarcoidosis *
CA> TP>	Sarcoidosis or multiple myeloma
CA>> TP<	Hyperparathyroidism

Carbon Dioxide (CO_2)

CO_2< (< 10 mEq/liter) K=N	Probable metabolic acidosis
CO^2> (> 35 mEq/liter) K=N	Probable metabolic alkalosis

Cholesterol (CHOL)

CHOL< GLU< SGOT> UA<	Administration of salicylates *
CHOL< GLU> UA>	Administration of nicotinic acid *
CHOL<< (< 150 mg/dL)	Malnutrition, liver damage, administration of cortisone, hyperthyroidism (check the diet, also check for exposure to chemicals, drugs, or alcohol)
CHOL<> GLU> UA<	Administration of corticoids *
CHOL>	Slight elevation in normal pregnancy
CHOL> GLU< LDH> SGOT> TP> + lipemic serum	Hypothyroidism *
CHOL> GLU> UA> + lipemic serum	Hyperlipoproteinemias *
CHOL> GLU> UA>	Gout (an elevated UA is essential) *
CHOL>> (> 400 mg/dL)	Biliary obstruction (if BILI is greater than 1.5 mg and ALB is normal), hypothyroidism, nephrosis, pancreatic disease, psoriasis, use of ether anaesthesia

Chloride (Cl)

CL< CO_2> K<	Hypochloremia, associated with hypokalemia and alkalosis
CL> CO_2< K< NA<	Hyperchloremia – most frequently associated with renal tubular acidosis, decreased CO_2 combining power, and hypokalemia

Creatinine (CREA)

CREA<	Low meat consumption, protein inavailability (Possibly, the kidneys are not functioning as well as they could. Check the ALB, A/G ratio and TP, in addition to the BUN/CREA ratio.)
CREA>	Meat-rich diet, muscle degeneration, or kidney disorder (It is best to consider the BUN/CREA ratio before making any conclusions regarding the health of the kidneys.)

Gamma Globulin (GG)

GG<	Protein is being depleted from cellular structures
GG>	Insufficient antibodies necessary to fight infection

Globulin (GLOB)

GLOB>	Hypochlorhydria (if 2.7-3.5 gm/dL), achlorhydria (if > 3.5 gm/dL)

Glucose (GLU)

GLU<	Possible hypoglycemia (check potassium in the blood, as well as ALB; also check the levels of chromium, manganese, and zinc in a hair mineral analysis)
GLU>	Possible diet rich in refined carbohydrates (check chromium, copper, manganese, potassium, and zinc levels in a hair mineral analysis)
GLU> (120-130 mg/dL) CHOL<	Probable hyperthyroidism
GLU> NA>	Possible hypothalamic lesion, head trauma, or hyperosmolar state
GLU>> (300-500 mg/dL)	Diagnostic for diabetes mellitus
GLU>>> (> 500 mg/dL)	Serious hyperglycemia with oxidative phosphorylation uncoupling (indicates interference with mitochondrial function)

Immunoglobulins (Ig)

IgA< IgG< IgM< TP<	Heavy chain disease
IgA> IgG> TP=N	Possible polyarteritis nodosa
IgM>> TP>	Macroglobulinemia

Iron (Fe)

FE< MCHC < 30 MCV < 80 micon^3	Iron deficiency anemia
FE< MCHC < 30 MCV < 95 micron^3	Pernicious anemia
FE< MCHC < 30 MCV=N	Normochromic anemia
FE> MCHC > 30 MCV=N	Hemolytic anemia
FE> SGOT> SGPT>	Acute liver damage

Lactic Dehydrogenase (LDH)

LDH> SGOT>	Seizures or muscular diseases (dystrophy, dermatomyositis, etc.) *
LDH> SGOT> SGPT> TRIG>	Myocardial infarction, possible malignancy or metal poisoning
LDH>>	Hemolytic disorder (check FE, MCHC, MCV, RBC), aluminum, lead, or nickel poisoning (check these levels in a hair mineral analysis), or possible malignancy (check the level of selenium in the hair)

Lipids (LIPID)

LIPID<	Possible hyperthyroidism (see T4, CHOL)
LIPID>	Find primary disorder that is causing hyperlipidemia, modify diet on a long-term basis

Phosphorus (P, PO_4)

P<	Periodontal disease (if P below 3.0 mg) increased susceptibility to caries, renal tubular acidosis (see BUN, CREAT, CO_2), malabsorption (see mineral levels in the hair), or hyperinsulinism

Potassium (K)

K> NA<	Dehydration, (check fluid intake, A/G ratio, TP), results in poor circulation and nervousness or sluggishness

Protein-Bound Iodine (PBI/I_2 Ratio)

PBI/I2 (<< 2.0)	True hypothyroidism
PBI/I2) (> 4.0)	True hyperthyroidism

Serum Glutamate Pyruvate Transferase (SGPT)

SGPT> (> 50 units)	Cirrhosis, extra biliary metastatic carcinoma of the liver (see the other possible liver damage – AP, BILI, LDH, SGOT)

Sodium (Na)

NA> (> 145)	Hypoproteinemia (check TP), congestive heart failure, administration of salt solutions, Cushing's syndrome, lower nephron nephrosis, administration of ACTH or cortisone

Sodium/Potassium Ratio (Na/K)

NA/K>	Poor circulation and nervousness

Total Protein (TP)

TP<	Possible malabsorption or liver disease
TP> UA>	Infection *

Triglycerides (TRIG)

TRIG<	Congenital alpha-beta lipoproteinemia or malnutrition

Uric Acid (UA)

UA<	Salicylate, ACTH, or cortisone therapy, Wilson's disease (check the level of copper in a hair mineral analysis)
UA=N	This does not rule out gout
UA> + elevated alpha lipoprotein	Rheumatoid arthritis
UA>	Gout possible (Any value of > 5 mg/dL for women and > 6 mg/dL for men is pathologic and indicates a wide variety of possible conditions. The level of UA varies in response to stress, emotional state, and to season.)

Condition vs. Possible Test Pattern

In this section, conditions are listed in the left column, with possible associated test patterns listed in the right column. These are adapted from Table 3, Reese, R. L. and Hobbie, R. K., *Computer evaluation of chemistry values: a reporting and diagnostic aid, American Journal of Clinical Pathology,* 57:664-675, 1972.

Condition	Possible Test Pattern
Alcohol ingestion or alcoholic hepatitis	Low CA
	Low TP
	Low ALB
	High CA
	High P
	High UA
	High TP
	High LDH
	High SGOT
	High BILI
	High AP
	Lipemic serum

Circulatory/Blood/Lymph: Hemolysis from venipuncture, serum on clot, or hemolytic anemia	High BUN High UA High CHOL High TP High LDH High SGOT High BILI Hemolyzed specimen essential
Circulatory/Blood/Lymph: Infectious mononucleosis	High UA High CHOL High LDH High SGOT High BILI High AP
Circulatory/Blood/Lymph: Leukemia or other myeloproliferative disorders	Low CA Low TP Low ALB High CA High UA High TP High LDH High BILI

Circulatory/Blood/Lymph: Lipemic serum (non-fasting, hyperlipoproteinemia, etc.)	Low P High CA High GLU High BUN High UA High CHOL High TP High LDH High SGOT High ALB High AP Lipemic serum essential
Circulatory/Blood/Lymph: Lymphoma (Hodgkin's disease)	Low TP Low ALB High CA High UA High TP High LDH
Circulatory/Blood/Lymph: Pernicious anemia or other macrocytic anemia	Low AP High UA High LDH essential High SGOT High BILI Low CHOL
Circulatory/Blood/Lymph: Plasma cell myeloma	High CA High P High BUN High UA High TP essential High AP Lipemic serum

Circulatory/Blood/Lymph: Myocardial infarction	Low ALB High GLU High BUN High UA High CHOL High LDH High SGOT essential High AP
Circulatory/Blood/Lymph: Vascular disease, degenerative (heart failure, generalized arteriosclerosis, hypertension, obesity)	Low ALB High GLU High BUN High UA High CHOL High LDH High SGOT High BILI High AP
Digestive: Gastrointestinal bleeding	Low ALB Low P High BUN High UA High BILI
Digestive: Hyperlipoproteinemias	High GLU High UA High CHOL Lipemic serum

Digestive: Malabsorption or malnutrition	Low CA Low P Low GLU Low BUN Low UA Low CHOL Low TP Low ALB High GLU
Digestive: Pancreatitis	Low CA Low TP Low ALB High GLU High BUN High LDH High SGOT High AP Lipemic serum
Digestive: Peptic ulcer	Low P Low TP Low ALB
Digestive: Regional enteritis	Low CA High AP High SGOT Low CHOL Low TP Low ALB
Digestive: Steatorrhea	Low CA Low P High AP

Digestive: Ulcerative colitis, intestinal obstruction, etc.	Low CA Low P Low CHOL Low TP Low ALB High GLU High AP
Drug Use: Hepatic or biliary damage from drugs (hepatitis or cholecystitis)	Low CHOL Low TP Low ALB High LDH High SGOT High BILI High AP
Drug Use: Nicotinic acid	Low CHOL High GLU High UA
Eating: Milk alkali syndrome	High CA High P High BUN High UA
Eating: Recent ingestion of high protein meal, borderline high values	High GLU High BUN High UA High CHOL High ALB
Eating: Strict diet with rapid weight loss	High GLU High UA High BILI High SGOT
Endocrine: Adrenal insufficiency	Low GLU High CA

Endocrine: Cushing's syndrome	High CA High GLU High BUN
Endocrine: Hyperparathyroidism	Low P High CA essential High BUN High AP High UA
Endocrine: Hyperthyroidism	Low P Low CHOL Low ALB High CA High AP
Endocrine: Hypoparathyroidism	Low CA High P
Endocrine: Pseudohypoparathyroidism	Low CA High P High AP
Hypertension: Certain cases	High CA High BUN High UA
Immobilization: Paraplegia, fracture, Paget's disease	High CA High P High AP Low ALB
Immobilization: Prolonged	Low TP Low ALB High CA High AP
Infection: Pneumonia, abcesses, etc.	High UA High TP

Infection: Rheumatic fever	Low ALB High TP High LDH High UA
Infection: Tissue necrosis (abscess, gangrene, peritonitis)	High P High UA High LDH High SGOT High BILI High AP
Laboratory Artifact: BSP dye use	High TP High ALB
Laboratory Artifact: Contamination of test tubes by detergent	High CA High TP High ALB
Laboratory Artifact: Nonfasting specimen	Low P High GLU High BUN High ALB High AP
Laboratory Artifact: Serum may be old, overheated, or too long on clot	Low GLU High P High TP High LDH High SGOT High ALB High AP
Laboratory Artifact: These tests may be falsely high if BILI is high	High CHOL High TP High ALB High BILI essential

Liver: Acute or chronic viral hepatitis	Low GLU Low BUN Low CHOL Low TP Low ALB High TP High LDH High SGOT essential High BILI High AP
Liver: Cirrhosis	Low BUN Low TP Low ALB High GLU High UA High TP High LDH High SGOT High BILI essential High AP
Liver: Hepatic disease (fatty metamorphosis)	Low BUN Low TP Low ALB High P High CHOL High TP High LDH High SGOT High BILI High AP

Liver: Hypersensitivity cholestatic hepatitis from drugs	High CHOL High LDH High SGOT essential High BILI High AP
Liver: Metastatic tumor in liver	Low TP Low ALB High CA High P High UA High TP High LDH High SGOT High BILI High AP essential
Liver: Obstructive hepatic disease	Low TP Low ALB High CHOL High LDH High SGOT High BILI High AP Lipemic serum
Liver: Subacute hepatitis of biliary cirrhosis	Low BUN Low ALB High CHOL High TP High LDH High SGOT essential High BILI High AP
Medications: Alkaline antacids	Low CA Low P

Medications: Corticoids	Low UA Low CHOL High GLU High CHOL
Medications: Salicylates	Low GLU Low UA Low CHOL High SGOT
Medications: Thiazide diuretics	Low P High CA High GLU High BUN High UA essential
Musculoskeletal: Bone metastases	Low TP Low ALB High CA High P High UA High LDH High SGOT High AP
Musculoskeletal: Muscle disease (dystrophy, dermatomyositis, etc.)	High LDH High SGOT
Musculoskeletal: Osteomalacia	Low CA Low P High AP
Musculoskeletal: Paget's disease	High CA High AP
Reproductive: Estrogens or oral contraceptives	Low CA Low TP Low ALB Low AP High CHOL

Reproductive: Pregnancy	Low CA Low BUN Low TP Low ALB High AP High GLU High CHOL Lipemic serum
Reproductive: Toxemia of pregnancy	Low CA Low TP High GLU High BUN High UA High AP
Respiratory: Pulmonary embolism or infarction	High UA High LDH High SGOT High BILI High AP
Sensory: Seizures	High LDH High SGOT
Sensory: Stroke	Low ALB High GLU High BUN High CHOL High LDH High SGOT

Systemic: Carcinoma	Low TP Low ALB High CA High P High UA High LDH High SGOT High BILI High AP
Systemic: Collagen disease, especially lupus and lupus hepatitis	Low ALB High TP High LDH High SGOT High BILI High AP
Systemic: Dehydration from enemas for X-ray studies	High CA essential High TP essential High ALB essential
Systemic: Dehydration of patient (or evaporation of specimen)	High CA High P High GLU High BUN High UA High CHOL High TP essential High ALB High BILI High AP High LDH High SGOT

Systemic: Diabetes mellitus	High GLU essential High BUN High UA High CHOL High LDH High SGOT High AP Lipemic serum
Systemic: Excessive fluid	Low CA Low P Low BUN Low UA Low CHOL Low TP Low ALB
Systemic: Gout	High GLU High UA essential High CHOL
Systemic: Sarcoidosis	Low P High CA High TP
Thyroid: Hypothyroidism	Low GLU High CHOL High LDH High TP High SGOT Lipemic serum
Treatment: Transfusions, following many	Low CA High BUN High UA
Urinary: Acute renal failure	High CA High BUN essential High UA

Urinary: Nephrotic syndrome	Low TP Low ALB High GLU High BUN High CHOL Lipemic serum
Urinary: Prerenal azotemia (CHF, shock, etc.)	Low CA Low TP Low ALB High P High GLU High BUN essential High UA High LDH High SGOT High AP
Urinary: Renal infarction	High BUN High LDH High SGOT
Urinary: Renal insufficiency	Low CA Low TP Low ALB Low CHOL High P High GLU High BUN essential High UA High LDH High SGOT High AP

Vitamin Use: Hypervitaminosis D	Low P High CA essential High P High BUN High AP
Vitamin Use: Vitamin D deficiency, rickets	Low CA Low P High AP

15 Urinalysis

The specific gravity of water is 1.000, and the specific gravity for urine runs from 1.010 to 1.030 (normal range). If it drops below 1.010, this means that fluid intake is high or salt intake is low. **The low value also indicates possible Diabetes insipidus and chronic nephritis.** The tubules have been damaged, so therefore they are having trouble with the water that effects the concentrations of the urine.

If the specific gravity of the urine is above 1.030, it is because water has been lost by sweating, vomiting, diarrhea or it could be that one just doesn't drink enough water. The average person should drink from 8-10 glasses of fluid on a daily basis. **The higher the value gets above 1.030, we have to think of diabetes mellitus, acute glomerulonephritis, fever, sweating, vomiting, and diarrhea.**

Urinary pH

Remember that a food that lowers the pH of the urine is classified as an acid-forming food. If it raises the pH, it is an alkaline-forming food. We like to see urine pH between 5.5 and 6.0, but never above, as in acidosis, diabetes mellitus, gout, or kidney stones. A pH below 5.5 is more strongly acidic and may suggest acidosis, diabetes mellitus, gout, lithiasis, or even a high protein diet or the taking of certain medicines such as mandelic acid, ammonium chloride, ammonium mandelate, or nitrates.

A pH above 6.0, although acidic, may indicate a shift toward the alkaline. A reaction of 6.0 becomes alkaline on standing, owing to the formation of ammonia from the urea. Urine pH may be alkaline after ingesting salts of organic acids and alkaline carbonates, during anemias, and in certain cases of debility.

Occult Urinary Blood

Blood is not a normal constituent of the urine of a healthy person. However, its presence may indicate several diagnostic possibilities. If you find red blood cells, first rule out menstrual blood. If the patient uses a catheter, you have to make sure that you always check in the urethra to make sure that you didn't create a trauma that caused the bleeding. Hematuria occurs in glomerulonephritis, infections, tuberculosis of the kidneys, the ureters and bladder, polycystic kidneys, and hemorrhagic diseases.

- If you find white blood cells (a few are found in the normal urine) they are increased in arthritis, cystitis, prostitis, pyelitis, pyelonephritis, salmonella vasiculitis, tuberculosis of the kidneys, and following trauma of catheterization.
- If you find casts, you're thinking, in terms of leukocytes of cellular casts, as In acute pyelonephritis, or the calcium oxalates. The large number of the calculi are indicative of the development of calcium stones.
- If you find a big increase in squamous epithelial calls in the urine, this indicates a pathological process at the site of the exfoliation. If it has casts with it, you can rest assured that there is nephrosis.

Urinary Aldosterone

Aldosterone is the most metabolically-active mineralocortocoid hormone, which is secreted bs the adrenal cortex. It is involved with maintaining the balance of sodium, potassium, and chloride, the levels of which are critical in the stabilization of blood volume and pH.

A high blood concentration of aldosterone causes retention of sodium, loss (through the urine) of potassium, and alkalosis. A chronic low serum potassium may be suggestive of primary or secondary (non-adrenal caused) aldosteronism.

- Primary aldosteronism is related to hyperfunction of the adrenal glands. It is often called Conn's syndrome. Symptoms may include high serum sodium, low serum potassium, alkalosis, tetany, weakness, paralysis, hypertension, cardiac dysrhythmia, polyuria, and polydipsia.
- Secondary aldosteronism is often associated with a diet low in sodium, cirrhosis of the liver (with ascites), congestive heart failure, malignant hypertension, nephrosis, and eclampsia.

A low urinary aldosterone level may be associated with hypoadrenalism or panhypopituitarism.

Urinary Acetone

Acetone is not a normal constituent of the urine of a healthy person. Its presence is indicative of a state of ketoacidosis; this may be confirmed by demonstration of the presence of ketones in the blood. The presence of acetone in the urine is termed "acetonuria" and may indicate diabetes mellitus, eclampsia, starvation (generates ketone bodies), cachexia, digestive disturbances, febrile disease in which carbohydrate intake is limited, and vomiting. Acetonuria may follow ether or chloroform anaesthesia.

Kidney Stones

You know, there's one area in the western part of Pennsylvania where over 113 hospital beds are filled with patients suffering from kidney stones. I know what it is, because I got one, too, while I was living there; they are the most painful things that you will ever see or ever feel. So far, none of the urologists that I worked with in that area can tell you why. They have never done any research to find out why that one particular area, a circle of about 50 miles, has such a high proportion of kidney stone patients. They don't care; all they are interested in is the butchery of going in there and cutting them out.

You can dissolve alkaline stones but you can't dissolve uric acid stones. Uric acid stones are the multicolored ones; when you do an X-ray you will find they have a very opaque shadow; you can identify them very easily. For alkaline stones, when you look at an X-ray, you see just a faint shadow; they are the calcium type, and if you load your patient with magnesium and phosphorus and then give him some castor oil, they can usually pass them. It works very well.

For Women

One other thing; it is especially important in women that we check for budding, yeast. We are seeing more and more yeast infections in women. It is a good idea for them to get away from the synthetics and the nylons especially with panty hose. These are one of the greatest mediums for growing a yeast infection within the vagina because they don't breathe.

16 Hair Mineral Analysis

The difference between the hair mineral analysis and the well-accepted urine and blood analyses lies in what the information is expected to indicate. **Even with expert interpretation, one cannot derive a specific diagnosis of health or disease from minerals in the hair, although general tendencies or conditions can frequently be determined. One thing is very clear; you cannot just supplement to a low level of a certain mineral. Supplementing minerals according to a hair mineral analysis is more complicated.**

We started doing hair analysis in 1969. By 1982, we assay 19 minerals from the hair. All of the while, we are learning how to correlate what we find from bloodwork with hair mineral levels. For instance, we are finding out that, if you have an elevated hair level of aluminum, certain other minerals may be pulled out of the bloodstream and accumulated in the tissues. Or, some minerals may pull other minerals out of the tissues and put them back into the bloodstream.

One of these days, I hope that we get up to where we are doing all 34 minerals that we know something about. We don't know enough about their correlation and their ratios to one another, to do that many. We're doing 19, we know how to do 22 right now, we're working on the rest of them.

Editor: Dr. Ellis followed closely the work of Henry A. Schroeder, M.D. (1906-1976) and Paul Eck, Ph.D. biochemist (1925-1996). The text of *Trace Minerals and Man* by Dr. Schroeder may be found online at http://spexspeaker.com/Documents/61-06_SPEXSpeaker.pdf. This was originally published in the *SPEX Industries Speaker* newsletter, Volume VI, No. 2, June, 1961. Dr. Eck lived eight years after Dr. Ellis' passing, carrying forward his research and discovering more about the dynamics of minerals in the hair. His work is being continued by a former colleague, Lawrence Wilson, M.D., of The Center for Development (see http://www.drlwilson.com/articles/hair_analysis_controversy.htm).

Hair is a tissue made of dried cells, consisting almost entirely of a protein called keratin. These cells are descended from stem cells in the scalp. Minerals are organically bound in the cells while the hair is growing. These minerals stay in the hair cells after they dry. Hair mineral levels reflect an average tissue level spanning the time during which the hair was growing, and the interpretation of one's physiological state on the basis of an accurate estimation of hair mineral levels is very reliable.

An imbalance characteristic of some pathological condition usually persists for some time before any problems develop, and it may disappear without having been treated. In some cases, however, what changes is only the specific sign (deviation from an accepted normal value range). For example, prediabetic impairments of pancreatic function may be indicated by an excess or a scarcity of chromium; disappearance of either sign may mean a transition between different prediabetic states. It is the underlying physiology and pathology that you must evaluate and not the signs. For this reason, clinical examination and other types of test are valuable.

Minerals can also be deposited into the hair from shampoos, conditioners, and colorings. Some of these compounds contain aluminum, selenium, phosphorus, and lead. After superficial dust and oils are removed, the minerals in the hair shaft itself are difficult to remove. Lithium and sodium can be leached out to some extent with strong detergents; several minerals can be partially removed with chelating agents, such as EDTA.

Collecting a Hair Sample

The objective is to get the most recent information concerning your patient's current physiological state; therefore, the sample of hair should be cut close to the scalp. Each centimeter of hair growth represents about three weeks of tissue mineral levels. It is actually an advantage to have the mineral levels averaged over time, because the temporary excess and deficiencies even out, leaving only the long-range values apparent.

The minimum sample necessary for accurate measurement is three packed tablespoons. Why so much hair? Small samples are prone to sampling errors. Further, since the hair is dissolved and sprayed into a flame in a photoelectric flame photometer, more starting material is needed, because the liquid sample is usually very small.

Colors are produced from the flames and analyzed with the use of prisms, light detectors, and a computer. Each mineral in the flame produces certain colors characteristic of the particular mineral, and the computer program is designed to take the data from the measuring instrument (atomic absorption spectrophotometer), analyze it, and express what mineral is present and its concentration in the sample.

Bell Curve

A standard bell curve is a typical statistical depiction of the distribution of a characteristic within a normal population, which may be a small or large group under study. The six-section area under the bell-shaped curve represents the total population, and the normal range, which includes 95% of the population, is considered to be the area included within the two large middle and two adjacent sections under the curve. The remaining 5% is located in the areas to the outside of the four middle areas. The numbers on the vertical axis are for illustration only. The mean (average) of the distribution is labeled mu, and sigma is the symbol for a unit of standard deviation from the mean.

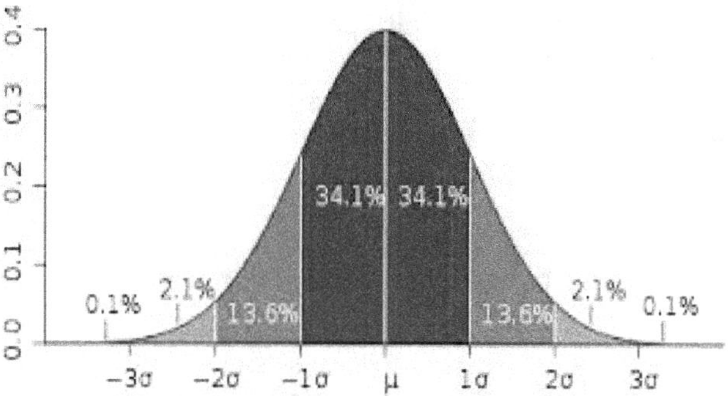

Figure 22: A standard bell curve.

When considering the mineral distribution in the hair of a population of individuals, it is customary to consider values to the left of the mean to be lower than the values to the right of the mean. Numerical values for mineral levels are considered normal if they fall within the middle four sections; these are within two standard deviations from the mean. However, values to the left of the mean in this area are termed low normal, and those to the right of the mean are termed high normal.

Values in the outer two sections of the normal range (more than one standard deviation from the mean) are still considered normal, but they are termed scarce (left) or excessive (right). Values in these sections are significant if you are interested in the ratios between two different minerals. Values in the farthest two sections from the normal range (more than two standard deviation from the mean) are low and high, respectively.

Brief Summary of Minerals

The chart below is compiled from information published on the website of Analytical Research Labs, Inc., 2225 W. Alice Avenue, Phoenix, Arizona 85021 USA, the company founded by Dr. Paul Eck. The values, although universal, are most relevant to their laboratory because of the standard protocols they use to prepare and test hair samples. **The tables below are very brief and should be subjects for further study.** Units are in mg%, meaning "milligrams of mineral assayed per 100 grams of hair."

Editor: Dr. Paul C. Eck, to correctly interpret a tissue mineral analysis, combined a number of modern biological, physiological, and biochemical concepts including the stages of stress discovered by Dr. Hans Selye, sympathetic and parasympathetic balancing as taught by Dr. Melvin Page, oxidation types as taught by Dr. George Watson, and mineral balancing as taught by Dr. William Albrecht and others. Dr. Eck pioneered many innovations in the study of trace mineral deficiencies and excesses and their relationship to various metabolic dysfunctions associated with disease. Dr. Eck was regarded as an authority on the science of balancing body chemistry through hair tissue mineral analysis. Because Dr. Ellis indicated his preference for Dr. Eck's teachings, Analytical Research Labs is considered to be the most closely aligned with Dr. Ellis' objectives. Much work has been done to refine hair analysis since his passing. Therefore, in the spirit of Dr. Ellis' belief that a health physician should constantly revise his working knowledge, the following newer material is presented. An overview of minerals by Dr. Lawrence Wilson is online at http://drlwilson.com/Articles/MINERALS%20FOR%20LIFE.htm.

Table 12: Macrominerals in Hair

Name	Normal Range mg%
Calcium Ca	40
Magnesium Mg	6
Phosphorus P	16-17
Potassium K	10
Sodium Na	25
Sulfur S	4,500

Table 13: Microminerals (Trace Minerals) in Hair

Name	Normal Range mg%
Boron Bo	0.05-0.08
Chromium Cr	0.06
Cobalt Co	0.002
Copper Cu	2.5
Germanium Ge	0.003
Iodine I	0.1
Iron Fe	2
Lithium Li	0.002
Manganese Mn	0.03-0.04
Molybdenum Mo	0.002
Rubidium Rb	0.06
Selenium Se	0.12
Vanadium V	0.004
Zinc Zn	15
Zirconium Zr	0.005

Table 14: Toxic Minerals in Hair

Name	Ideal Range mg%
Aluminum Al	0.65-1.0
Arsenic As	0.005-0.008
Cadmium Cd	0.005-0.007
Lead Pb	0.06-0.09
Mercury Hg	0.03-0.04
Nickel Ni	0.02-0.04
Other toxic metals (that are much less well researched	
Name	**mg%**
Antimony Sb	0.005-0.01
Barium Ba	0.03-0.05
Beryllium Be	0.001-0.002
Bismuth Bi	0.05-0.1
Platinum Pt	0.008-0.01
Silver Ag	0.08-0.1
Strontium Sr	0.008-0.01
Thallium Tl	0.004-0.006
Thorium Th	0.004-0.006
Tin Sn	0.02-0.04
Titanium Ti	0.05-0.07
Uranium U	0.002-0.004

Mineral Synergy/Antagonism

Editor: Issue 27-29 of the *Healthview Newsletter*, 1981, was devoted to educating the public about the effect of minerals in the body, according to Dr. Paul Eck. This publication may be found online at http://freedom-school.com/health/healthview-newsletter-27-29.pdf.

In the preliminary interview, Dr. Eck stated that fatigue was one of the major health problems of all time. He observed that there was no reliable or predictable method for increasing a person's energy and suggested that there should be a systematized, organized approach for the correction of fatigue. In the rest of the newsletter, Dr. Eck explained the interaction of minerals and the complexity involved when attempting to supplement individual minerals based only on their levels, as determined by hair mineral analysis.

The classic mineral chart, as shown in Figure 23, shows some important mineral elements that the body needs. It is an attempt to illustrate how the level on one mineral affects others. To do this, lines and arrows have been placed between minerals, each of which can be synergistic or antagonistic to another, called the counterpart of the first mineral.

Unfortunately, supplementing individual minerals indicated as low may not yield the desired results and increase the vitality of the individual. One reason is that, if the body has too much or to little of a particular mineral, it affects its counterpart, causing an excess or deficiency that can be toxic. In this graphic, an arrow that points to a particular mineral means that an excess of the mineral may cause a deficiency of the mineral that the arrow comes from (its counterpart). For example, too much calcium can cause decreased absorption of phosphorus, zinc, magnesium, and manganese (calcium's counterparts).

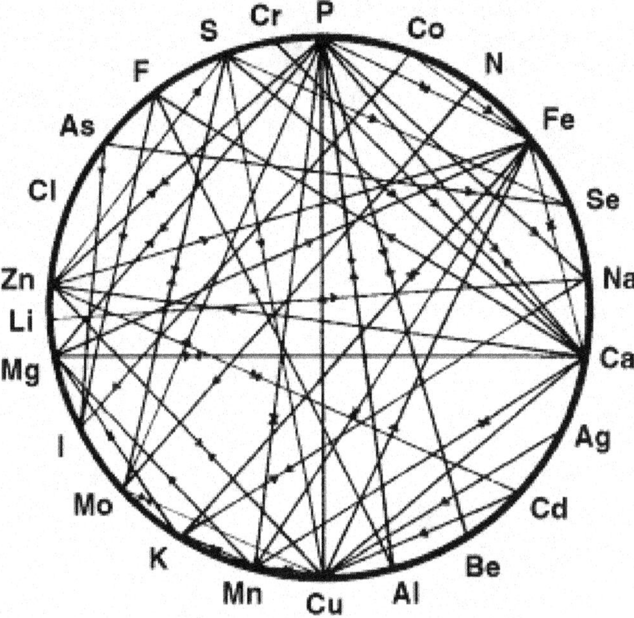

Figure 23: Mineral antagonisms

Editor: Further study may be necessary to develop a reliable way to supplement minerals for individuals, taking into account complex interactions. See http://www.drlwilson.com/articles/LABS.htm and http://www.arltma.com/.

Significant Hair Mineral Values/Patterns

Persons low in a particular mineral vary widely in how much they are affected. Some show no ill effects, while others may show signs of deficiency, even though their level is within the normal range. Scarcities of the toxic minerals are not true deficiencies. Some persons with an excess of a mineral may tolerate it, while others with less extreme levels may show toxic symptoms. We can't say in advance who will be affected or what symptoms they will exhibit, only that certain effects are likely or unlikely. For example, all high calcium levels are not necessarily associated with arthritis and all low zinc levels are not necessarily associated with diabetes!

Editor: The following patterns are taken from Dr. Ellis' personal, handwritten notes, which were not in strict alphabetic order. If you arrange the names and deviations of actual test results in alphabetical order first; for example, Ca, Mg, Na, and Zn, rather than Mg, Ca, Zn, and Na, it may be easier to compare them to the patterns listed below.

Table 15: Hair Mineral Level Patterns and Their Significance

Mineral Pattern < = Below, > = Above Acceptable Values	**Possible Tendencies/Conditions**
Ca< Mg<	The low levels of calcium and magnesium indicate a tendency to nervousness and irritability. Low calcium may indicate reduced insulin production. Supplemental magnesium has a calming or quieting effect on the nervous system.
Ca< Mg< Cu< Zn> Cd>	Disruption of several minerals indicate hyperlipidemic tendencies. Low calcium may indicate reduced insulin production.
Ca< Mn< Zn<	Monoamine oxidase inhibitors in food or drugs are especially undesirable in a person with low manganese. Low calcium may indicate reduced insulin production. Low manganese suggests reduction of libido and cholesterol. A zinc level below 20 mg% suggests a reduction in hydrochloric acid and pancreatic enzymes.
Ca< P>	Excess phosphorus may be interfering with calcium metabolism, with possible adverse effects on bones, teeth, nerves, and muscle. Low calcium may indicate reduced insulin production.
Ca< Zn<	This pattern suggests a lowering of activity of monoamine oxidase. Foods high in phenylethylamine, such as chocolate, and cheese, may trigger headaches. Low calcium may indicate reduced insulin production. A zinc level below 20 mg% suggests a reduction in hydrochloric acid and pancreatic enzymes.
Ca>	A high calcium level, in relation to those for other minerals, could provide a physical basis for tics, tremors, palpitations, tachycardia, confusion, disorientation, excitability, apprehensiveness, or depression. If symptoms such as these exist, they may not be psychogenic. Even if a psychological explanation can be formulated, the real cause may be in calcium consumption or calcium metabolism. Correction of the calcium level could reduce the incidence or severity of any symptoms of an abnormal calcium concentration in the tissues.

Mineral Pattern < = Below, > = Above Acceptable Values	Possible Tendencies/Conditions
Cr<	The low level of chromium suggests a possible tendency toward hypoglycemia, sometimes misleadingly called low blood sugar. Blood sugar is glucose, while ordinary table sugar is sucrose, something the blood does not need at all. Eating table sugar temporarily relieves symptoms of weakness, headaches, depression, or vertigo in persons in whom the hypoglycemic tendency is strong, but within a few hours, it makes matters worse. Brown sugar is the same chemically as white sugar, with brown coloring or molasses added. Like white sugar, it traumatizes kidneys, adrenals, and the pancreas. If a hypoglycemic does not follow a proper regimen, Diabetes mellitus may develop. In addition to a good diet, supplements may be of some value.
Cr< Mn< Cu>	There may be a possibility for schizophrenia.
Cr< Mn=N	Some signs of a hypoglycemic tendency are present, but others are absent. Possibly the tendency can be slowed or reversed.
Cu< Mg< Na> Ca> Cd>	This pattern may signal a tendency to develop cardiovascular problems, and the person may benefit from a preventive, heart-healthy regimen.
Cu< Mn< Li< Pb>	A high level of lead may be blocking cellular energy and suggests a tendency to lack energy and feel depressed. Paradoxicallly, a syndrome of hyperactivity appears in some cases of lead poisoning.
Cu< Mn< Zn> K>	This pattern suggests a hypothyroid tendency.
Cu< Pb>	Lead interferes with copper and may impair mitochondrial electron transport, blood formation, and resistance to radiation.
Cu< Zn> Hg>	Mercury may be interfering with blood formation, aerobic respiration, and nervous system functioning.
Cu> Mn>	Excess manganese may aggravate emotional symptoms of other mineral imbalances.
Fe<	A low iron level suggest that this person may suffer from shortness of breath, constipation, undue fatigue, or other signs of a generally sluggish metabolism. One should suspect iron deficiency anemia if the appearance is pale and the hair and nails are brittle and lusterless.
Fe< Cr>	An elevated level of chromium may interfere with iron transport to the tissues.

Mineral Pattern < = Below, > = Above Acceptable Values	Possible Tendencies/Conditions
Fe< Cu<	A low copper level may be a contributing factor in iron deficiency anemia.
Fe< Cu< Zn<	There may be difficulty in catalyzing a number of cellular oxidations and reductions. Also, there may be difficulty in producing blood. A zinc level below 20 mg% suggests a reduction in hydrochloric acid and pancreatic enzymes.
Fe< Cu>	An elevated copper level may contribute to an iron deficiency anemia.
Fe< Cu> Zn>	The body may be unable to use iron in its tissues.
Fe< Hg>	An unacceptable level of mercury suggests the tendency to fatigue.
Fe< Mn< Pb>	Lead may be interfering with both iron and manganese metabolism. Low manganese suggests reduction of libido and cholesterol.
Fe< Zn<	The level of zinc may contribute to an iron deficiency anemia. A zinc level below 20 mg% suggests a reduction in hydrochloric acid and pancreatic enzymes.
Fe< Zn< Ca< Cu>	The balance between zinc and copper is an index of the balance between anabolic and catabolic processes. This pattern shows catabolism as found in anemia, cachexia, hypochlorhydria, pancreatitis, starvation, malabsorption and old age. The low levels of iron and calcium suggest prolonged loss of blood and bone material from the body. A zinc level below 20 mg% suggests a reduction in hydrochloric acid and pancreatic enzymes. Low calcium may indicate reduced insulin production.
Fe< Zn< Pb>	Lead is high enough to impair synthesis of hemoglobin, especially with the low level of zinc. In this situation, there is a tendency for the body's iron reserve to become depleted. A zinc level below 20 mg% suggests a reduction in hydrochloric acid and pancreatic enzymes.
Fe> Cd>	Levels of iron and cadmium suggest the possibility of hypertension. High iron is indicative of rheumatoid arthritis and cirrhosis.
Fe> Cu> Cd>	Many pressor (atrial wall stretching) hormones require copper as a cofactor. High iron is indicative of rheumatoid arthritis and cirrhosis. This pattern also suggests the possibility of hypertension.

Mineral Pattern < = Below, > = Above Acceptable Values	Possible Tendencies/Conditions
K< Mg< Na> Ca>	This pattern shows a tendency toward anxiety and depression that could develop together or separately. It is common for either or both of these tendencies to match the other.
K< Na>	These electrolyte levels indicate a tendency or susceptibility to weakness, apathy, abnormal EKG, or chronic fatigue. Fluid is being held between cells.
K< Na> Cu> Mg>	The low level of potassium compared with other electrolytes may indicate a general depression of potassium functioning inside and outside the cells. There may be a difficulty with neuromuscular or cardiac function.
K< Rb<	The effects of potassium deficiency tend to be worse when rubidium is also low.
K< Zn< Cr=N Ca>	Some signs of a hypoglycemic tendency are present, but others are absent. A zinc level below 20 mg% suggests a reduction in hydrochloric acid and pancreatic enzymes. Possibly the tendency can be slowed or reversed.
K< Zn< Mn< Ca>	Low potassium and calcium levels add to the possibility of a hypoglycemic or prediabetic tendency or state. A zinc level below 20 mg% suggests a reduction in hydrochloric acid and pancreatic enzymes. Low manganese suggests reduction of libido and cholesterol.
K< Zn< Mn=N Ca>	Some signs of a hypoglycemic tendency are present, but others are absent. A zinc level below 20 mg% suggests a reduction in hydrochloric acid and pancreatic enzymes. Possibly the tendency can be slowed or reversed.
Mg> Fe> Cd>	The high level of magnesium adds to the probability of hypertension. High iron is indicative of rheumatoid arthritis and possible cirrhosis.
Mg< Mn< Cr< Zn<	Depressed levels of magnesium, manganese, and zinc suggest a tendency toward a prediabetic or diabetic state. Low manganese suggests reduction of libido and cholesterol. A zinc level below 20 mg% suggests a reduction in hydrochloric acid and pancreatic enzymes.
Mg< P<	Tissue magnesium levels may not be sufficient to support phosphorus metabolism.

Mineral Pattern < = Below, > = Above Acceptable Values	Possible Tendencies/Conditions
Mg< Zn< Mn> Pb>	Disturbance of the minerals in this pattern may tend to create a learning disorder. A zinc level below 20 mg% suggests a reduction in hydrochloric acid and pancreatic enzymes.
Mn<	Sugar consumption is deleterious, especially with the low level of manganese. This level suggests possible problems in the functioning of many enzyme systems, including those necessary for proper metabolism of carbohydrates and fats. Low manganese suggests reduction of libido and cholesterol.
Mn< Cr< Zn<	Zinc is needed for the function of insulin and glucose metabolism. This pattern is similar to that found in diabetes. Low manganese suggests reduction of libido and cholesterol. A zinc level below 20 mg% suggests a reduction in hydrochloric acid and pancreatic enzymes.
Mn< Cr=N	Some signs of a hypoglycemic tendency are present, but others are absent. Possibly the tendency can be slowed or reversed. Low manganese suggests reduction of libido and cholesterol.
Mn< Pb>	The level of lead suggests problems in synthesizing cartilage. A good diet, with increased consumption of vitamin C and manganese may be of some value. Low manganese suggests reduction of libido and cholesterol.
Mn>	An excess of manganese may aggravate neuromuscular disorders. Low manganese suggests reduction of libido and cholesterol.
Na< K<	This indicates adrenal insufficiency and is typical of a slow oxidizer.
Na< K>	The abnormal ratio of sodium to potassium suggests impairment of adrenal function. This indicates fluids held within cells.
Na< K>	This electrolyte imbalance is typical of adrenal insufficiency, which if present, is manifested as insomnia, vertigo (especially upon arising), craving for salt, excessive thirst, morning fatigue, or in other ways. Adrenal insufficiency is sometimes related to use of nicotine, caffeine, amphetamines, sugar, or other drugs. These over stimulate the adrenals and, in the long run, impair them with deleterious effects on the body as a whole. This imbalance includes features of a kind sometimes associated with multiple sclerosis.

Mineral Pattern < = Below, > = Above Acceptable Values	Possible Tendencies/Conditions
Na> K>	This indicates adrenal hyperactivity and is typical of a fast oxidizer.
Na< Mn< Pb> Ca>	There is some indication of lead and calcium contributing to a breakdown of synovial fluid, a characteristic of arthritis. Low manganese suggests reduction of libido and cholesterol.
Na< P< Mg< Zn> Cd>	Disruption of several minerals indicate possible nervous tendency.
Na< P< Mn< Cr<	This pattern is similar to the diabetic pattern for tissue factors and monovalent electrolytes. Low manganese suggests reduction of libido and cholesterol.
Na< Zn< Ca> Cd>	Hypertensive tendencies may be present. A zinc level below 20 mg% suggests a reduction in hydrochloric acid and pancreatic enzymes.
Ni<	This level suggests under consumption of foodstuffs rich in nucleic acids.
Ni< P<	Concomitant low level of phosphorus supports the suggestion of under consumption of foods rich in nucleic acids.
Ni>	An excess of nickel could reflect exposure to carcinogens, such as nickel carbonyl or nickel suboxide, or ingestion of hydrogenated vegetable oils contaminated by the nickel catalyst. Overconsumption of yeast prepared in stainless steel vessels is another possibility.
P< Al>	Excess aluminum may interfere with phosphorus metabolism, with possible effects on bones, teeth, nerves, muscles, and other tissues. Fluorides may be detrimental in amounts that would not matter if phosphorus were at a normal level.
Rb<	A depressed rubidium level may be a sign of aging.
Se<	A depressed selenium level may be related to the inability to protect unsaturated fats in the body from rancidification.
Se< Cu< Zn<	Low levels in selenium and the mineral cofactors for superoxide dismutase suggest sensitivity to radiation. Exposure to radiation may be less tolerable than usual. A zinc level below 20 mg% suggests a reduction in hydrochloric acid and pancreatic enzymes. Supplementation of copper, zinc, and selenium, along with vitamins may be of value.

Mineral Pattern < = Below, > = Above Acceptable Values	Possible Tendencies/Conditions
Zn<	Low tissue zinc is associated with impairment of the chemical senses – taste and smell. A zinc level below 20 mg% suggests a reduction in hydrochloric acid and pancreatic enzymes.
Zn< Ca< Cu>	This pattern may reflect a loss of calcium from the tissues, a consequence of a generally catabolic state, as indicated by an imbalance among the blood metals, calcium and copper. A zinc level below 20 mg% suggests a reduction in hydrochloric acid and pancreatic enzymes. Low calcium may indicate reduced insulin production.
Zn< Ca< Fe< Cu>	The balance between zinc and copper is an index of the balance between anabolic and catabolic processes. In this case, there is some indication of an imbalance in the direction of catabolism; the body's material may be breaking down faster than it is being replenished. No specific disease is uniquely associated with this kind of imbalance. It is often found in conditions as varied as anemia, starvation, pancreatitis, cachexia, hypochlorhydria, malabsorption, insufficiency of pancreatic digestive enzymes, chronic subclinical scurvy, and old age. In addition, the levels of iron and calcium suggest prolonged loss of vital substances from the body. A zinc level below 20 mg% suggests a reduction in hydrochloric acid and pancreatic enzymes. Low calcium may indicate reduced insulin production.
Zn< Ca>	A high level of calcium may block absorption and the activity of zinc. For unknown reasons, this pattern occurs in many with arteriosclerosis. A zinc level below 20 mg% suggests a reduction in hydrochloric acid and pancreatic enzymes. An increased intake of zinc may be of value in this case.
Zn< Ca> Cu>	This pattern may reflect a loss of calcium from the tissues, a consequence of a generally catabolic state, as indicated by an imbalance among the blood metals, calcium and copper. A zinc level below 20 mg% suggests a reduction in hydrochloric acid and pancreatic enzymes.

Mineral Pattern < = Below, > = Above Acceptable Values	Possible Tendencies/Conditions
Zn< Cd>	Cadmium further interferes with the activity of zinc-containing enzymes. A zinc level below 20 mg% suggests a reduction in hydrochloric acid and pancreatic enzymes. Taste, smell, and mental functions may be affected. A high cadmium level, when considered in relation to other minerals, may tend to inhibit growth, healing of wounds, formation of new blood, immune responses to infection and tumors, and sexual maturation and functioning. Urogenital disorders may be caused by the level of cadmium not being controlled by an adequate level of zinc. One possible symptom is retention of fluids.
Zn< Cu>	When copper is elevated or zinc is depressed, activity of monoamine oxidase or carbonic anhydrase could lead to depletion of the normal levels of biogenic amines and other neurotransmitters. Mental dysfunction, emotional instability, or headaches may result. A zinc level below 20 mg% suggests a reduction in hydrochloric acid and pancreatic enzymes. The relative levels of copper and zinc are like those sometimes observed in cases of neoplasms, especially in the urinary or digestive tract. A zinc level below 20 mg% suggests a reduction in hydrochloric acid and pancreatic enzymes. Zinc is important to normal repair of tissue.
Zn< Fe< Cu> Ca>	The balance between zinc and copper is an index of the balance between anabolic and catabolic processes. Possible causes are as varied as anemia, cachexia, hypochlorhydria, pancreatitis, starvation, malabsorption, and old age. A zinc level below 20 mg% suggests a reduction in hydrochloric acid and pancreatic enzymes.
Zn< Mn<	This pattern is indicative of possible current or future reproductive difficulties. A zinc level below 20 mg% suggests a reduction in hydrochloric acid and pancreatic enzymes. Low manganese suggests reduction of libido and cholesterol.
Zn< Mn< P<	Low level of phosphorus may contribute to current or future reproductive difficulties. A zinc level below 20 mg% suggests a reduction in hydrochloric acid and pancreatic enzymes. Low manganese suggests reduction of libido and cholesterol.
Zn< Pb> Fe>	Lead may be blocking synthesis of hemoglobin. High iron is indicative of rheumatoid arthritis and cirrhosis. It is possible that the high level reflects losses of iron that the body is not ready to use.

Mineral Pattern < = Below, > = Above Acceptable Values	Possible Tendencies/Conditions
Zn< Mn>	Excess manganese may aggravate emotional symptoms of other mineral imbalances.

Hair Mineral Level Ratios - Balance

A mineral level ratio is a unitless number resulting from dividing the assayed level of one mineral by that of another. Along with a physical examination, a CBC, a blood chemistry analysis, a urinalysis, and a diet journal, hair mineral levels and their ratios, we can get a better idea about a patient's health. **Ratios are not diagnostic to any disease condition, but they may indicate associations or trends that direct our attention to the results of other tests.** These ratios may help us predict future problems and chart the course of treatment.

When you are reviewing a hair analysis report, in addition to deviations of individual mineral levels from the normal range and patterns of multiple deviations, it is important to be concerned with the five important ratios described below.

Editor: For information about factors that have an influence on interpretation of these ratios, see the original article, *Basic Ratios and Their Meaning*, by Dr. Paul C. Eck and Lawrence Wilson, M.D., Copyright © 1987, The Eck Institute of Applied Nutrition and Bioenergetics, Ltd., that may be found at http://www.advancedfamilyhealth.com/ratios.html#_minratio. Also, see http://www.arltma.com/Newsletters/SuppMinHighNews.htm.

Mineral Ratio	Ideal Value	Possible Tendencies/Conditions	
		High	Low
Ca/Mg "Blood Sugar Ratio"	6.67	6.67-10 - Good 10-12 - Hypoglycemia 12+ - Diabetes Ellis: Don't mix these two in the same supplement or when taking both. If the ratio is 8.4 and higher, these people are highly nervous and irritable. A high value may also be associated with arteriosclerosis, hypothyroidism, arthritis, and mental disorders.	3.3-6.67 - Good 3-3.3 - Hypoglycemia 1-3.3 - Diabetes Also, a very high (greater than 16.0) or very low calcium/magnesium ratio (less than 2.0) is associated with mental or emotional disturbances. If the ratio is too low, less than 4.1, it may indicate muscle cramps, weakness, fatigue, and may be associated with vitamin D deficiency, malabsorption, osteoporosis, bone-cancer, or dilantin therapy. Ellis: Epileptics are very low in Mg and B6. The best tranquilizer is Mg and B6 with niacinamide.

Mineral Ratio	Ideal Value	Possible Tendencies/Conditions	
		High	Low
Ca/K "Thyroid Ratio"	4	4-8 - Mildly sluggish thyroid activity 10-25% energy loss 8-16 - Moderately sluggish thyroid 25-50% energy loss 16-32 - Sluggish thyroid 50-75% energy loss 32+ - Severe low thyroid activity 75%+ energy loss Fast Oxidizer: Ca/K < 4:1 and Na/Mg > 4.17:1 Slow Oxidizer: Ca/K > 4:1 and Na/Mg < 4.17:1 Mixed Oxidizer: Ca/K > 4:1 and Na/Mg > 4.17:1 or Ca/K < 4:1 and Na/Mg < 4.17:1	2-4 - Mildly fast thyroid activity 10-25% energy loss 1-2 - Moderately fast thyroid activity 25-50% energy loss Below 1 - Excessive thyroid activity 50% or more energy loss

Mineral Ratio	Ideal Value	Possible Tendencies/Conditions	
		High	Low
Na/K "Life-Death Ratio"	2.5	2.5-4 - Mild elevation - good adrenal function 4-6 - Moderate elevation - tendency towards inflammation 6+ - Severe elevation - inflammation and adrenal imbalance. High ratio can also be associated with asthma, allergies, kidney, and liver problems. A high sodium/ potassium ratio is considered preferable to a low sodium/potassium ratio. Ellis: Sodium is high on the inside of blood vessel walls, potassium is high on the outside. Any deviation from the ideal is important: if above 6, chronic fatigue, chronic constipation, and cystic fibrosis may be associated.	2-2.5 - Mild inversion - beginning of adrenal exhaustion 1-2 - Moderate inversion - kidney and liver dysfunction, allergies, arthritis, adrenal exhaustion, digestive problems, deficiency of hydrochloric acid Below 1- Severe inversion - tendency towards heart attack, cancer, arthritis, kidney and liver disorders Ellis: If the ratio is 2 or less, it may be associated with a low salt diet or postural hypotension.

Mineral Ratio	Ideal Value	Possible Tendencies/Conditions	
		High	Low
Na/Mg "Adrenal Ratio"	4.17	4.17-8 - Mild excessive adrenal activity 10-25% energy loss 8-16 - Moderate excessive adrenals 25-50% energy loss 16+ - Extremely overactive adrenals 50% or more energy loss Fast Oxidizer: Ca/K < 4:1 and Na/Mg > 4.17:1 Slow Oxidizer: Ca/K > 4:1 and Na/Mg < 4.17:1 Mixed Oxidizer: Ca/K > 4:1 and Na/Mg > 4.17:1 or Ca/K < 4:1 and Na/Mg < 4.17:1	2-4.17 - Mild sluggish adrenal activity 10-25% energy loss 1-2 - Moderate sluggish adrenals 25-50% energy loss Below 1 - Adrenal insufficiency 50% or more energy loss If the ratio is above 6:l, chronic fatigue, chronic constipation, cystic fibrosis may be associated. If the ratio is too low, a low salt diet, postural hypotension may be involved. The blood tests may be normal, but the tissue mineral test will show abnormal adrenal function. Symptoms, however, usually correlate well with the hair analysis.

Mineral Ratio	Ideal Value	Possible Tendencies/Conditions	
		High	Low
Zn/Cu	8	8-16 - Copper deficiency or unavailability 16+ - Severe copper deficiency or bio-unavailability of copper	4-8 - Copper toxicity 2-4 - Severe copper toxicity - Excessive breakdown, emotional instability A low ratio may be associated with skin problems (acne, psoriasis, slow healing, eczema), emotional instability, spaciness, detached behavior, schizophrenia, PMS, reproductive problems, prostatitis, menstrual difficulties depression and fatigue. Zinc deficiency problems such as impotence, slow healing, loss of taste, smell, appetite, and hair loss Ellis: A low ratio is also associated with arteriosclerosis, hypoglycemia, and diabetes.
Zn/Cr			Ellis: This ratio must be closely watched. If it is too low, lung disorders, allergies, and asthma are possible.

Detoxication of Selected Minerals (Cu, Pb, Strontium 90)

Editor: Suggestions about detoxicating selected metals are given in a humorous context below, as found in Dr. Ellis' notes. The reader is directed elsewhere for other detoxication methods. A chlorophyll-based general detoxicator of as many as 12 heavy metals is Chelazyme, offered by Biotics Research Corporation, but others may be listed on the internet.

Aluminum

Aluminum can be removed using methionine, alginates, and a lot of vitamin C.

Arsenic (As)

The best chelation for arsenic is with vitamin C.

Copper

For copper, the best thing is home-made apple sauce (pectin). Take the top of the core and the calyx out and use everything else, including the seeds and the skin. Cut it up and put it into a pan with a very small amount of water on low temperature. Keep the apple on the heat until it gets soft. Take it out and mash it all up. Eat a dish a day, and it will take out the copper.

Lead

At the Florida State Chiropractic Convention, Dr. Miller was telling about lead and how to neutralize it. He said what you want to do to get your lead out is to eat a dish of baked beans everyday. That didn't go over well until some fellow in the back hollered, "That a way, Doc, you tell 'em how to shoot it out." The sulfhydryl groups (-SH) in beans captures the lead. That is a way to get the lead out that you are exposed to from various products, including hair dyes. One of the worst is Grecian Formula; it's loaded with something like 3,800 parts per million of lead.

Strontium 90 (Sr)

The best chelation for strontium is with vitamin C.

Editor: See also the article, *The Use of Hair Tissue Mineral Analysis in Clinical Decision-Making Regarding Heavy Metal Chelation*, Explore! Volume 19, Number 3, 2010, George J. Georgiou, Ph.D., N.D., D.Sc (AM)., MSc., BSc, Cyprus at http://detoxmetals.com/wp-content/uploads/pdf/Georgiou.pdf. Also, *How To Detox Heavy Metals: A Highly Effective & Safe Chemical and Heavy Metals Detox* is a website devoted to detoxication of heavy metals from the body, found at http://www.howtodetoxheavymetals.com/chelate/.

Appendix A: Additional Reading

Editor: This appendix contains articles and abstracts of articles related to points made by Dr. Ellis in previous chapters. **The opinions stated therein belong solely to the authors and may not all be congruent with the beliefs of Dr. Ellis, but they may shed light on the rationale that Dr. Ellis used in formulating some of his opinions.** Again, anyone afflicted with a serious disorder should seek a thorough evaluation by a licensed health practitioner and follow sound medical advice.

We thank Dr. Alan Cantwell for permission to print the following article in its entirety. Dr. Ellis held Dr. Livingston in high regard, and he believed that bacterial organisms in intracellular form were causative agents for many diseases and likely provided a focus for cancer in various tissues, unless treated and eradicated.

Dr. Alan Cantwell is a retired dermatologist and the author of *The Cancer Microbe* and *Four Women Against Cancer,* both available from Aries Rising Press, PO Box 29532, Los Angeles, CA 90029 (www.ariesrisingpress.com). Email: alancantwell@sbcglobal.net. Abstracts of 30 published papers can be found at the PubMed website (type in Cantwell AR). Many of his personal writings can be found on www.google.com by using key words "alan cantwell" + articles. His books are also available on www.amazon.com and through Book Clearing House @ 1-800-431-1579.

Virginia Livingston, M.D.: Cancer Quack or Medical Genius?

by Alan Cantwell, M.D., Los Angeles, California

Cancer is the most frightening human disease and its cause remains elusive. Therefore, it seems inconceivable that the discovery of a germ cause of cancer would provoke such hostility among the cancer establishment. But, in truth, the belief in a cancer germ has always been the ultimate scientific heresy.

In the long history of cancer research there was never a physician more outspoken and controversial than Virginia Wuerthele-Caspe Livingston (1906-1990). For more than 40 years, she championed the revolutionary idea that bacteria caused cancer and devised a treatment to try and combat these microbes by immunotherapy.

Sixteen years after her death she is now largely forgotten but still condemned by such powerful organizations as the American Cancer Society and blacklisted on Quackwatch, a self-proclaimed "non-profit corporation dedicated to combating health-related frauds, myths, fads, and fallacies."

Livingston's Cancer Research

Beginning in the late 1940s, Livingston was able to grow bacteria from cancer tumors; and when she and her associates injected cancer bacteria into laboratory animals, some developed cancer. Other animals developed degenerative and proliferative diseases, and some animals remained healthy. Livingston believed the "immunity" of the host was an important factor in determining whether cancer would develop.

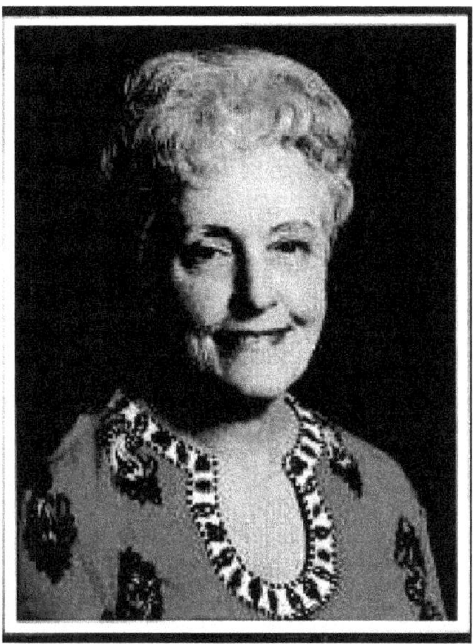

Figure 24: Virginia Livingston M.D. (1906-1990)

In 1969 at a meeting at the New York Academy of Sciences, Livingston and her colleagues proposed that cancer was caused by a highly unusual bacterium which she named Progenitor cryptocides, Greek for "ancestral hidden killer." Nevertheless, Livingston claimed elements of the microbe were present in every human cell. Due to its biochemical properties, she believed the organism was responsible for initiating life and for the healing of tissue and for killing us with cancer and other infirmities. Critics of this research continued to insist there was no such thing as a cancer germ.

In her attempt to use a variety of modalities (diet, supplements, antibiotics, as well as traditional methods) to treat cancer, she utilized an 'autogenous' vaccine derived from the patient's own cancer bacteria found in the urine and blood. Livingston explained it was not an anti-cancer vaccine, but rather a vaccine to stimulate and improve the patient's own immune system. The administration of this unapproved vaccine caused a furor in the cancer establishment and eventually legal action was undertaken against her and the Livingston-Wheeler Clinic in San Diego. In spite of all her legal troubles, she continued seeing patients until her death at 83.

In March 1990, the year of her death, a highly critical article on the Livingston-Wheeler therapy appeared in the American Cancer Society-sponsored CA: A Cancer Journal for Physicians. (No authors were listed.) The report advised patients to stay away from the San Diego clinic and claimed: "Livingston-Wheeler's cancer treatment is based on the belief that cancer is caused by a bacterium she has named Progenitor cryptocides. Careful research using modern techniques, however, has shown that there is no such organism and that Livingston-Wheeler has apparently mistaken several different types of bacteria, both rare and common, for a unique microbe. In spite of diligent research to isolate a cancer-causing microorganism, none has been found. Similarly, Livingston-Wheeler's autologous vaccine cannot be considered an effective treatment for cancer. While many oncologists have expressed the hope that someday a vaccine will be developed against cancer, the cause(s) of cancer must be determined before research can be directed toward developing a vaccine. The rationale for other facets of the Livingston-Wheeler cancer therapy is similarly faulty. No evidence supports her contention that cancer results from a defective immune system, that a whole-foods diet restores immune system deficiencies, that ascorbic acid slows tumor growth, or that cancer is transmitted to humans by chickens." (The full report is on-line at: http://caonline.amcancersoc.org/cgi/reprint/40/2/103.)

Bacteria As a Cause of Cancer

The recognition of disease-producing bacteria allowed medical science to emerge from the dark ages into the era of modern medicine. In the late nineteenth century when diseases like tuberculosis (TB), syphilis, and leprosy were proven to be caused by bacteria, some doctors also suspected human cancer might have a similar cause.

The idea that bacteria cause cancer is considered preposterous by most physicians. However, despite the antagonistic view of the American Cancer Society and medical science, there is ample evidence in the published peer-reviewed literature that strongly suggests that "cancer microbes" cause cancer.

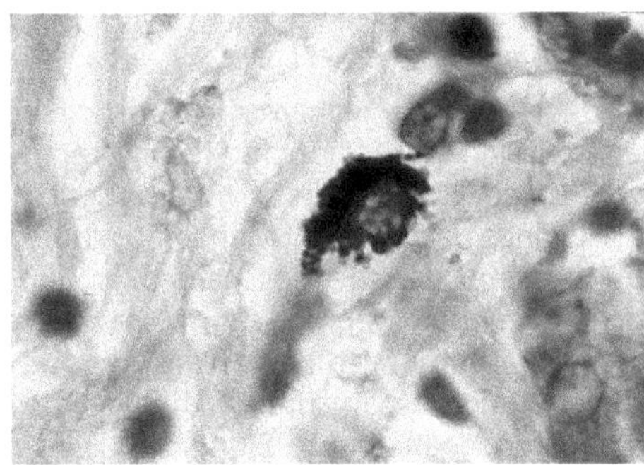

Figure 25: Intracellular variably-sized coccoid forms in breast cancer. Acid-fast; x1,000.

According to reports by Livingston and various other researchers, cancer is caused by pleomorphic, cell wall-deficient bacteria. The various forms of the organism range in size from submicroscopic virus-like forms, up to the size of bacteria, yeasts, and fungi. In culture and in tissue the bacterial forms are variably 'acid-fast' (having a staining quality like TB bacteria). These bacteria are ubiquitous and exist in the blood and tissues of all human beings (yet another "heresy"). In the absence of a protective immune response, these cell wall-deficient bacteria may become pathogenic and foster the development of cancer, autoimmune disease, AIDS, and certain other chronic diseases of unknown etiology.

Needless to say, all of this research fell on dead ears because bacteria were totally ruled out as the cause of all cancers in the early years of the twentieth century. Thus, bacteria observed in cancer were simply dismissed as elements of cellular degeneration, or as invaders of tissue weakened by cancer, or as 'contaminants' of laboratory origin.

Livingston and Progenitor Cryptocides

Beginning in 1950, in a series of papers and books, Livingston and her co-workers claimed the cancer microbe was a great imitator whose various pleomorphic forms resembled common staphylococci, diphtheroids, fungi, viruses, and host cell inclusions. Yet if the germ were studied carefully through all its transitional stages, it could be identified as a single agent. She was the first to suggest that the acid-fast stain was the key to the identification of the cancer microbe in tissue and in culture; and also demonstrated its appearance in the blood of cancer patients, by use of dark-field microscopy.

Anyone who takes the time to read Livingston's reports in the medical literature will quickly recognize that she was a credible research scientist, who allied herself with other experts-and was certainly not the quack doctor pictured by her detractors. Her achievements in cancer microbiology can also be found in her autobiographical books: Cancer, A New Breakthrough (1972); The Microbiology of Cancer (1977); and The Conquest of Cancer (1984). Her research has been confirmed by other scientists, such as microbiologist Eleanor Alexander-Jackson, cell cytologist Irene Diller, biochemist Florence Seibert, and dermatologist Alan Cantwell, among others.

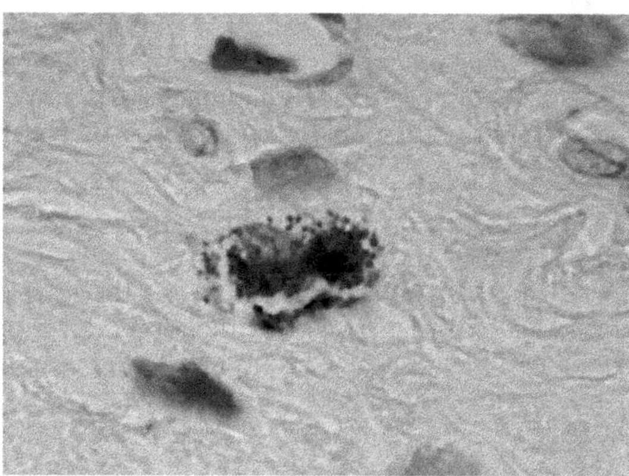

Figure 26: Intracellular bacteria in prostate cancer. Acid-fast; x1,000,

The Cancer Microbe and Bacterial Pleomorphism

Microbiologists have long resisted the idea of bacterial pleomorphism, and do not recognize or accept the various growth forms and the bacterial 'life cycle' proposed by various cancer microbe workers. Most bacteriologists do not accept the idea of a bacterium changing from a coccus to a rod, or to a fungus. Depending on the environment, the microbe in its cell wall-deficient phase may attain large size, even larger that a red blood cell. Other forms are submicroscopic and virus-sized. Electronic microscopic studies and photographs of filtered (bacteria-free) cultures of the cancer microbe show virus-size elements of the cancer microbe that can revert into bacterial-sized microbes.

The cancer microbe has adapted to life in man and animals by existing in a mycoplasma-like or cell wall-deficient state. In tissue sections of cancer stained for bacteria with the special acid-fast stain, the microbe can be seen as a variably acid-fast (blue, red, or purple-stained) round coccus or as barely visible granules. At magnifications of one thousand times (in oil), these forms can be observed within and also outside of the cells.

Careful study and observation of the tiny round coccoid forms in cancer tissue indicate they can enlarge progressively up to the size of so-called Russell bodies, which are well-known to pathologists. Russell bodies can attain the size of red blood cells, and even larger.

William Russell was a well-respected Scottish pathologist who in 1890 first reported the finding of 'cancer parasites' in the tissue of all of the cancers he studied. However, modern pathologists deny that Russell's bodies are microbial in origin. For more information on Russell bodies and Russell's 'cancer parasite' (and its intimate relationship to cancer microbes), Google: The forgotten clue to the bacterial cause of cancer; or go to: http://www.joimr.org/phorum/read.php?f=2&i=50&t=50.

Overlooking Hidden Bacteria in Cancer

Once bacteria were eliminated as a cause of cancer a century ago, it became dogma and impossible to change medical opinion. In this current era of medical science, one would think it impossible for infectious disease experts and pathologists to not recognize bacteria in cancer. However, bacteria can still pop up in diseases in which they were initially overlooked.

When a new and deadly lung disease broke out among legionnaires in Philadelphia in July 1976, 222 people became ill and 34 died. The cause of the killer lung disease remained a medical mystery for over five months until Joe McDade at the Leprosy Branch of the CDC detected unusual bacteria in guinea pigs experimentally infected with lung tissue from the dead legionnaires. Further modification of bacterial culture methods finally allowed the isolation of the causative and previously overlooked bacteria, now known as Legionella pneumophila.

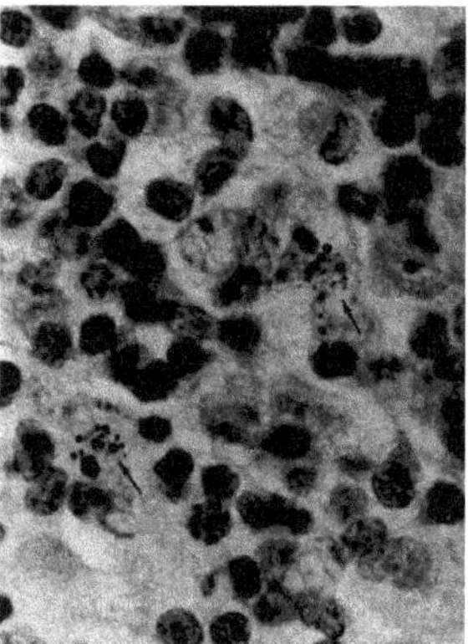

Figure 27: Lymph node showing Hodgkin's lymphoma. Gram stain; x1,000.

Arrows point to variably-sized round coccoid forms and larger Russell bodies.

Yet another example of dogma-defying research is provided by recent studies proving that bacteria (Helicobacter pylori) are a common cause of stomach ulcers, which can sometimes lead to stomach cancer and lymphoma. For a century, physicians refused to believe bacteria caused ulcers because they thought bacteria could not live in the acid environment of the stomach. In 2005 the Nobel Prize in Medicine was awarded to two Australian researchers for their 1982 discovery. These stomach bacteria could only be detected by use of special tissue stains. The CDC now claims that H. pylori causes more than 90% of duodenal ulcers and 80% of gastric ulcers. Approximately two-thirds of the world's population is infected with these microbes.

In the past four years there have been medical reports of newly discovered bacteria in serious lymph node disease; in Hodgkin's lymphoma; in cancer of the mouth; and in prostate cancer, to name only a few.

All of these studies prove bacteria can pop up in diseases where they are least expected. Such a caveat is appropriate for doctors who think they know everything about cancer and who pooh-pooh all aspects of cancer microbe research.

A Century of Cancer Microbe Research

Livingston never claimed that she was the discoverer of the microbe of cancer. In her writings she always gave credit to various scientists, some dating back to the nineteenth century, who attempted to prove that bacteria cause cancer. Some of these remarkable researchers include the long-forgotten cancer microbe studies of Scottish obstetrician James Young, Chicago physician John Nuzum, Montana surgeon James Scott, the infamous psychiatrist and cancer researcher Wilhelm Reich, microscopist Raymond Royal Rife, and others too numerous to mention.

This cancer microbe research has been explored in my books *The Cancer Microbe: The Hidden Killer in Cancer, AIDS, and Other Immune Diseases,* 1990 and in Four Women Against Cancer: Bacteria, Cancer, and *The Origin of Life*, 2005 - the story of Livingston, Alexander-Jackson, Diller and Seibert - four outstanding women scientists who attempted to bring the cancer microbe to the attention of a disinterested medical establishment. I was privileged to have met all of these remarkable women, who greatly influenced my own cancer research.

Why is research exploring bacteria in cancer so strongly opposed? Perhaps it poses a threat to the money interests involved in the established and orthodox treatment for cancer. Various forms of cancer treatment include surgery, radiation and chemotherapy. These therapies might have to be reevaluated if it were proven that cancer was an infectious disease.

Suggestions for Further Internet Study

Further information pertaining to cancer microbe research (both pro and con) can be found by Googling: cancer microbe; bacterial pleomorphism; cell wall-deficient bacteria; "alan cantwell"; "virginia livingston"; "Eleanor Alexander-Jackson"; as well as other names and key words mentioned in this communication.

For a list of scientific publications pertaining to the microbiology of cancer, go to the PubMed website hosted by the National Institute of Health (www.ncbi.nlm.nih.gov) and type in "Cantwell AR", "Livingston VW", "Alexander-Jackson E", "Diller IC", "Seibert FB", etc. in the search box.

This short communication is unlikely to convince many health professionals that bacteria cause cancer. However, after four decades of studying cancer microbes in cancerous tissue, I am personally convinced that Dr. Virginia Livingston will one day be vindicated and recognized as one of the greatest medical geniuses of the twentieth century.

Ralph W Moss, cancer advocate and author of The Cancer Industry, notes her passing was "a major loss to the cancer world." In the *Cancer Chronicles #6*, 1990, he writes, "Virginia Livingston was a great person and a great scientist. Sadly, she never received the recognition she deserved in her lifetime. The true scope of her achievements will only become known in years to come."

This report honors the centennial of her birth which takes place on December 28, 2006.

Bibliography (for Dr. Cantwell's article only)

Alexander-Jackson E. A specific type of microorganism isolated from animal and human cancer: bacteriology of the organism. Growth. 1954 Mar;18(1):37-51.

Cantwell AR. Variably acid-fast cell wall-deficient bacteria as a possible cause of dermatologic disease. In, Domingue GJ (Ed). Cell wall-deficient Bacteria. Reading: Addison-Wesley Publishing Co; 1982.pp. 321-360.

Cantwell A. The Cancer Microbe. Los Angeles: Aries Rising Press; 1990.

Cantwell A. Four Women Against Cancer. Los Angeles: Aries Rising Press; 2005.

Diller IC, Diller WF. Intracellular acid-fast organisms isolated from malignant tissues. Trans Amer Micr Soc. 1965; 84:138-148.

Greenberg DE, Ding L, Zelazny AM, Stock F, Wong A, Anderson VL, Miller G, Kleiner DE, Tenorio AR, Brinster L, Dorward DW, Murray PR, Holland SM. A novel bacterium associated with lymphadenitis in a patient with chronic granulomatous disease. PLoS Pathog. 2006 Apr;2(4):e28.Epub 2006 Apr 14.

Hooper SJ, Crean SJ, Lewis MA, Spratt DA, Wade WG, Wilson MJ. Viable bacteria present within oral squamous cell carcinoma tissue. J Clin Microbiol. 2006 May;44(5):1719-25.

Nuzum JW. The experimental production of metastasizing carcinoma of the breast of the dog and primary epithelioma in man by repeated inoculation of a micrococcus isolated from human breast cancer. Surg Gynecol Obstet. 1925; 11;343-352.

Russell W. An address on a characteristic organism of cancer. Br Med J. 1890; 2:1356-1360.

Russell W. The parasite of cancer. Lancet. 1899;1:1138-1141.

Sauter C, Kurrer MO. Intracellular bacteria in Hodgkin's disease and sclerosing mediastinal B-cell lymphoma: sign of a bacterial etiology? Swiss Med Wkly. 2002 Jun 15;132(23-24):312-5.

Scott MJ. The parasitic origin of carcinoma. Northwest Med. 1925;24:162-166.

Seibert FB, Feldmann FM, Davis RL, Richmond IS. Morphological, biological, and immunological studies on isolates from tumors and leukemic bloods. Ann N Y Acad Sci. 1970 Oct 30;174(2):690-728.

Shannon BA, Garrett KL, Cohen RJ. Links between Propionibacterium acnes and prostate cancer. Future Oncol. 2006 Apr;2(2):225-32.Review.

Wuerthele Caspe-Livingston V, Alexander-Jackson E, Anderson JA, et al. Cultural properties and pathogenicity of certain microorganisms obtained from various proliferative and neoplastic diseases. Amer J Med Sci. 1950; 220;628-646.

Wuerthele-Caspe Livingston V, Livingston AM. Demonstration of Progenitor cryptocides in the blood of patients with collagen and neoplastic diseases. Trans NY Acad Sci. 1972; 174 (2):636-654.

Young J. Description of an organism obtained from carcinomatous growths. Edinburgh Med J. 1921; 27:212-221.

Intracellular Parasites

Modified from Wikipedia, Online version: http://en.wikipedia.org/wiki/Intracellular_parasite, various references cited.

Intracellular parasites are parasitic microorganisms that are capable of growing and reproducing inside the cells of a host. Facultative types can live and reproduce both inside and outside host cells. Some examples are given below

Bacteria	Fungi	Protozoa
Francisella tularensis	Histoplasma capsulatum	Plasmodium
Listeria monocytogenes	Cryptococcus neoformans	Toxoplasma gondii
Salmonella typhi		
Brucella		
Legionella		
Mycobacterium		
Nocardia		
Rhodococcus equi		
Yersinia		
Neisseria meningitidis		

Obligate intracellular parasites cannot reproduce outside host cells; they must depend on factors within a cell to reproduce. This category includes viruses, but other examples are listed below.

Bacteria	Fungi	Protozoa
Chlamydia	Pneumocystis jirovecii	Apicomplexans, such as Plasmodium species
Rickettsia		Toxoplasma gondii
Coxiella		Cryptosporidium parvum
Mycobacterium, such as Mycobacterium leprae		Trypanosomatids, such as Leishmania species
		Trypanosoma cruzi

Bacteria and cancer: cause, coincidence or cure?

by D L Mager (dmager@forsyth.org), *Journal of Translational Medicine* 2006, 4:14 doi:10.1186/1479-5876-4-14. (electronic version online: http://www.translational-medicine.com/content/4/1/14.

Research has found that certain bacteria are associated with human cancers. Their role, however, is still unclear. Convincing evidence links some species to carcinogenesis while others appear promising in the diagnosis, prevention or treatment of cancers. The complex relationship between bacteria and humans is demonstrated by Helicobacter pylori and Salmonella typhi infections. Research has shown that H. pylori can cause gastric cancer or MALT lymphoma in some individuals. In contrast, exposure to H. pylori appears to reduce the risk of esophageal cancer in others. Salmonella typhi infection has been associated with the development of gallbladder cancer; however S. typhi is a promising carrier of therapeutic agents for melanoma, colon and bladder cancers. Thus bacterial species and their roles in particular cancers appear to differ among different individuals. Many species, however, share an important characteristic: highly site-specific colonization. This critical factor may lead to the development of non-invasive diagnostic tests, innovative treatments and cancer vaccines....

It is estimated that over 15% of malignancies worldwide can be attributed to infections or about 1.2 million cases per year. Infections involving viruses, bacteria and schistosomes have been linked to higher risks of malignancy. Although viral infections have been strongly associated with cancers, bacterial associations are significant. For example, convincing evidence has linked Helicobacter pylori with both gastric cancer and mucosa-associated lymphoid tissue (MALT) lymphoma, however other species associated with cancers include: Salmonella typhi and gallbladder cancer, Streptococcus bovis and colon cancer, and Chlamydia pneumoniae with lung cancer. Important mechanisms by which bacterial agents may induce carcinogenesis include chronic infection, immune evasion and immune suppression.

It has been shown that several bacteria can cause chronic infections or produce toxins that disturb the cell cycle resulting in altered cell growth. The resulting damage to DNA is similar to that caused by carcinogenic agents as the genes that are altered control normal cell division and apoptosis....

The immune system is an important line of defense for tumor formation of malignancies that express unique antigens. Certain bacterial infections may evade the immune system or stimulate immune responses that contribute to carcinogenic changes through the stimulatory and mutagenic effects of cytokines released by inflammatory cells....Chronic stimulation of these substances along with environmental factors such as smoking, or a susceptible host appears to contribute significantly to carcinogenesis.

How bacteria could cause cancer: one step at a time

Alistair J. Lax and Warren Thomas, Dept of Oral Microbiology, King's College London, Guy's Hospital, London, UK SE1 9RT, *Trends in Microbiology*, Volume 10, Issue 6, 293-299, 1 June

2002, doi:10.1016/S0966-842X(02)02360-0,

Abstract

Helicobacter pylori highlighted the potential for bacteria to cause cancer. It is becoming clear that chronic infection with other bacteria, notably Salmonella typhi, can also facilitate tumour development. Infections caused by several bacteria (Bartonella spp., Lawsonia intracellularis and Citrobacter rodentium) can induce cellular proliferation that can be reversed by antibiotic treatment. Other chronic bacterial infections have the effect of blocking apoptosis. However, the underlying cellular mechanisms are far from clear. Conversely, several bacterial toxins interfere with cellular signalling mechanisms in a way that is characteristic of tumour promoters. These include Pasteurella multocida toxin, which uniquely acts as a mitogen, and Escherichia coli cytotoxic necrotizing factor, which activates Rho family signalling. This leads to activation of COX2, which is involved in several stages of tumour development, including inhibition of apoptosis. Such toxins could provide valuable models for bacterial involvement in cancer, but more significantly they could play a direct role in cancer causation and progression.

Editor: Thanks to Helen Faria, Admin, HaciendaPublishing.com, Former Managing Editor, *Medical Sentinel* for permission to include the following article in this section. The article is available online at http://www.haciendapub.com/medicalsentinel/mycoplasmal-infections-chronic-illnesses-fibromyalgia-and-chronic-fatigue-syndromes-.

Mycoplasmal Infections in Chronic Illnesses: Fibromyalgia and Chronic Fatigue Syndromes, Gulf War Illness, HIV-AIDS and Rheumatoid Arthritis

Author: Garth L. Nicolson, PhD, Marwan Y. Nasralla, PhD, Joerg Haier, MD, PhD, Robert Erwin, MD, Nancy L. Nicolson, PhD, Richard Ngwenya, MD

This article was published in the *Medical Sentinel,* Volume 4, Number 5, September/October 1999, pp. 172-175, 191

Abstract

Invasive bacterial infections are associated with several acute and chronic illnesses, including: aerodigestive diseases such as Asthma, Pneumonia, Inflammatory Bowel Diseases; rheumatoid diseases, such as Rheumatoid Arthritis (RA); immunosuppression diseases such as HIV-AIDS; genitourinary infections and chronic fatigue illnesses such as Chronic Fatigue Syndrome (CFS), Fibromyalgia Syndrome (FMS) and Gulf War Illnesses (GWI). It is now apparent that such infections could be (a) causative, (b) cofactors or (c) opportunistic agents in a variety of chronic illnesses. Using Forensic Polymerase Chain Reaction we have looked for the presence of one class of invasive infection (mycoplasmal infections) inside blood leukocyte samples from patients with CFS (Myalgic Encephalomyelitis), FMS, RA, and GWI. There was a significant difference between symptomatic CFS, FMS, GWI, and RA patients with positive mycoplasmal infections of any species (45-63%) and healthy positive controls (~9%) (P<0.001). This difference was even greater when specific species (M. fermentans, M. hominis, M. penetrans, M. pneumoniae) were detected. Except for GWI, most patients had multiple mycoplasmal infections (more than one species of mycoplasma). Patients with different diagnoses but overlapping signs and symptoms often have mycoplasmal infections, and such mycoplasma-positive patients generally respond to multiple cycles of particular antibiotics (doxycycline, minocycline, ciprofloxacin, azithromycin, and clarithromycin). Multiple cycles of these antibiotics plus nutritional support appear to be necessary for successful treatment. In addition, immune enhancement and other supplements appear to help these patients regain their health. Other chronic infections may also be involved to various degrees with or without mycoplasmal infections in causing patient morbidity in various chronic illnesses.

Introduction: Chronic Illnesses

There is growing awareness that many chronic illnesses may have an infectious nature that is either responsible (causative) for the illness, a cofactor for the illness or appears as an opportunistic infection(s) that is responsible for aggravating patient morbidity.(1) There are several reasons for this notion, including the nonrandom or clustered appearance of an illness, often in immediate family members, the course of the illness, and its response to therapies based on infectious agents. Since chronic illnesses are often complex, involving multiple, nonspecific, overlapping signs and symptoms, they are difficult to diagnose and even more difficult to treat. Most chronic illnesses do not have effective therapies, and patients rarely recover from their conditions,(2) causing in some areas of the world catastrophic economic problems.

Some chronic illnesses, such as Rheumatoid Arthritis (RA), are well established in their clinical diagnosis,(3) whereas others, such as Chronic Fatigue Syndrome (CFS, sometimes called Myalgic Encephalomyelitis), Fibromyalgia Syndrome (FMS), and Gulf War Syndrome or Gulf War Illnesses (GWI), have rather nonspecific but similar complex, multi-organ signs and symptoms that overlap or are almost identical.(1) In the case of CFS, FMS and GWI these include: chronic fatigue, headaches, muscle pain and soreness, nausea, gastrointestinal problems, joint pain and soreness, lymph node pain, cognitive problems, depression, breathing problems and other signs and symptoms.(4) The major difference between these illnesses appears to be in the severity of specific signs and symptoms. For example, FMS patients have as their major complaint muscle and overall pain, soreness and weakness, whereas CFS patients most often complain of chronic fatigue and joint pain, stiffness and soreness, but otherwise their complaints usually overlap. Often these patients have increased sensitivities to various environmental irritants and enhanced allergic responses. Although chronic fatigue illnesses have been known for several years, most patients with CFS, FMS, GWI and in some cases RA have had few treatment options. This may have been due to the imprecise nature of their diagnoses, which are based primarily on clinical observations rather than laboratory tests, and a lack of understanding about the underlying causes of these illnesses or the factors responsible for patient morbidity.(1) These illnesses could have different initial causes or triggers but similar cofactors or similar opportunistic infections that cause significant morbidity.

Chronic Illnesses: Overlapping Signs and Symptoms

The multiple signs and symptoms of FMS, CFS and GWI are complex, nonspecific and completely overlapping (Figure 1), suggesting that these illnesses are related and not completely separate syndromes.(1,6) In this figure only differences in the signs and symptoms after the onset of illness are shown, and the data for FMS and CFS have been combined, because previous studies indicated that with the exception of muscle pain and tenderness, there was essentially no difference in patient signs.(4) Illness Survey Forms were analyzed to determine the most common signs and symptoms at the time when blood was drawn from patients. The intensity of patient signs and symptoms prior to and after onset of illness was recorded on a 10-point rank scale (0-10, extreme). The data were arranged by 38 different signs and symptoms and were considered positive if the value after onset of illness was two or more points higher than prior to the onset of illness. The data in Figure 1 indicate that patients diagnosed with CFS or FMS had complex signs and symptoms that were similar to those reported for GWI. In addition, the presence of rheumatoid signs and symptoms in each of these disorders indicates that there are also similarities to RA.(7) Moreover, it is not unusual to find immediate family members who display similar signs and symptoms. For example, there is evidence that GWI has slowly spread to immediate family members,(8) and it is likely that it has also spread to some degree in the workplace.(1) A preliminary survey of approximately 1,200 GWI families indicated that approximately 77% of spouses and a majority of children born after the war had signs and symptoms similar or identical to veterans with GWI.(8)

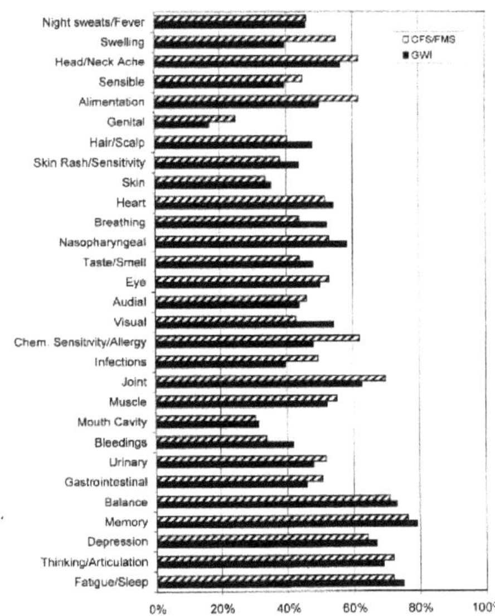

Figure 28: Incidence of increase in severity of signs and symptoms in 203 patients with CFS/FMS compared in GWI after the onset of illness.

Severity was assessed using a Patient Illness Survey Form that included 114 signs and symptoms. The intensity was scored by patients on a 10-point scale (0, none; 10, extreme) prior to and after the onset of illness. Scores were determined in each category (3-9 questions) as the sum of differences between values prior to and after onset of illness divided by the number of questions in the category. Changes in score values of 2 or more points were considered relevant.

In the absence of laboratory tests to the contrary, chronic illnesses are often misdiagnosed as somatoform disorders caused by stress and other nonorganic factors.(9) Patients with CFS, FMS and GWI usually have cognitive problems, such as short term memory loss, difficulty concentrating and other problems, and physicians who find psychological or psychiatric problems in these patients often decide that these conditions are caused by somatoform disorders, not organic problems.(1) Stress is often mentioned as an important factor or the important factor in these disorders. Indeed, GWI patients are often diagnosed with Post Traumatic Stress Disorder (PTSD) in veterans' and military hospitals.(10) The evidence that has been offered as proof that stress or PTSD is the source of GWI sickness is the assumption that veterans must have suffered from stress by virtue of the stressful environment in which they found themselves during the Gulf War,(10) but the veterans themselves do not feel that stress-related diagnoses are an accurate portrayal of their illnesses. Most testimony to date refutes the notion that stress is the major factor in GWI,(11) suggesting that stress, albeit important, is not the cause of GWI.(12) But most physicians would agree that stress can exacerbate chronic illnesses and suppress immune systems, suggesting that stress plays a secondary not primary role in chronic illnesses, such as GWI, CFS, and FMS.(1) However, in the absence of physical or laboratory tests that can identify possible origins of FMS, CFS or GWI, many physicians accept that stress is the cause of these chronic illnesses. It has been only recently that other causes were seriously considered, including chronic infections.(13)

Mycoplasmal Infections in CFS, FMS and GWI

We have been particularly interested in the association of certain chronic infectious agents in CFS, FMS and GWI, because these microorganisms can potentially cause most or essentially all of the signs and symptoms found in these patients.(1,14) One type of infection that elicited our attention was microorganisms of the class Molecutes, small bacterial mycoplasmas, lacking cell walls, that are capable of invading several types of human cells and are associated with a wide variety of human diseases.(14)

We have examined the presence of mycoplasmal blood infections in GWI, CFS, and FMS patients. The clinical diagnosis of these disorders was obtained from referring physicians according to the patients' major signs and symptoms. Since the signs and symptoms of CFS and FMS patients completely overlapped, these patients were therefore considered together (CFS/FMS).(1) Blood was collected, shipped over night at 4°C and processed immediately for PCR after purification of DNA using a Chelex procedure.(1,7) Patients' blood was analyzed for the presence of mycoplasmal infections in blood leukocytes. Positive PCR results were confirmed if the PCR product was 717 base pairs in size using the genus-specific primers (or 850 base pairs for M. fermentans specific primers, etc.) along with a positive control of the same size in the same gel, and if a visible band was obtained after hybridization with the internal probe.(15) The sensitivity and specificity of the PCR methods were determined by examining serial dilutions of purified DNA of M. fermentans, M. pneumoniae, M. penetrans, M. hominis and M. genetalium. Amounts as low as 10 fg of purified DNA were detectable for all species using the genus primers. The amplification with genus primers produced the expected fragment size in all tested species, which was confirmed by hybridization with an inner probe.(16)

Mycoplasma tests were performed on all patients as described previously (1,7,17) either from Chelex-purified DNA or DNA prepared from whole blood using a commercial kit. The targeted Mycoplasma spp. sequence was amplified from DNA extracted from the peripheral blood of 144/203 CFS or FMS patients (~70%). In 70 healthy subjects positive results for Mycoplasma spp. were obtained in 6 samples (<9%). The difference between patient and control groups was significant ($p<0.001$).(17) In addition, two of the 70 controls were positive for M. fermentans. The ratio between positive and negative patients was comparable in female and male patients. These results are quite similar to the results recently published by others.(18) Similarly, using Nucleoprotein Gene Tracking to analyze the blood leukocytes from GWI patients we found that 91/200 (45%) were positive for mycoplasmal infections.(19,20) In contrast, in nondeployed, healthy adults the incidence of mycoplasmal infections was 4/62 (~6%).(19,20)

Patients with FMS or CFS often have multiple mycoplasmal infections and probably other chronic infections as well. When we examined CFS/FMS patients for M. fermentans, M. pneumoniae, M. penetrans, M. hominis infections, multiple infections were found in over one-half of 93 patients (Figure 2). CFS/FMS patients had double (over 30%) or triple (over

20%) mycoplasmal infections, but only when one of the species was M. fermentans or M. pneumoniae.(17) Higher score values for increases in the severity of signs and symptoms were also found in patients with multiple infections. CFS/FMS patients infected with different mycoplasma species generally had a longer history of illness, suggesting that patients may have contracted additional infections with time.(17)

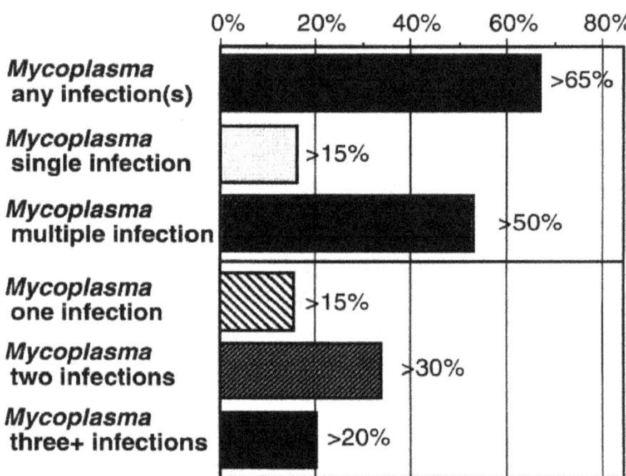

Figure 29: Incidence of multiple mycoplasmal infections in 93 CFS/FMS patients. Patients were examined for M. fermentans, M. pneumoniae, M. penetrans, or M. hominis blood infections by Forensic PCR.

In the course of our studies we found that DNA preparation and blood storage was extremely important in preserving the test samples. Storage of blood frozen or at 0-4°C resulted in reproducible assay results, whereas storage at room temperature resulted in loss of PCR signal over time. Within 1-2 days at room temperature, most of the positive samples reverted to negative results.(1) Also, blood drawn in tubes (blue-top) containing citrate and kept at 0-4°C before the assay yielded better results than other anticoagulants, unless the samples were frozen in EDTA (purple-top) tubes.

Mycoplasmal Infections in Rheumatoid Diseases

The underlying causes of rheumatoid diseases are not known, but RA and other autoimmune diseases could be triggered or exacerbated by infectious agents. It has been known for some time that infectious diseases in some animal species result in remarkable clinical and pathological similarities to RA and other rheumatoid diseases. Aerobic and anaerobic intestinal bacteria, viruses and mycoplasmas have been proposed as important agents in RA.(21) Recently there has been increasing evidence that mycoplasmas may play a role in the initiation or progression of RA.(22) Mycoplasmas have been proposed to interact nonspecifically with B-lymphocytes, resulting in modulation of immunity, autoimmune reactions and promotion of rheumatoid diseases.(23) M. pneumoniae, M. salivarium and U. urealyticum have also been found in the joint tissues of patients with rheumatological diseases, suggesting their pathogenic involvement.(24)

When we examined RA patients' blood leukocytes for the presence of mycoplasmas, we found that approximately one-half were infected with various species of mycoplasmas.(7) The most common species found was M. fermentans, followed by M. pneumoniae and M. hominis and finally M. penetrans. Similar to what we found in CFS/FMS patients, there was a high percentage of multiple mycoplasmal infections in RA patients when one of the species was M. fermentans.(7)

Although the precise role of mycoplasmas in RA and other rheumatoid inflammatory diseases remains unknown, mycoplasmas could be important cofactors in the development of inflammatory responses and for progression of the disease. As an example of the possible role of mycoplasmas in rheumatological diseases, M. arthritidis infections in animals can trigger and exacerbate autoimmune arthritis.(25) This mycoplasma can also suppress T-cells and release substances that act on polymorphonuclear granulocytes, such as oxygen radicals, chemotactic factors, and other substances.(26) Mycoplasmal infections can increase proinflammatory cytokines, such as Interleukin-1, -2, and -6,(27) suggesting that they are involved in the development and possibly progression of rheumatological diseases.

In addition to mycoplasmal infections, other microorganisms have been under investigation as cofactors or causative agents in rheumatological diseases. The discovery of EB virus(28) and cytomegalovirus(29) in the cells of the synovial lining in RA patients suggested their involvement in RA, possibly as a cofactor. There are a number of bacteria and viruses that are candidates in the induction of RA or its progression.(30) In support of bacterial involvement in RA, it has been known for some time that antibiotics like minocycline can alleviate the clinical signs and symptoms of RA.(31) Although this has been proposed to be due to their anti-inflammatory activities, these drugs are likely to be acting to suppress infections of sensitive microorganisms like mycoplasmas.

Mycoplasmal Infections in Immunosuppressive and Autoimmune Diseases

Mycoplasmas have been implicated in the progression of HIV-AIDS. It has been known for some time that some species of mycoplasmas are associated with certain terminal human diseases, such as an acute fatal illness found with certain Mycoplasma fermentans infections in non-AIDS patients.(32) Recently, mycoplasmal infections have attracted attention as a major source of morbidity in AIDS patients. For example, M. fermentans can cause renal and CNS complications in patients with AIDS,(33) and M. penetrans has also been found in the respiratory epithelial cells of AIDS patients.(34) Other species of mycoplasmas have also been found in AIDS patients where they have been associated with disease progression, such as M. prium and M. hominis.(32) Blanchard and Montagnier(35) have proposed that mycoplasmas are cofactors in HIV-AIDS, accelerating progression and accounting, at least in part, for increased susceptibility of AIDS patients to additional infections. In addition to immune suppression, some of this increased susceptibility may be the result of mycoplasma-induced host cell membrane damage from toxic oxygenated products released from intracellular mycoplasmas.(36) Also, mycoplasmas may regulate HIV-LTR-dependent gene expression,(37) suggesting that mycoplasmas may play an important regulatory role in HIV pathogenicity.

There is some preliminary evidence that mycoplasmal infections could be associated with autoimmune diseases. In some mycoplasma-positive GWI cases the signs and symptoms of Multiple Sclerosis (MS), Amyotrophic Lateral Sclerosis (ALS or Lou Gehrig's Disease), Lupus, Graves' Disease and other complex autoimmune diseases have been seen. Such usually rare autoimmune responses are consistent with certain chronic infections, such as mycoplasmal infections, that penetrate into nerve cells, synovial cells and other cell types. These autoimmune signs and symptoms could be caused when intracellular pathogens, such as mycoplasmas, escape from cellular compartments and incorporate into their own structures pieces of host cell membranes that contain important host membrane antigens that can trigger autoimmune responses. Alternatively, mycoplasma surface components ('superantigens') may directly stimulate autoimmune responses,(38) or their molecular mimicry of host antigens may explain, in part, their ability to stimulate autoimmunity.(39)

Mycoplasmal Infections in Other Clinical Conditions

Asthma, airway inflammation, chronic pneumonia and other respiratory diseases are known to be associated with mycoplasmal infections. For example, M. pneumoniae is a common cause of upper respiratory infections,(40) and severe asthma is commonly associated with mycoplasmal infections.(41) Recent evidence has shown that certain mycoplasmas, such as M. fermentans (incognitus strain), are unusually invasive and often found within respiratory epithelial cells.(34)

Heart infections (myocarditis, endocarditis, pericarditis and others) are often due to chronic infections, such as Mycoplasma,(42,43) Chlamydia(44) and possibly other infectious agents.

Other species of mycoplasmas are also associated with various illnesses: M. hominis infections were first found in patients with hypogammaglobulinemia, and M. genitalium was first isolated from the urogenital tracts of patients with nongonococcal urethritis.(45,46) Although mycoplasmas can exist in the oral cavity and gut as normal flora, when they penetrate into the blood and tissues, they may be able to cause or promote a variety of acute or chronic illnesses. These cell-penetrating species, such as M. penetrans, M. fermentans and M. pirum among others, can probably result in complex systemic signs and symptoms. Mycoplasmas are also very effective at evading the immune system, and synergism with other infectious agents can occur.(14) Similar types of chronic infectious agents may occur.(14) Similar types of chronic infections caused by Chlamydia, Brucella, Coxiella or Borrelia may also be present either as single agents or as complex, multiple in

Mycoplasmal Infections: Treatment Suggestions

Once mycoplasmal infections have been identified in the white blood cell fractions of subsets of CFS, FMS, GWI, RA and other patients, they can be successfully treated. Appropriate treatment with antibiotics should result in patient improvement and even recovery.(6,19,20) The recommended treatments for mycoplasmal blood infections require long-term antibiotic therapy, usually multiple 6-week cycles of doxycycline (200-300 mg/day),(47) ciprofloxacin (1,500 mg/day), azithromycin (500 mg/day) or clarithromycin (750-1,000 mg/day).(48) Multiple cycles are required, because few patients recover after only a few cycles, possibly because of the intracellular locations

of mycoplasmas like M. fermentans and M. penetrans, the slow-growing nature of these microorganisms and their relative drug sensitivities. For example, of 87 GWI patients that tested positive for mycoplasmal infections, all patients relapsed after the first 6-week cycle of antibiotic therapy, but after up to 6 cycles of therapy 69/87 patients recovered and returned to active duty.(19,20) The clinical responses that were seen were not due to placebo effects, because administration of some antibiotics, such as penicillins, resulted in patients becoming more not less symptomatic, and they were not due to immunosuppressive effects that can occur with some of the recommended antibiotics. Interestingly, CFS, FMS and GWI patients that slowly recover after several cycles of antibiotics are generally less environmentally sensitive, suggesting that their immune systems may be returning to pre-illness states. If such patients had illnesses that were caused by psychological or psychiatric problems or solely by chemical exposures, they should not respond to the recommended antibiotics and slowly recover. In addition, if such treatments were just reducing autoimmune responses, then patients should relapse after the treatments are discontinued.(1)

Patients with CFS, FMS, RA or GWI usually have nutritional and vitamin deficiencies that must be corrected.(48) These patients are often depleted in vitamins B, C, and E and certain minerals. Unfortunately, patients with these chronic illnesses often have poor absorption. Therefore, high doses of some vitamins must be used, and others, such as vitamin B complex, must be given sublingual. Antibiotics that deplete normal gut bacteria can result in over-growth of less desirable flora, so Lactobacillus acidophillus supplementation is recommended. In addition, a number of natural remedies that boost the immune system are available and are potentially useful, especially during antibiotic therapy or after therapy has been completed.(48) One of us (R.N.) has been involved in the development of ancient African and Chinese natural immune enhancers and cleansers help to restore natural immunity and absorption. Although these products are known to help AIDS patients, their clinical effectiveness in GWI/CFS/FMS/RA patients has not been carefully evaluated. They appear to be useful during therapy to boost the immune system or after antibiotic therapy in a maintenance program to prevent relapses.(48)

Why aren't physicians routinely treating mycoplasmal and other chronic infections? In many cases they are treating these infections, but it has been only recently that such infections have been found in so many unexplained chronic illnesses. These infections cannot be successfully treated with the usual short courses of antibiotics due to their intracellular locations, slow proliferation rates and inherent insensitivity to most antibiotics. In addition, a fully functional immune system may be essential to overcoming these infections, and this is why vitamin and nutritional supplements are so important.

Conclusions

We have proposed that chronic infections are an appropriate explanation for the morbidity seen in a rather large subset of CFS, FMS, GWI and RA patients, and in a variety of other illnesses. Not every patient will have this as a diagnostic explanation or have the same types of chronic infections, and additional research is necessary to clarify the role of such infections in chronic diseases.(1,7) Some patients may have chemical or radiological exposures or other environmental problems as an underlying reason for their chronic signs and symptoms. In these patients, chronic infections may be opportunistic. In others, somatoform disorders or illnesses caused by psychological or psychiatric problems may indeed be important. However, in these patients antibiotics, supplements and immune enhancers should have no lasting effect whatsoever, and they should not recover on such therapies. **The identification of specific infectious agents in the blood of chronically ill patients may allow many patients with CFS, FMS, GWI or RA and other chronic diseases to obtain more specific diagnoses and effective treatments for their illnesses. Finally, patients with cardiopathies, AIDS, respiratory illnesses, and urogenital infections are often infected with Mycoplasma, Chlamydia, Brucella or other chronic, invasive bacterial and parasitic infections, and these patients could benefit from appropriate antibiotic and neutraceutical therapies that alleviate morbidity.**

References

1. Nicolson GL, Nasralla M, Haier J, Nicolson NL. Biomed. Therapy 1998;16:266-271.

2. Hoffman C, Rice D, Sung H-Y. (1996) JAMA 1996;276:1473-1479.

3. Hochberg MC, et al. Arthritis Rheumatol. 1992;35:498-502.

4. Nicolson GL, Nicolson NL. J. Occup. Environ. Med. 1996;38:14-16.

5. Murray-Leisure K. et al. Intern. J. Med. 1998;1:47-72.

6. Nicolson GL. Intern. J. Med. 1998;1:42-46.

7. Haier J, Nasralla M, Nicolson GL. Rheumatol 1999;38:504-509.

8. Senate Committee on Banking, Housing and Urban Affairs, U. S. Congress (1994) U.S. chemical and biological warfare-related dual use exports to Iraq and their possible impact on the health consequences of the Persian Gulf War, 103rd Congress, 2nd Session, Report: May 25, 1994.

9. N.I.H. Technology Assessment Workshop Panel. The Persian Gulf experience and health. JAMA 1994;272:391-396.

10. Nicolson GL, Nicolson NL. Med. Confl. Surviv. 1997;13:140-146.

11. House Committee on Government Reform and Oversight, U. S. Congress (1997) Gulf War veterans': DOD continue to resist strong evidence linking toxic causes to chronic health effects, 105th Congress, 1st Session, Report: 105-388.

12. U. S. General Accounting Office (1997) Gulf War Illnesses: improved monitoring of clinical progress and reexamination of research emphasis are needed. Report: GAO/SNIAD-97-163.

13. Nicolson GL, Nicolson NL. Townsend Lett. Doctors 1996;156:42-48.

14. Baseman JB, Tully JG. Emerg. Infect. Dis. 1997;3:21-32.

15. Van Kuppeveld FJM, et al. Appl. Environ. Microbiol. 1992;58:2606-2615.

16. Erlich HA, Gelfand D, Sninsky JJ. Science 1991;252:1643-1651.

17. Nasralla M, Haier J, Nicolson GL. Clin. Microbiol. Infect. Dis. 1999; in press.

18. Vojdani A, Choppa PC, Tagle C, Andrin R, Samimi B, Lapp CW. FEMS Immunol. Med. Microbiol. 1998;22:355-365.

19. Nicolson GL, Nicolson NL. Intern. J. Occup. Med. Immunol. Tox. 1996;5:69-78.

20. Nicolson GL, Nicolson NL, Nasralla M. Intern. J. Med. 1998;1:80-92.

21. Midvedt T. Scan. J. Rheumatol. Suppl. 1987;64:49-54.

22. Schaeverbeke T, et al. Rev. Rheumatol. 1997;64:120-128.

23. Simecka JW, Ross SE, Cassell GH, Davis JK. Clin. Infect. Dis. 1993;17 (Supp. 1):S176-S182.

24. Furr PM, Taylor-Robinson D, Webster ADB. Ann. Rheumatol. Dis. 1994;53:183-184.

25. Cole BC, Griffith MM. Arthritis Rheumatol. 1993;36:994-1002.

26. Kirchhoff H, et al. Rheumatol. Int. 1989;9:193-196.

27. Mühlradt PF, Quentmeier H, Schmitt E. Infect. Immunol. 1991;58:1273-1280.

28. Fox RI, Luppi M, Pisa P, Kang HI. J. Rheumatol. 1992;32:18-24.

29. Takei M, et al. Int. Immunol. 1997;9:739-743.

30. Krause A, Kamradt T, Burnmester GR. Curr. Opin. Rheumatol. 1996;8:203-209.

31. Tilley BC, et al. Ann. Intern. Med. 1995;122:81-89.

32. Savio ML, et al. New Microbiol. 1996;19:203-209.

33. Bauer FA, Wear D J, Angritt P, Lo S-C. Hum. Pathol. 1991;22:63-69.

34. Stadtlander CT, Watson HL, Simecka JW, Cassell GH. Clin. Infect. Dis. 1993;17 (Suppl. 1):S289-S301.

35. Blanchard A, Montagnier L. Ann. Rev. Microbiol. 1994;48:687-712.

36. Pollack J D, Jones MA, Williams MV. Clin. Infect. Dis. 1993;17 (Suppl. 1):S267-S271.

37. Nir-Paz R, Israel S, Honigman A, Kahane I. FEMS Microbiol. Lett. 1995;128:63-68.

38. Kaneoka H, Naito S. Jap. J. Clin. Med. 1997;6:1363-1369.

39. Baseman JB, Reddy SP, Dallo SP. Am. J. Respir. Crit. Care Med. 1996;154:S137-S144.

40. Balassanian N, Robbins FC. N. Engl. J. Med. 1967;277:719.

41. Gill JC, Cedillo RL, Mayagoitia BG, Paz MD. Ann. Allergy 1993;70:23-25.

42. Prattichizzo FA, Simonetti I, Galetta F. Minerva Cardioangiol. 1997;45:447-450.

43. Hofner G, et al. Zeit. Kardiol. 1997;86:423-426.

44. Bowman J, et al. J. Infect. Dis. 1998;178:274-277.

45. Tully JG, Taylor-Robinson D, Cole RM, Rose DL. Lancet 1981;1:1288-1291.

46. Risi GF Jr, Martin DH, Silberman JA, Cohen JC. Mol. Cell. Probes 1987;1:327-335.

47. Nicolson GL, Nicolson NL. JAMA 1995;273:618-619.

48. Nicolson GL. Intern. J. Med. 1998;1:115-117 and 123-128.

Prof. Garth L. Nicolson, Drs. Marwan Nasralla, Joerg Haier, Robert Erwin and Nancy L. Nicolson are affiliated with The Institute for Molecular Medicine, 15162 Triton Lane, Huntington Beach, CA 92649-1401, (714) 903-2900, Fax (714) 379-2082, website: www.immed.org, email: gnicimm@ix.netcom.com; Dr. Richard Ngwenya is affiliated with the James Mobb Immune Enhancement Clinics, 132 Josiah Chinamano Ave., Harare, Zimbabwe, Fax: +263-4-739-832.

Dr. Nicolson et al's article is hereby published as one view of the possible cause(s) of the Gulf War Syndrome and other chronic illnesses and because a federal grant has been earmarked to evaluate his thesis, but its publication should not be construed as an endorsement of that thesis by the Medical Sentinel or the AAPS---Editor.

Appendix B: Tips for a Successful Practice

What you pick up in your everyday practice is what is going to make you a doctor. It is that practical knowledge that you pick up, not the book learning, that makes all of the difference in the world if you are to be a good or bad practitioner. Get in there, show your patients that you love them and that you are trying to help them. If you do this in your practice and in life, believe me, I don't care what town you go into, within three months, you will have a successful practice.

When your clinical research goes against the consensus of medical opinion – and nobody can describe what is the consensus of medical opinion – you are in for a tough time. In other words, if you have a hundred medical doctors down the street that are all practicing the same, their opinions are worth more than yours because you're different than they are. You will have to be well-studied and strong in your commitment to continue helping your patients according to your beliefs.

Keep Complete and Accurate Records

Hundreds of well-educated, dedicated practitioners have been intimidated for their beliefs, investigated closely, and brought before boards and into courts to answer for how they treated their patients. Even when you think you are in the right, you still must:

- Have well-founded reasons for the tests that you recommend, the conclusions that you draw from examinations and testing, the supplements and medications that you use, and the written and verbal statements that you make to each and every patient. **In almost every instance in which a practitioner was censured, lost a license, or was convicted, it was partly because of inadequate patient records.**
- Always ensure that the patient states unequivocally why he or she has sought your services and understands completely your diagnosis and treatment plan. and what outcomes to anticipate. It is vital that these elements are put into writing at the outset; many such legal document templates are available. The patient must sign off on 100% of your intentions before any of your work begins.
- **Never get so busy that you can't go out and learn more.** Over my years of practice, I always took six weeks off every year, five of those weeks to study and

one week to rest. If you can find entry into some place, get into all of the research centers you can.

Engage Patients Sincerely

Many times when a patient comes in, you're not quite sure of what to do. Go somewhere private in your office, close your eyes, and have a little meditation to yourself, and ask God for direction, "What should I do?", "How should I do it?" You'd be surprised as you develop this particular technique, how the answers will come to you. To me this has been one of the great things as far as my own life is concerned.

I never get on a platform without having said this type of prayer that the words will come from Him, through me, to give you something that you can use in your everyday lives. That to me is the important thing; what I do, what I say; because I feel that God has been so wonderful to me as far as my life is concerned. I don't care what religion you are, just so you have a religion. I don't believe in atheism; I think God was the one that created us. He created the earth. As long as I feel that way, I'm going to continue to talk that way.

Cultivate Diagnostic Sensitivity

I was fortunate to be trained by Dr. John B. Deaver, a famous clinician and surgeon and President of the American College of Surgeons. While examining a patient, he never touched him. Rather he stood at the foot of his bed observing him. He never looked at the chart, but he could gave the patient's temperature, respiration, pulse, and blood pressure – all exactly as written on the chart. How did he do it? By observation.

John Blair Deaver, Philadelphia surgeon, was born on 25 July 1855 near Buck, Lancaster County, Pennsylvania. He was the son of Joshua Montgomery and Elizabeth Moore Deaver. He received his M.D. from the University of Pennsylvania in 1878.

Dr. Deaver served internships at Germantown Hospital and Children's Hospital of Philadelphia. In 1886, he also became Surgeon to Lankenau (then German) Hospital. He became Chief of the Surgical Department in 1896 and was noted for his skill and physical endurance as well as for abdominal surgery, in particular, appendectomies.

Dr. Deaver returned to the University of Pennsylvania in 1911 as Professor of the Practice of Surgery. In 1918, he became the John Rhea Barton Professor of Surgery and held this post until retiring in 1922.He died of a progressive anemia at his home in Wyncote, Pennsylvania, on 25 September 1931.

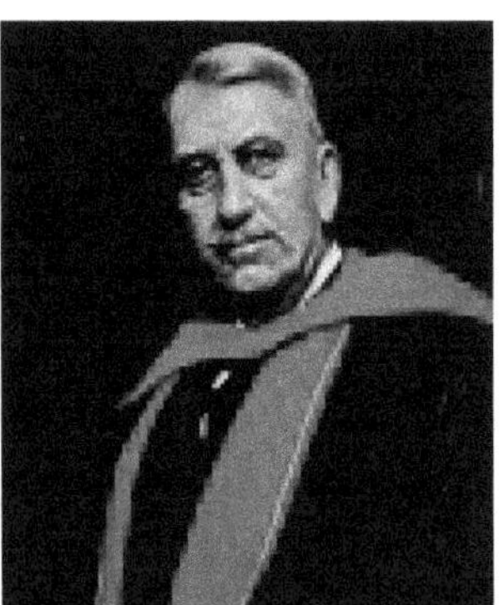

John Blair Deaver, 1855-1931, Adolphe Borie, artist,1877-1934

I want you to be observant, so watch the skin texture. When patients are lying down, watch the jugular vein – the way it comes up. You can tell what their blood pressures and pulse rates are. If you watch the lobes of the ears, the nares of the nose and around the eyes, you can tell what their temperatures are.

A variation of 10 degrees in pulse rate over normal corresponds to one degree of temperature. For examples, see Table 16.

Table 16: Relationship Between Pulse Rate and Body Temperature

Pulse Rate	Corresponding Temperature (degrees F)
60	98
70	99
80	100
90	101
100	102
110	103

You can watch the chest move up and down to get their respiration rate. Then observe skin textures. These are the most important things to observe. I would note all of my observations of the patients; then, in surgery, I would see which pathologies they had and match my observations with their pathologies.

Develop your palpation. I can feel a hair through 26 pages in a textbook. Make your fingers that sensitive to tissue, because when you put your hands on a person, you want to know what's underneath it; you want to know what those muscles are doing, what those ligaments are doing, and what the blood vessels are doing, because if you don't understand that, then you have no business doing a manipulation on anybody.

One of the biggest problems chiropractors have is the use of force in technique, because they never palpated to know what the tissues were doing. You can use force and tear ligaments and get some symptomatic results, but the long lasting results are worse than if you hadn't even treated them in the first place. So learn to be observant of all things, especially what you feel with your hands.

The palm of the left hand has a negative magnetic charge. The right hand has a positive charge. I cannot picture images In my mind from touching someone, so I do it through the magnetic forces of my body, by going around the patient and feeling the auras. The break in the aura will tell me what is wrong with that particular patient. It is the same when treating a patient. The left hand receives; therefore use the left hand to palpate the patient's spine. Run two fingers down the spine and note the thermal changes. The hottest spot is your key lesion (not the cold spots).

Use Antibiotics, Drugs, and Medicines Sensibly

In your practice, you must always use your own judgement with respect to the use of antibiotics in each individual situation, but do not neglect to build up the immune system and detoxify the body. If I did have to use an antibiotic, I would go with penicillin. I don't think I used four bottles in my whole years of practicing because I just didn't believe in it. But if I had to give an antibiotic, I'd always detoxify the patient first and then get all of the vitamins and minerals into the body. Then I might give one shot of penicillin; most of the time it was half a cc instead of a full one, just to show that I had given it and had it on my record. And all it did was act like the proverbial bullwhip on a tired horse to make it run. I had the ingredients in there to stimulate production of more antibodies, and as long as they had the antibodies, they were going to destroy the bacteria.

We who are the believers in the manipulative phase of our work are not in with the group that is giving us these drugs and medicines. Sure, I believe in certain acute cases of using some drugs and medicines to help us over the hump. But I know one thing about all of the infections like children's diseases, if you give them the proper supplementation and do the cleansing job that we recommend, you often don't have to use antibiotics. I have taken children with measles, chicken pox, and scarlet fever, cleared them up in three to four days, and had them back to school in a week. Clean them out first, then give them the vitamins and minerals they need to form their own antibodies to fight their infections.

Use Colonic Irrigation Routinely

A lot of people don't understand what a colonic irrigation is. It is a glorified enema. Instead of using two quarts of water, you use from five to 30 gallons of water. But you want to be very careful where you go to have colonic irrigations. If you really want to do something in your offices, put in a colonic irrigator. Get a nurse to do the job for you. You can make $10 to $15 per patient every 30 minutes over an eight-hour period; that's the easiest money you're going to make and one of the finest things that you will ever do for that patient. Even if your patients take vitamins, minerals, drugs, or medicines, if they do not have a bowel that can do the job of digesting and assimilating food to make it usable, they are wasting their money. That's where so many of these doctors are wrong.

If done correctly, colonic irrigations are probably the finest detoxifying agents that we have. They are absolutely the finest therapy I know for high blood pressure; with colonic irrigations, you don't need anything else.

To me a Dierker Colonic is, by far, the ideal one. I do not like gravitational types because you have to depend upon a sick bowel to tell you how much pressure you have before you try to expel it. The Dierker has a great big tube that they put some aloe vera gel on, which is what I try to get them to do instead of the KY jelly, because that helps them a little bit more, and a little small tube that lets the water in. The bigger tube lets the fecal material and gas out. If you watch in this particular machine, they have about a 12" glass or plastic tube which is clear. If you get curious, you can tip your head a little and watch everything that comes out of that bowel. They have a quart container with a level on it, and while the operator has this on, one for the water going in and out, they have this other one because all of a sudden, if they see something like undigested food or a worm or a parasite, they twist what goes into the collection tube and they can open up and let the water go in or out. In this way, you can analyze it, and find out what is going on.

The Dierker also has a mercury column on it, so if the pressure goes in and you hit a fecal impaction or a gas pocket your mercury column will climb. That being the case, you reverse the flow and let it come out. If you start sucking it out too much, the mercury column will drop, and you reverse the flow and put it back in again. So you can operate in this manner of in and out. At the very end of your colonic, if you will fill the bowel with water then take the lever and bang it in and take it out as fast as you can work that lever, you will give them one of the greatest peristaltic massages they have ever had in the colon. And you can take a lazy colon and, by this method, you can normalize the activity of that musculature in the colon. So it's a case again of learning how to do it.

These are wonderful instruments to have in your office, because even with a lot of the manipulation which we do, these toxic muscles are like rubber bands when you feel them. When you go over that back, when you go over that leg or over their ankles or their knees, test out that tissue. If it feels rubbery to you, be very careful of how you manipulate because you can do a lot of damage. When you find it, just say, "You're so toxic I'm going to have to see that you get cleaned out first." And detoxify. Then you won't have any trouble doing the manipulating. One of the most valuable things that we do is make sure tissues are acceptable for manipulation. If they are not, manipulation can be harmful.

Editor: The Dierker closed system colonic machine is no longer being manufactured under that name. Some used units are available on the internet. The reader may refer to the International Association for Colon Hydrotherapy publication, *Colon Therapy, 2 Edition*, found at https://www.cga.ct.gov/2013/phdata/tmy/2013SB-00873-R000220-International%20Assoc%20for%20Colon%20Therapy%20(I-ACT)-TMY.PDF.

Treat Children with Love and Respect

Always express love, so I tell you one little thing for you to do when you get into practice. It is one of the biggest practice builders that I know of. Every child that comes into your office; always give them a bear hug and a kiss. Don't be gruff with them.

You will be surprised what happens to the parents when they see you get down on one knee and put your arms around their small child, give him or her a big bear hug and say "I'm going to give you a bear hug and a kiss." This in itself shows the love that you have for people. When you show it to children first, you will never have any trouble treating those children.

After that, the next thing I said to a little boy was, "First of all we're going to make you a big man like me." So, of course, with the Ritter table you have automatic rise, so I brought him up to the same height that I am.

Here's another little trick. Let them see what you're doing, and you be the patient, because what I did was to take my stethoscope out and say, "Now you're going to be the doctor and you tell me what it is. When you look in my ear, it's supposed to have something gray down at the bottom of it. When I look in yours, I want to see if I can see anything gray in there, too."

So I put it up to my ear, turned it on, and let him look through it. He said, "Yeah, I can see that gray thing in there." I said, "Well, that's the drum. That's how clean your ears should bet so that you can see the gray, not red. If it's red, there's something wrong." He said, "Okay." So I looked in his ear; no problem at all, his mother didn't hold him at all.

Shorten Recovery Times Intelligently

I don't believe in giving blood as a transfusion; I don't believe that the body needs somebody else's blood. However, I do believe that, if you were to give a patient some amino acids intravenously, the body will take care of itself and do what It has to do in the rebuilding of every cell and tissue of the body.

When I used to admit patients in the hospital, they never could understand how they recovered so quickly. The reason is that I insisted that, on the night before surgery (I wrote the orders to make sure it was done.) we administer one bottle of amino acids with 3,000 mg of ascorbic acid in it. My patients never had shock, they never had pneumonia, they were up within hours after they got back from the recovery room. They would heal quickly, their stitches would be out on the fourth day, and they would be out on the fifth day. Do you think that I could get the other doctors in the hospital to follow that sort of a routine? No. They did not want to do it, because nobody else in the hospital was doing it either.

Support Pregnancy and Birthing Nutritionally

Now one of the other big factors in protein metabolism actually starts at the time of conception, because if the mother does not have sufficient proteins in the body she does not have sufficient minerals in the body. If she were to become pregnant, she wouldn't know it until about the sixth week. If she does not have enough zinc in her body at that time, her child can have a hair lip, a cleft palate, or both.

I have taken women that have previously given birth to such babies, put them on our program for five or six months, let them get pregnant, and they have the most beautiful children that you've ever seen and the easiest deliveries that they've ever had. Also, if the woman is properly balanced nutritionally, she should not experience long labor.

I have put over 800 pregnant women on the program, I have delivered over 350 of the babies myself; I have never lost a mother, and I have never lost a child, I have never had a malformed child, and my average delivery time is 2 hours and 20 minutes. I'll put this record against anybody's.

Take my own daughter and daughter-in-law, for instance. They had each two children. Their labors for their first children ranged from 39 to 45 hours under their chosen doctors. I blew my top and said, "Look, this is my specialty, why do you go to somebody else? Let me lay out your program, I'll pay for it, but you must follow it the way that I want you to do it, if you will do it." So they both agreed to try. Each one of them had the easiest nine months carrying the child. When it came time, I said, "Now the next thing that I want you to do is when you go into the labor room, I don't want you to bear down; just take deep breaths any time that you get any pain, just relax, your being in balance will start the peristaltic activity of the uterus. It shrinks when you have your labor pain; it'll do the work, because you're balanced. So, without any pressure of bearing down, my daughter delivered in 44 minutes, and my daughter-in-law delivered in 45 minutes. Then they decided they weren't going to have any more children.

We have done this many times. Another recent case involved a mother with only half a kidney on one side; a bunch of auxiliary junk up above, because it never developed right; and a tortuous ureter. We took care of her and put her in shape; then she got married and, within a short time, she was pregnant. She delivered this 9-pound, 2-ounce baby boy in a little more than three hours.

I'll tell you something that everybody gets a kick out of when I tell them. This grandmother, Dolly Ware, is a nutritionist in Houston. She is a multi-millionairess in her own right, and her hobby is nutrition. She takes all of the doctors' failures – about 90 patients a year – and takes care of them, showing them how to get straightened out. Dolly, being the insightful grandmother, four times every day, would take the baby's diapers off, put him on a pot, and hold him there. At the end of six weeks, that baby was completely pot-trained. He never had a dirty diaper after the sixth week.

Now believe it. I did not believe it either, until I saw them doing it. The child has never had so much as a sniffle; it has never had any cow's milk. In a *Science News* article of August 17, 1974, the author, Joan Arehart-Treichel, states, "The junk you eat during pregnancy may make your child susceptible to diseases later in life." This is documented, and much of the information that I share with practitioners and the public in my lectures comes from *Science News* and other similarly-credible sources.

Learn About Magnetism in Healing

Albert Roy Davis has written four books about magnetism. These are:

- *Anatomy of Biomagnetism*
- *The Magnetic Effect*
- *Magnetism and Its Effects on Living Tissue*
- *Rainbow in Your Hands*

His collaborator, Walter Rawls, Ph.D., assisted in research and updated Davis' books over the years. The books are very good, although the English may not be the best. Davis describes how to use north pole and south pole magnets and what they do the tissues. Each one has its own particular effects; the south pole liquefies, for example, in pneumonia of the lungs, you put 4,000-8,000 gauss south pole magnet on the chest for 15 minutes to liquefy the congestion. Then, you turn it around to the north pole and lay it on the chest to help heal it. The north pole magnet will take the soreness out of muscles in a hurry.

Editor: The gauss is the unit of measurement of a magnetic field; it is also called the magnetic flux density or the magnetic induction. The current source for magnets and books from those trained by Davis and Dr. Rawls is http://www.magnetage.com/Home_Page.html. Some of Davis' out of print books are listed on amazon.com.

Dr. Harold Brownlee has done a lot of work on magnetism with Albert Roy Davis. He has spent his whole career with monopole magnets, using the north or south pole by itself, as opposed to the U-type. I can say this, that I saw an experiment in Georgia, involving growing corn. One group of corn plants was treated with the north pole magnet, another with the south pole, another with both poles, and the control group with no magnets. Other groups were irrigated with water treated by the corresponding magnet. The corn treated with the south pole magnet and watered with water treated by this magnet had a 6-22% increase in protein content and a 25-30% increase in growth. Corn treated with the north pole grew very poorly – worse than the control group. Now some farmers are magnetizing their irrigation water and getting good results.

Editor: Dr. Harold Brownlee, Ottawa, Canada, was an attendee at Dr. Ellis' lecture. He has worked in the field of diagnosing human ailments utilizing two separate and distinct magnetic energies. It started with Ralph Seaira, D.C. in Puerto Rico. He has a magnet on a pulley that generates 24,000 gauss. He manipulates this magnet with the pulley down onto the knee or shoulder to heal the joint.

For people, we use the north pole magnet. For example, in treating infections, such as dental abscesses, a south pole magnet will worsen the condition. We use a bar 6"X 2"X 5/8" with 3,500-4,000 gauss. In a case of pneumonia we would use the south pole to liquefy the area, then the north pole to heal the tissues. How many of you know what the lymphatic pump is? In all my years of practice I have never lost a case of pneumonia, because of that lymphatic pump. With proper manipulation you won't have any problems, because the body's natural drainage system will work. Detoxification is important also (coffee or vitamin C enemas).

A Visit to Albert Roy Davis' Lab

It was fascinating to see Davis' original place. You would open the front door and, if you weren't instructed in what you would see, you would turn around and walk right out of the place. You never saw a place like this in your life because this man didn't believe in caging the animals he used in research; they were all over. But the one room where he did his research was spic and span. The first thing he did was put you in a chair and talk to you. You didn't realize it, but you had a video camera on you; then he played your conversation back to you. He has people from all over the world coming, to visit him, and he has them all on videotape.

Davis has devoted his entire life to the use of south and north pole magnets for what they do in the human body. He developed a magnet six feet long, three feet wide, and one foot thick, with 100,000 gauss capacity. He states that he has been finding that, if he can put somebody under the magnet twice a day for 20 minutes, he can take stop almost any disease in its tracks and make the patient better by using that high amount or gauss.

The Dotto Ring

Magnetic flux will stop a bruise or sprain immediately if you have that much energy. The only other instrument that comes close to this is the Dotto Ring. The Dotto Ring was devised by Gianni Dotto in Dayton Ohio. It is a big circular thing with a copper-core; you can stand on the inside of the ring, because it has to go up and down over you. Half of this one-inch thick copper core is so hot that it will burn you if you touch it, the other half is so cold it will burn you from freezing; they pass these electromagnetic forces through this copper core through the heat and cold then run this thing up and down over. you. They run it so many times up over you for the type of disease that you have.

The famous actress and health advocate, Gloria Swanson thought it was so good and what he was doing with it that she took Dotto to Italy. He is now (as of 1982) in a small town just north of Venice, treating over 100 people every day and getting very wonderful results. But the AMA did something typical of what they try to do. Dotto had his windows wired up to en electric seeing eye. He caught two top medical doctors of Dayton opening his window and coming in, taking the various animals and switching the animals charged with the Dotto ring with the control animals that were not so treated. This was an attempt to show that the Dotto ring was no good. That is how low these people can get to try and stop you when you have something that may work out pretty good for people.

Editor: Read the history of the Dotto Ring at http://www.keelynet.com/biology/dotto.htm. Also, read the 1973 newspaper article at http://news.google.com/newspapers?nid=2002&dat=19730127&id=i7IiAAAAIBAJ&sjid=Y7MFAAAAIBAJ&pg=4153,3187962.

Appendix C: Manipulation Notes

To be effective and minimize pain for your patients, you must learn proper manipulative techniques. I treat the total body because I think that if only one lesion is left untreated, it is going to reset everything else in the body.

Many types of medical professionals are employing manipulation in their practices. However, most never learn good manipulation; they don't know the basic principles. Yet under physical medicine, they are doing manipulation. Orthopedic surgeons are doing a lot of manipulation today and most of them are using forced techniques that are wrong.

One of the situations that teaches you the great respect that you must have for manipulative technique is when you try to do manipulation with the patient under anesthesia. When you first start doing that kind of work, and we've done plenty of it over the years, chills run up and down your spine. When you start breaking adhesions loose under manipulation with anesthesia, you have to have a stout heart.

I remember the first one that I did was breaking loose a frozen shoulder on a young girl. I'll tell you I sweated worse than the patient when she came out of the anesthesia because I really thought I had torn everything loose. But by constant treating afterwards, by using the proper minerals, we were able to straighten out that frozen shoulder so it wasn't frozen anymore. But all those fibrous adhesions were a challenge; we had to break them because it's the only way you can do It when they are bad.

That reminds me of another story. This little kid, if he stood up or sat up for 30 minutes, he would fall over completely blacked out. So his father had a watch built for him so that every 28 minutes, it buzzed and regardless of where he was he would immediately lie right down and stay there for two or three minutes. When he got up, he would be alright again. He had been examined by several orthopedics in St. Louis. We went in unknown to the doctors in charge. The supervising woman was very much interested in the kids, so she invited us in to check them. When I saw this one kid and heard the story, I immediately checked behind the angle of the jaw to find out how the cervical vertebrae were doing; man, were they out of position! Then I put my hand in back and found, for the first time in my life, the odontoid process off-center to one side.

This child had been in several close calls with cars from running out into the street. His parents told him he would be punished. One day, a car did hit him, and he was so scared at what would happen, he just got up and ran. His condition developed after that incident. He wouldn't tell anybody because it would get back to his parents. I got a hold of his parents and told them what we had discovered. His parents took him back to the same orthopedics that missed the diagnosis in the first place. Fortunately for the kid, they were able to put him to sleep and take that dislocation and put it back where it belonged. He had a very fine recovery with no more blackout spells. So you see these are the kinds of things you see if you really go looking for the unusual.

These key lesions will affect other areas from the cuboid all the way up to the spheno-basilar junction. Key lesions are central to many techniques: reflexology, zone therapy, Fitzgerald work, and acupuncture. The trouble with acupuncture is that too many practitioners do not know their 1,100 acupuncture points, and if they don't get results, they give it all up.

Editor: The following procedures derive from notes taken during Dr. Ellis' demonstrations to a group of students. In the absence of pictures and hands-on instruction, they are not intended to be comprehensive or complete. Consequently, these techniques are directed only toward professionals that have been previously trained in diagnosis and good manipulative techniques. The suggestions are supplemental and should be tried and incorporated only if completely understood.

Spine and Upper Body

A handy technique was shown to me by a Edgar O. Heist, D.O. of Hamilton, Ontario, during the American Osteopathic Association convention in Cleveland in 1934. I was Director of Research of Musebeck shoe company, and we had a booth at that convention where I used to treat 150-200 peoples' feet daily.

One day, I had a man on the table and was struggling at the adjustment of his feet. This little man, Dr. Heist, came along and said, "Hey, doctor, it looks like you're having a little trouble. May I show you something?" I said, "Sure, I'd be pleased!" (remember that you can always learn something from someone else). **He demonstrated correction of a lesion of the anterior third rib, using the anterior thoracic roll technique, and cautioned me to be more gentle, and by so doing, I corrected everything in the feet.** The key was the anterior third rib lesion. It locks the cuboid, the head of the fibula, L5, T12, the third rib, occiput, and the spheno-basilar junction.

Never use force without making use of proper leverage. Lesions are produced in a flexed or extended position. Take out the slack and have the patient take a deep breath and exhale. Thrust at the point of relaxation, even if it is only halfway through exhalation. Be relaxed when doing your techniques. See Basic (Anterior Thoracic) Roll Technique on page 395.

I believe that, unless the third anterior rib is in the proper position, adjustments do not hold as well. I always observe the relative levels of the clavicles; if one is higher than the other, I check the anterior ribs to see if they are aligned with each other at the medial aspect. **In approximately 85% of all cases, the left third anterior rib is out of position; in the other 15%, the right third anterior rib is out of position. It is the third anterior rib**

that controls the motion of the twelfth thoracic and fifth lumbar vertebrae; so, it is easy to understand how important the proper positioning of the third rib is to low back pain. See Third Rib Lesion on page 396.

Always reinforce your treatment by putting a positive thought into the patient's mind, such as, "Feel how much it is now." Tell your patient never to crack his own joints. This activity produces a hypermobility causing inflammation that develops into an arthritic condition. For arthritis, supplement with calcium, magnesium, manganese, phosphorus, and protein.

Head and Neck (Whiplash)

This manipulation is for posteriority of the occiput on atlas en masse.

Treatment: Have your patient sit facing you.

1. Placing both of your thumbs in front of the patient's ears, contact the rim of the occiput with the full length of both of your index fingers.
2. Pull the patient's head to your chest and have him drop his shoulders and arms.
3. Take out the slack and thrust with extension and traction.

Note: Expect to strain a few necks before perfecting this move.

Basic (Anterior Thoracic) Roll Technique

This is a simple and effective technique. Often no thrust is required to correct a lesion, only having to roll the supine patient, whose arms are folded across the chest. The forearms are not crossed. **A lesion to me is a limitation of movement in its normal plane.** I want to gap it; to allow the synovial fluid to get in there and grease the joint.

Treatment: Have your patient place the hand of the side of the lesion on his opposite shoulder and his other hand over the elbow of the first arm. The hand will be stabilized in the doctor's infraclavicular fossa.

1. Make a fist with your contact hand, and place this on the spine, just below the joint you want to adjust.
2. With your other hand, support the patient's head and neck, lift him forward, curling him upward and flexing the spine. Lift with your legs to avoid straining your back.
3. Roll the patient downward, taking out the slack and feeling the lesion underneath your contact hand.

   The lesion will show itself by its lack of joint play or springiness under your contact. Don't let up the slack and rock the patient. Too many doctors let up the slack and then bang 'em. That's the worst technique in the world!
4. Ask the patient to inhale, then to exhale.
5. Mobilize the lesion with a thrust, dropping your shoulder, at a certain point in the exhalation – a point of relaxation.

Note: In a case of scoliosis, we use the same technique but only on the convex side of the curves in order to straighten them. To treat, rotate the patient to one side to straighten out the curve you are going to work on. Make your corrective aojustment and bring the patient back. With the patient that has an S curve, rotate him to the other side and work on the higher curve.

From this point on, you must practice. You may hurt a few people, but once you master it, your other techniques will be much easier to do. Remember that you must make your hands sensitive to tissue. Be gentle!

First Rib Move

This manipulation is similar to that for the T1, but with a different contact point.

Treatment: Have the patient lie prone.

1. Contact the first rib with the base of your first finger.
2. Roll the patient's head back over the contact with rotation to the side of involvement.
3. Take out any slack and thrust.

Third Rib Lesion

I would say that 90% of lesions in the areas of the cuboid, the head of the fibula, L5, T12, the third rib, occiput, and spheno-basilar junction begin at the third rib. If you remove this lesion, the others will all be very simple to correct. If you use this technique before doing any other manipulation, subsequent manipulations will be much easier. The first purpose of manipulation is to open the joint and increase lubrication by the synovial fluid. If this technique does not unlock the cuboid and other areas previously mentioned, in 15% of the cases, look to one of these areas for the key lesion.

The medial end of the clavicle is raised on the affected side. The third rib interspace on that side will have tight, congealed, hypertonic muscles. There may also be tenderness at the insertion of tibialis anterior on the cuboid.

Treatment: The patient lies on a flat adjusting table, with his head at the end away from the headpiece. The fulcrum is the doctor 's thenar eminence, which is adducted across that hand.

1. Place your hand on the patient's back, parallel with the vertebral column and medial to the superior angle of the scapula.
2. Have your patient place the hand of the side of the lesion on his opposite shoulder and his other hand over the elbow of the first arm. (The hand will be stabilized in the doctor's infraclavicular fossa.)
3. Place your other hand over the patient's arms and contact the third rib at the midclavicular line with the base of the index finger.

   Keep your thumb as much out of the way as possible. This may be awkward. Your contact hand must always be over the patient's arms, not under, or else you won't get the proper positioning or leverage. (The reason for putting the patient's hand over his elbow is to make a cushion between the elbow and your infraclavicular fossa. You may use a small cushion instead, but you won't feel as much movement.)

4. Raise the patient's arm with the elbow padded by the patient's hand and tucked underneath your clavicle, at your midclavicular line. Raise to a point about 90° to the patient's body, until you feel the contact area begin to move away from you. (The movement is akin to going up a hill and down the other side. You stop at the top of the hill and make your corrective adjustment there. When you get into that position, take out the slack and hold it. Do not let the elbow slip out from under your clavicle.)
5. Ask the patient to inhale, then to exhale. At a point of relaxation during the exhalation, thrust, dropping your shoulder.
6. Recheck the diagnostic points on the feet. Move from the medial cuneiform to the sustentaculum tali to find reflex points related to the rest of the spine. Don't dig in with your thumb. Be light, because the more pressure you use, the less you feel.

Upper Dorsal (Thoracic) Vertrebrae Lesions

Treatment: Have the patient lie prone (face down).

1. Cup his chin in your cephalic hand.
2. Extend and side bend his head, using your forearm to rotate his head toward you. Take out any slack.
3. With your other hand, contact the opposite transverse processes of the upper dorsal vertebrae with the heel of your palm (a broad contact), take out the slack and thrust down and away.

Fifth Lumbar Vertrebra (See Sacroiliac Lesion, below)

Treatment: Have the patient lie in the side position on the side of his short leg. Face the patient.

1. Pull the lower shoulder forward and flex the upper leg at the hip. Let the straight leg dangle off of the table to take advantage of the weight of the leg for leverage.
2. Place your thumb on the fifth lumbar to feel the centering of torsion.
3. Take out the slack and thrust, using the lumbar roll technique. Work the patient to take out all directions of fixation.

Sacroiliac Lesion

If you suspect degenerated discs, always check for an anatomical short leg. What you're trying to balance is the base of the sacrum. Before using any manipulation, rule out rotation by checking the heights of the crests of the ilia and anterior superior iliac spine (ASIS) positions. **The one and only way to determine an anatomical short leg is in a standing position.** Also check the play of the fifth lumbar vertebra.

Measure the distance of the crest of the ilia and acetabula from the floor. If you want to do it accurately you do a standing anterior-posterior and lateral of the lumbar spine and pelvis to prove it. It is vital to know what you are working with. You can see the difference in the heights of the acetabula. Also, watch the difference in the ilia, to find out if one is broad and the other isn't because in this way you can also tell whether or not you have a rotation of the ilia on the sacrum. This also has to be corrected to check it out. **Just because you put somebody on a table and make a correction, getting their legs to appear of equal length, does not mean you have corrected the anatomical short leg.** You think you've done something, but you stand him up again, put your hands on the crests of the ilia and you still find that they are exactly the same as they were before you treated them. Then you know you're dealing with an anatomical short leg.

Treatment: If the patient does have a short leg, have him or her lie in the side position on the side of his short leg. Face the patient. The side of the longer leg is done last. Place a pillow under the neck to align the head with the spine.

1. Pull the lower shoulder forward and flex the upper leg at the hip. Let the straight leg dangle off of the table to take advantage of the weight of the leg for leverage.
2. Put the patient in sufficient rotation to immobilize the fifth lumbar vertebra.
3. Contact the ileum between your forearm, abdomen, and other hand.
4. Have the patient take a deep breath and exhale; take out the slack and thrust.
5. Once again, check for a short leg. If the hips are level, the legs are of similar length, and the adjustment has been successful.

Note: If there remains an anatomical short leg, build up the the sole and heel of the shoe on the short side. Patients will tell you that they feel a lot better as soon as they put in a heel and sole lift. In the use of your wedge, make sure you always use both a sole and a heel lift; don't put it on the heel only. To do so throws the body into torsion and that is worse than no lift at all. If you have a sacrum backward, the fifth lumbar comes in and turns the other way to try to compensate. That's the same pattern that destroys the discs. So you've got a relaxation of the capsular ligaments and when you're stretching them, all of a sudden you get a bang and you will pop the disc right through that weak area.

Shoulder

Most lesions in the shoulder occur at the acromio-clavicular articulation. Manipulation of the shoulder must include removal of any involvement of the second, third, or fourth rib first, using the technique described above for correcting the third rib lesion. Modify the position of your hands to accommodate the appropriate rib.

Treatment: The patient is in a standing position with his arm at his side. The doctor is standing behind the patient's opposite shoulder.

1. Flex his forearm and externally rotate the thumb to its end of motion.
2. Reach your arms around the patient, one in front and one behind, and cup your fingers onto the elbow.
3. Take out all slack.
4. Ask the patient to inhale deeply, then to exhale. At a point of relaxation during the exhalation, thrust straight upward to gap the acromio-clavicular joint.

Elbow and Wrist

Both tennis elbow and baseball elbow involve the wrist, as well.

Treatment of Elbow: Stand facing the patient and hold the arm in front of and perpendicular to the patient.

1. Rotate the hand and forearm externally, until the thumb points laterally.
2. Rest the patient's elbow in your hand while cupping your fingers over the olecranon; hold the patient's hand with your other hand.
3. Have the patient take a deep breath and relax; take out the slack and thrust upwards and outwards on the elbow at a 45° angle.
4. To adjust the radius, have the patient abduct the arm medially, then rotate the arm.
5. Contact the proximal head of the radius, take out the slack, and thrust.

Treatment of Wrist: Stand facing the patient and shaking hands.

1. Take your free hand and grasp the patient's wrist such that your thenar eminence is level with patient's carpals.
2. Roll the patient's carpals and metacarpals between your two hands using them as a rolling press. You can open up every joint this way.

Alternative Wrist Move: While facing the patient, interlock your fingers on the palmer surface of the patient's hand with your thumbs over the carpals on the dorsal surface.

1. With his arm hanging at his side, have patient raise his shoulder.
2. Have the patient take a deep breath and relax; take out the slack, follow the descent of arm, and thrust downwards at the end of the descent.

Asthma, Bronchitis, Emphysema

Treatment: Have your patient lie on his back with his head near the edge of the table. Stand on either side.

1. The contact point is a ligament halfway between the belly button and the xiphoid process of the sternum; then 2" to the left.
2. Place the tips of your fingers on this ligament, take out the slack, and thrust.

Pneumonia

Treatment: This technique involves use of a lymphatic pumping action. Have the patient lie on his back with his head near the the edge of the table. Stand at the head of the table.

1. Have the patient clasp his hands behind the front leg of the doctor, causing his chest to rise higher.
2. Overlap your hands on the chest, take up the slack, and gently apply and release pressure quickly or slowly. Slow pumping can be done for 15 minutes.

3. When finished, have the patient take a deep breath and pump all of the way down to the lower end of the ribs. This action will stir the liver, pancreas, and spleen and empty a lot of toxins.

Note: I have never lost a patient as long as I used this pump technique along with cleaning the bowels and giving the proper supplementation.

Sinus Drainage and Oral Cavity

When tonsils are removed, some portions of the adenoids may remain and form adhesions that can grow right over the eustacian opening into the oral cavity, causing ketoral deafness, dizziness, or middle ear infection.

This technique enhances sinus drainage and opens the oral cavity through turning upward and outward the maxilla and volmer bones. It is somewhat painful to the patient, because you are applying pressure to sensitive tissues at the junction of the soft and hard palates and laterally. Gagging is a possibility. Give the patient several tissues to use after treatment.

Treatment: Put a finger cot on your index finger to facilitate sliding. Have the patient sit facing you with his mouth open and begin breathing in a heavy, short panting manner to avoid gagging. Continue panting during the entire treatment.

1. Place the tip of your index finger on the hard palate, at the base of the upper front teeth (hard palate).
2. Apply pressure upwards, with the force directed toward the tip of the nose. When you feel separation take place, you know that you have done the job in front.
3. Continuing to apply the upward force, run your finger along the base of the teeth, all the way back to the soft palate. This is where it becomes tender.
4. When your finger reaches the pterygoid plate, move it over to the side.
5. Return to the midline between the hard and soft palates and direct the force to the external occipital protuberance.
6. Move your finger toward the eustacian opening behind the soft palate in the nasal pharynx and slide it down.
7. When approximately halfway down toward the lower jaw, thrust outward to break adhesions and clean out the eustacian tube.
8. Repeat the procedure for the opposite side of the mouth.
9. Withdraw your finger when finished and allow the patient to blow his nose on the tissues. Some bleeding may occur.

This procedure is sufficient to improve drainage in an average-sized infected sinus cavity. It is considered to be one of the finest therapies for the ear.

Temporomandibular Joint (TMJ) Correction

The temporal bone in the TMJ rotates, so the objective is to get one key where it locks this bone, and it is off of the zygomatic arch.

Treatment: Put a finger cot on your index finger to facilitate sliding. Have the patient sit facing you with his mouth open.

1. Place your index finger into the patient's open mouth, between the cheek and the base of the upper teeth.
2. Push your finger as far back as possible and direct it upwards, under the zygomatic arch. Make sure that your finger is flat in place.
3. Have the patient close his mouth and breathe deeply in and out.
4. When the patient is breathing out, turn your finger 90°; this will correct the TMJ on that side under the zygomatic arch.
5. Repeat the process for the other side.

The masseter muscle can hold the joint and keep it from being corrected. If you find that the TMJ has not moved, check the masseters. To loosen these muscles, put finger cots on your thumbs, insert them on either side between the cheeks and the teeth, take out the slack, and apply an outward thrust. If you recheck the TMJ, you will find that it was corrected.

Treatment for Acute Broken Nose

When using this technique, tell the patient that he won't have any pain for six weeks, at which time his nose will be back to normal.

Treatment: Put a pad on either side of the patient's nose and strap it down.

1. Place a finger cot on one of your fingers that is small enough to deeply penetrate the nares.
2. Lubricate the finger, place it into the nose and remodel it.

Feet and Knees

This section contains procedures for the correction of positions and articulations of the areas indicated.

Editor: This section is adapted from the booklet, *Foot Manipulation*, written by Dr. Ellis in 1934. In the Foreword, he credits Dr. George S. Rothmeyer of Philadelphia, Dr. Hubert J. Pocock of Toronto, Canada, and Mr. George E. Musebeck of Danville, Illinois for their contributions and encouragement. Even though the booklet is in the Public Domain, it is used by permission of the Foot-So-Port Shoe Company, successor to the Musebeck Shoe Company. **The reader is requested to forgive the poor quality of the accompanying pictures.** The only source found was a Xerox copy of a badly worn copy of the booklet. Should a booklet in better condition be obtained, the pictures will be replaced.

Metatarso-phalangeal Articulations

Two methods are necessary. The first uses the fingertips to correct all of the four lesser articulations at once; the other uses the thumb to correct the first phalangeal articulation. To begin, place the patient in the supine (face up) position on the manipulation table.

Multiple Correction of Four Lesser Phalanges

If the correction is needed on the left foot, stand to the right side of the table. Ask your patient to flex the left knee. Place the fingertips of your right hand on the heads of the metatarsals on the plantar surface. Lap your fingers over the toes so that the metacarpo-phalangeal articulations are in contact with the proximal (near) end of the proximal phalanx of each toe, as shown in Figure 30, below.

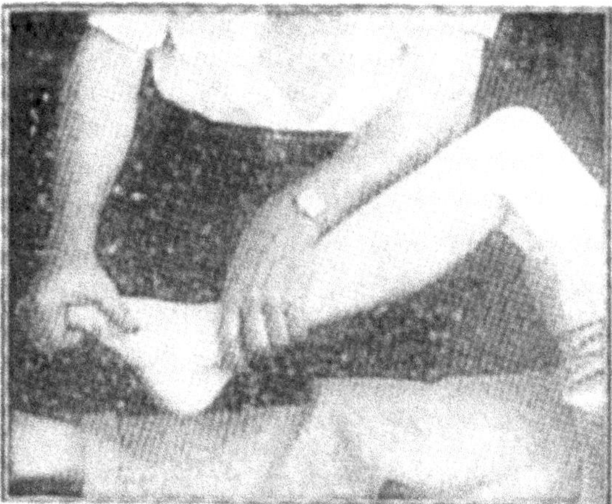

Figure 30: Method 1: Multiple correction, four lesser metatarso-phalangeal articulations.

Correction: With the left knee flexed, grasp the patient's left ankle with your left hand, flex the toes, and give a quick upward thrust with your right fingertips.

Single Correction of First Phalanx

With the patient's left knee flexed, grasp the left foot under the heel with your left hand. With your right hand, grasp the foot by the instep; with your right thumb contacting the head of the metatarsal on the plantar surface and the index finger on the proximal part of the first phalanx on the dorsal surface, as shown in Figure 31, below.

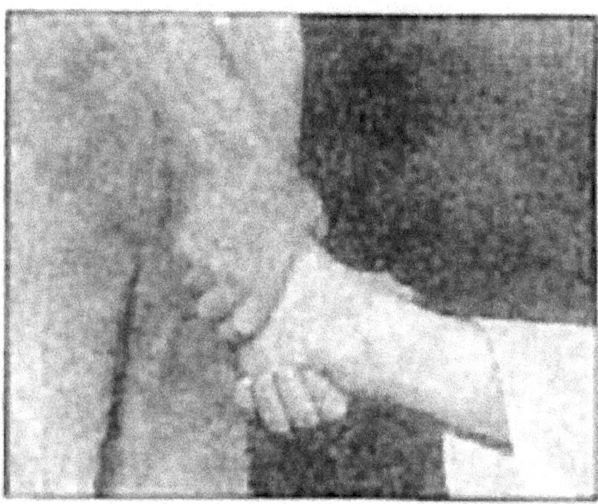

Figure 31: Method 2: Single correction of first metatarso-phalangeal articulations.

Correction: With your left hand, flex the toes, and give a quick upward thrust with your right fingertips.

Mid- and Hindfoot

The following procedures are helpful to:

- Raise the sustentaculum tali and inwardly rotate the calcaneus (os calcis)
- Rotate the head of the talus (astragalus) laterally
- Develop motion between the head of the talus and the navicular (scaphoid)
- Develop a separation strain in the calcaneo-cuboid articulation

Begin with the patient in a supine position. Assuming that the correction is on the left foot, ask the patient to flex the left knee. Face the patient at the left side of the table. With your left hand, grasp the lateral side of the calcaneus, with the thenar eminence of your left hand contacting, for the first thrust, the sustentaculum tali and, for the second thrust, the tuberosity of the navicular. Place your right hand on the dorso-lateral aspect of the left foot so that the proximal phalanx of your index finger contacts the cuboid, as shown in Figure 32, below.

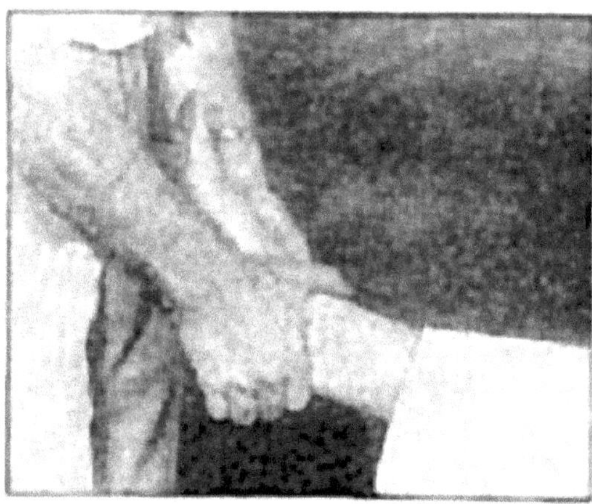

Figure 32: Starting position for multiple correction of midfoot bones.

Correction: Place the fingers of your left hand on the calcaneus and thrust medially. On the first thrust, your left thenar eminence moves the sustentaculum tali upward and laterally. On the second thrust, the thenar eminence moves the tuberosity of the navicular toward the prominence of the fifth metatarsal. For both actions, your right hand thrusts medially.

Your hands are not strong enough to complete this correction, so you must gain leverage from the strength of your legs. Position the dorsal aspect of each of your hands on the inner sides of your thighs, as shown below. When you thrust with your hands, push your knees together simultaneously, as shown in Figure 33, below.

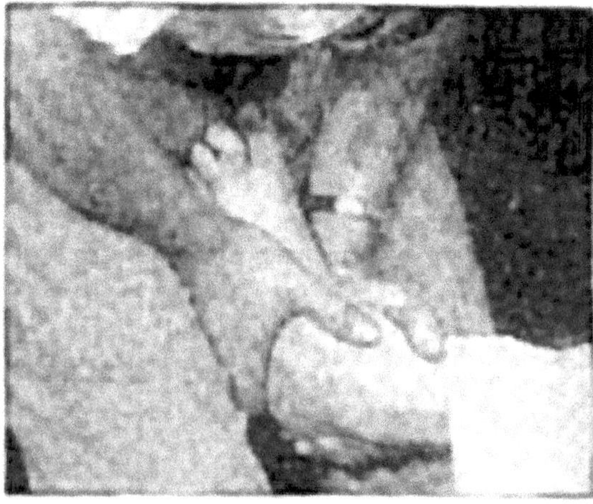

Figure 33: Augmenting thrust with pressure from thighs.

The resulting occurs:

- Because your right hand overlaps the outer part of the patient's left foot, including the cuboid, a separation develops between the cuboid and calcaneus.
- As the posterior part of the tuberosity of the navicular overlaps the medial side of the head of the talus, motion develops between the talus and the navicular, and the head of the talus is rotated laterally.
- The thrusts on the sustentaculum tali and the calcaneus raise the sustentaculum tali and inward rotation of the calcaneus.

Subastragaloid (Ankle Bone) Articulation

It is this joint that is most involved in sprained ankles. This correction can be done with the patient in either the prone (face down) or supine position. Let us assume that the patient's right foot needs correcting.

Patient in Prone Position

Face your patient's right foot. With your right hand, grasp the dorsolateral aspect of the foot, so that the proximal phalanx of your index finger contacts the superior surface of the talus (astragalus) anterior to its articulation with the tibia. Place the dorsum of your right hand on the table. Place the palm of your left hand on the planar surface of the calcaneus and apply sufficient pressure to eliminate slack, as shown in Figure 34, below.

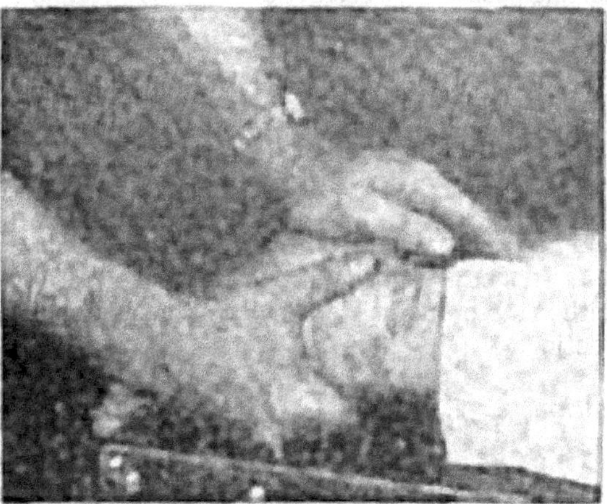

Figure 34: Starting position for correction of subastragaloid articulation (patient prone).

Correction: Thrust upward and forward on the calcaneus. This force reduces adhesions between the talus and calcaneus and between the talus and tibia.

Patient in Supine Position

Face the inside of the patient's flexed knee, which is allowed to drop off of the side of the table. Hold down the dorsum of the right foot to the surface of the table. Place the posterior of the palmar surface of your right hand on the medial side of the calcaneus, as shown in Figure 35, below.

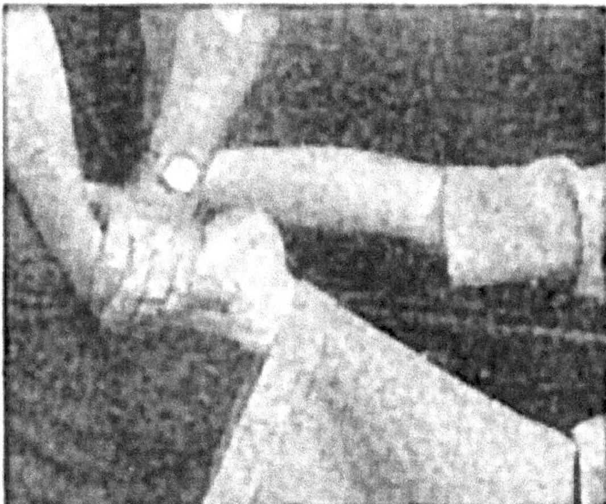

Figure 35: Starting position for correction of subastragaloid articulation (patient supine).

Correction: Use a firm thrust on the calcaneus toward the table surface. It is through this articulation that most of the inversion and eversion of the foot are accomplished.

Cuboid Rotation

A rotated cuboid bone can cause foot problems, postural problems, backaches, shoulder aches, and headaches. It can be a cause of atrophy to the feet. This procedure can be done with the patient in either the prone or standing position. Let us assume that the patient's right foot needs correcting.

Patient in Prone Position

Grasp the dorsum of the patient's right foot with the palmar surface of your right hand, so that the web between your thumb and index finger is positioned approximately at the talo-navicular articulation. Your thumb should extend along the lateral margin of the foot, with your index finger definitely beyond the prominence of the base of the fifth metatarsal. Then place the hypothenar eminence of your left hand on the prominence of the plantar end of the medial border of the cuboid. This location is about halfway across the plantar surface of the foot, from the posterior end of the base of the fifth metatarsal, as shown in Figure 36, below.

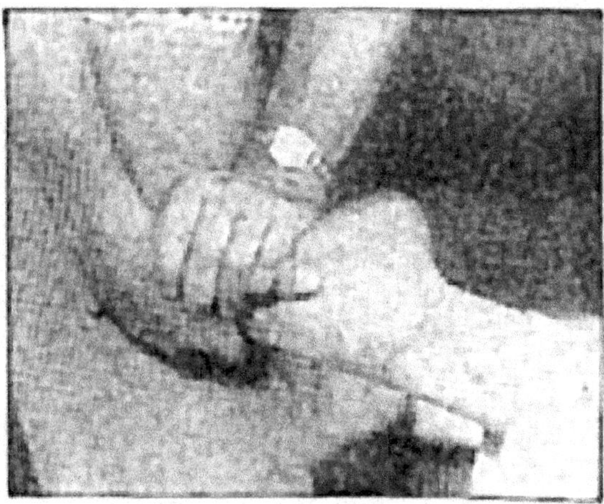

Figure 36: Starting position for correction of the cuboid (patient prone).

Correction: Supporting your right forearm and dorsum of your right hand on your right thigh, place the patient's foot in full extension. Keeping the foot straight in line with the leg, make a thrust with your straight left arm toward the dorsum of the articulation between the cuboid and the third cuneiform.

The resulting occurs:

- The third cuneiform moves, rotating the cuboid on its long axis so the the fifth metatarsal is lowered and the fourth metatarsal is raised.
- The third cuneiform moves upward in the arch caused by the friction between it and the cuboid and the slant at which the third cuneiform is placed in the transverse arch.

Patient in Standing Position

The same mechanics may be applied with the patient standing erect with his or her back to the doctor. Stand facing your patient's right leg. Grasp the dorsum of the patient's right foot with the palmar surface of your right hand, position the web between your thumb and index finger at the talo-navicular articulation. Your thumb should extend along the lateral margin of the foot, with your index finger beyond the prominence of the base of the fifth metatarsal. Then place the hypothenar eminence of your left hand on the prominence of the plantar end of the medial border of the cuboid. Apply a gentle circular motion to the leg to get the patient to relax. Bring the leg back in a straight line with the thigh, extend the leg, and completely extend the foot.

Correction: Keeping the foot straight, make a thrust with your straight left arm toward the dorsum of the articulation between the cuboid and the third cuneiform. The sudden stopping of the right hand gives the same effect as that produced by the thigh during the correction with the patient in the prone position.

Head of the Fibula

This procedure can be done with the patient in either the prone or supine position. Assume that the patient's right knee needs correcting.

Patient in Prone Position

Grasp the right ankle with your left hand and place your right hand in the bend of the knee joint, such that the metacarpo-phalangeal articulation of your index finger is behind the knee joint and proximal to the head of the fibula. Flex this leg on the thigh with the foot in a position of outward rotation until firm pressure is made by the head of the fibula against the metacarpo-phalangeal articulation of your right index finger., as shown in Figure 37, below

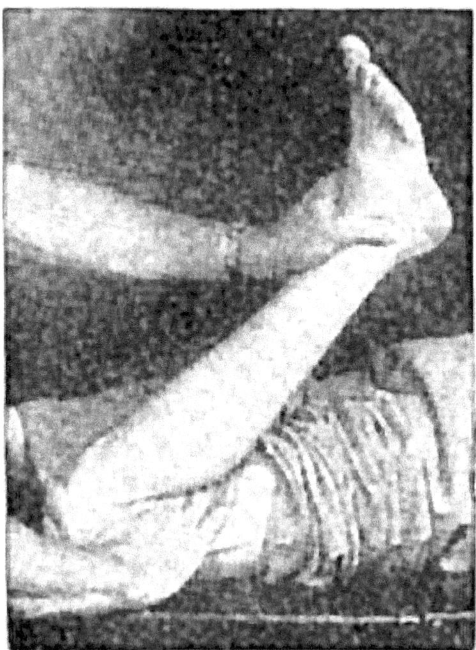

Figure 37: Starting position for correction of the fibula (patient prone).

Correction: Make a thrust by forcing the leg into extreme flexion until you feel the head of the fibula move.

Patient in Supine Position

Grasp the right ankle with your left hand and place your right hand in the bend of the knee joint, such that the metacarpo phalangeal articulation of your index finger is behind the knee joint and proximal to the head of the fibula. Flex the thigh onto the abdomen with the foot in a position of outward rotation until firm pressure is made by the head of the fibula again the metacarpo-phalangeal articulation of your right index finger.

Correction: Make a thrust by forcing the leg into extreme flexion until you feel the head of the fibula move.

Tibial and Cartilage Lesions

This procedure is best done with the patient in the prone position. Assume that the patient's right foot needs correcting. Grasp the ankle with your left hand and grasp the midfoot with your right hand. Start with the leg flexed to a comfortable position, as shown in Figure 38 and Figure 39, below.

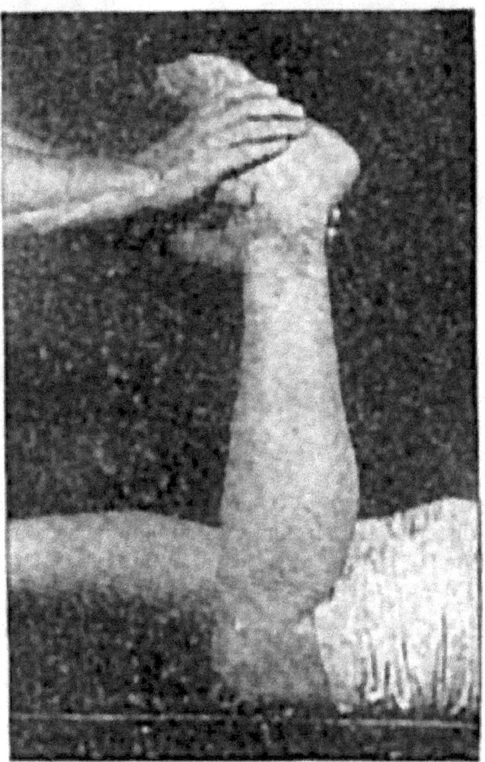

Figure 38: Inward rotation, correction of tibial and cartilage lesions (patient prone).

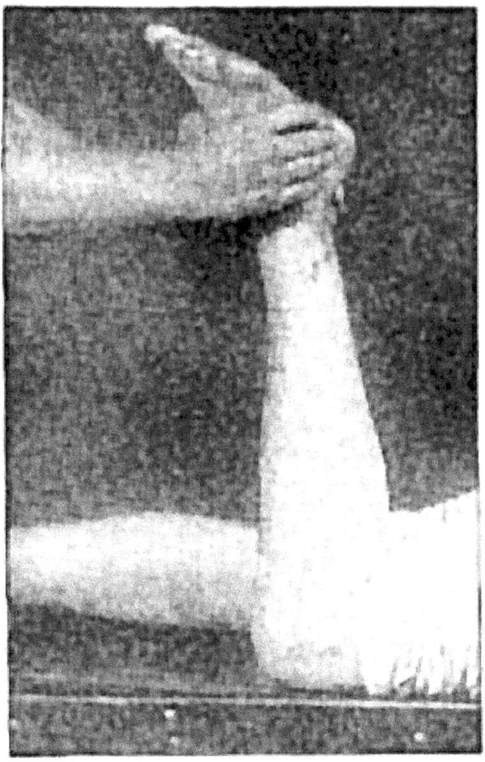

Figure 39: Outward rotation, correction of tibial and cartilage lesions (patient prone).

Correction: Flex and extend the right leg, alternating inward and outward rotation of the foot on the leg a short distance and gradually increasing this distance until full flexion and extension are accomplished.

Posterior-Transverse Arch

This procedure is best done with the patient in the supine position. Assume that the patient's left foot needs correcting. Interlock the fingers over the dorsum of the foot and place your palms on the medial and lateral sides of the foot so that the posterior-tranverse arch is in the center of each palm, as shown in Figure 40, below.

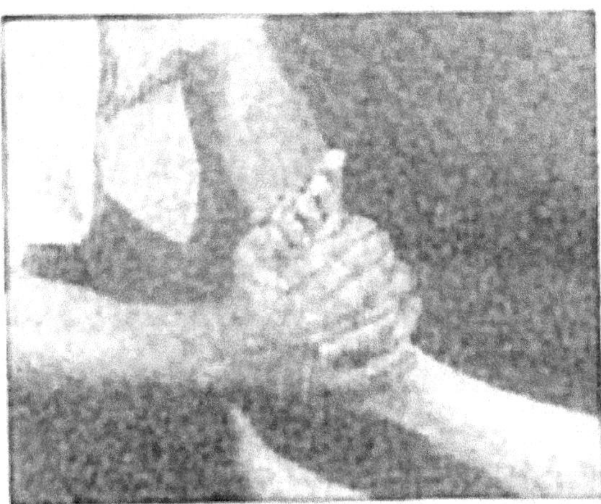

Figure 40: Starting position for raising the posterior-transverse arch (patient supine).

Correction: Gradually bring your hands together, using the interlocked fingers as a hinge. The friction produced by the pressure from your hands will cause the arch to be raised.

Taping of Foot After Corrections

To ensure that your treatments remain effective, your patient's feet should be strapped with tape for two days following correction. It is important to use the proper tape and not apply it so tightly as to impair circulation. Use two strips of adhesive tape 1 1/2" wide and of sufficient length to encircle the foot and overlap on the dorsal surface. If the patient has tender skin, apply tincture of benzoin to the feet before strapping.

Editor: In more recent times, Dr. Ellis recommended against adhesive tape in favor of less irritating, non-allergenic, non-waterproof micropore tape.

Place the first strip on the plantar surface of the foot so that the front edge of the tape is slightly in front of the head of the fifth metatarsal. Then, bring the tape up on the lateral side, over the dorsum, pulling it taut (not tight; do not stretch the skin). Bring up the tape on the medial side, overlapping the tape from the lateral side and pulling it taut, as well, as shown in Figure 41, below.

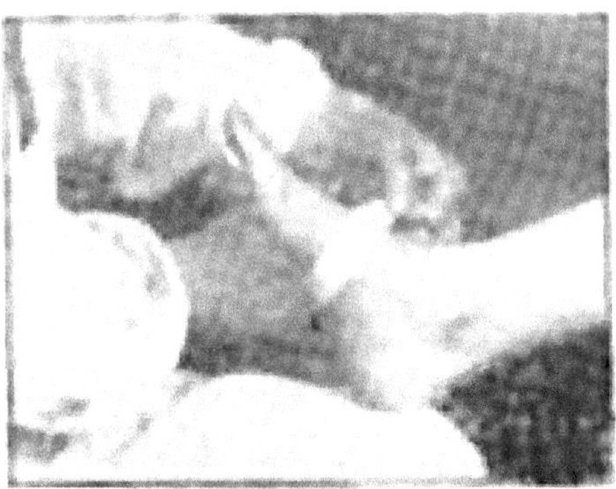

Figure 41: Application of first tape strip.

Place the second strip 3/4" forward from the first strip, applying it in the same way as the first strip. These two strips should cover the posterior transverse arch and the posterior metatarsal arch, as shown in Figure 42, below.

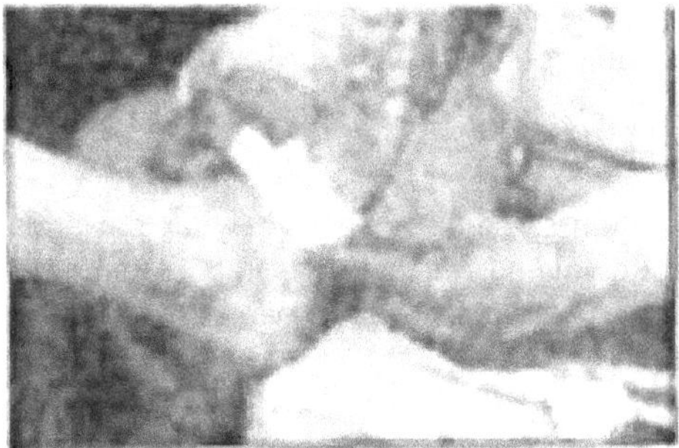

Figure 42: Application of second tape strip.

Instruct your patient not to remove the tape. Rather, remove the tape for your patient, loosening the end of the tape that was last applied. Draw this end back over the tape in the direction that it was applied, with the thumb of your other hand holding the skin taut, close to the tape being removed.

Exercises to Strengthen the Feet

There are several simple exercises that your patient can do at home to keep the feet flexible and strong. Some of these are listed below.

Extension-Flexion

To begin, have your patient completely extend his or her feet, curling the toes downward as far as possible. While keeping the toes curled, flex and extend (up and down) the feet on the ankles. Do this exercise for fifteen minutes, three times a day. See Figure 43, below.

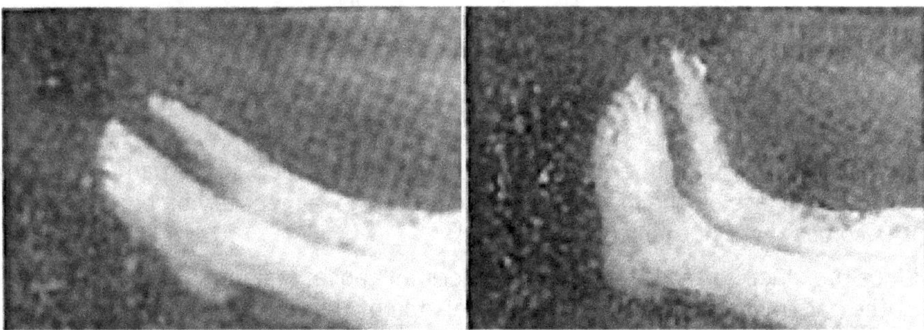

Figure 43: Alternating extension with flexion while keeping toes curled.

A cramp will develop in the feet and/or calves after doing this exercise for a couple of minutes. The patient should rest until the cramp disappears; then exercise again.

Bunching a Towel

Stand on the end of a Turkish towel, carrying the weight of the body on the heels that are in direct contact with the floor. By flexing the toes, bunch as much of the towel as possible under the feet.

Walking Modification

On a safe path, walk on the outside of the feet until the ankles become tired, being careful not to turn the ankles.

Installing Cuboid Pads in Shoes

Rotation of the cuboid bone causes atrophy of the foot and other problems, such as postural defects, backaches, shoulder pain, and headaches. To prevent downward rotation of the cuboid and and forward rotation of the calcaneus, we use a very simple, rectangular pad. We do not use metatarsal pads because they lift the metatarsals, causing hammer toes and denuding nerve centers going into the toes.

The pad that we use is a rectangle of hard felt and is approximately 3/16" thick, 1" wide, and 6" long. The edges on one side are beveled to avoid irritation. The objective of using the cuboid pad is to create a very shallow groove for the fifth metatarsal to drop down into. This groove is along the outside of the beveled cuboid pad which is directly under and supporting the fourth metatarsal. 1/8" too far forward or backward can make be difference between success and failure.

Follow these steps for correct size and placement of the cuboid pad into the shoe.

1. Trim a large cuboid pad to the proper size for the individual's foot. Bevel the edges from 1/8" to the edge at a 45° angle to ensure comfort.

   How long should the pad be? The posterior end of the trimmed pad is to be placed at a point 3/16" in front of the calcaneus (approximately 1/4" behind the breast of the heel of an average man's shoe) and end with the pad aligning with the anterior end of the fourth metatarsal. The breast of the heel is a shoe industry term to describe the location of the posterior end of the shank.

2. Take the sock lining out of the shoe and lay it aside. The pad will be attached to the insole below.
3. Spread quick drying rubber cement on the unbeveled side of the pad and on the adhering surface on the insole of the shoe. Let the cement dry on both surfaces until it becomes tacky but not runny.
4. Place the glued surfaces together as described above, making sure that the outer side of the pad aligns parallel with the lateral side of the fourth metatarsal.
5. To support the cuboid, insert an arch support to fill the cavity between the arch of the foot and the insole.
6. Replace the sock lining.

Appendix D: Vendors

This appendix lists as current information as possible about companies mentioned in the text and vendors that provide services described in the text.

Food Supplements

Name **Website** **Address** **Phone Numbers** **Online Contact** **Product List/Cross References**
Biotics Research Corporation http://www.bioticsresearch.com/landing/index.php?show=1 6801 Biotics Research Dr Rosenberg, TX 77471 800-231-5777 281-344-0909 Local 281-344-0725 Fax http://www.bioticsresearch.com/sfcontactus http://www.bioticsresearch.com/productlist
Enzyme Process http://www.enzymeprocess.co/index.php?option=com_content&view=article&id=100&Itemid=498 470 N. 56th Street Chandler, Arizona 85226 Toll Free: 800-521-8669 E-mail: info@enzymeprocess.co http://www.enzymeprocess.co/index.php?option=com_virtuemart&view=category&virtuemart_category_id=23&categorylayout=default&virtuemart_manufacturer_id=2&showcategory=1&showproducts=1&productsublayout=0&Itemid=561

Lily of the Desert http://www.lilyofthedesert.com/ 1887 Geesling Rd. Denton, TX 76208 940-566-9914 (800) 229-5459 Fax: 940-566-9925 http://www.lilyofthedesert.com/contact-us/ http://www.lilyofthedesert.com/our-products/
Life-Mate (Formerly Research Formula #2) http://lifematenutrition.com/ 351 W 6160 S Murray, UT 84107 888-600-1703 http://lifematenutrition.com/contact-us/ http://lifematenutrition.com/why-choose-life-mate/ingredients/
Miller Pharmacals http://www.millerpharmacal.com/index.php Miller Pharmacal Group 350 Randy Road, Suite 2 Carol Stream, IL 60188-1831 (800) 323-2935 Monday through Friday between 7:30 AM - 4:00 PM Central Time http://www.millerpharmacal.com/contact.html http://www.millerpharmacal.com/products.html
Standard Process Inc. http://www.standardprocess.com/ 1200 W. Royal Lee Drive Palmyra, WI 53156 800-848-5061 (toll free) 262-495-2122 (local) Customer Service (Orders) Phone: 800-558-8740 Fax: 800-438-3799 Email: info@standardprocess.com Email: SPOrders@standardprocess.com http://www.standardprocess.com/Standard-Process/Key-Ingredient-Cross-Reference
Vitaminerals http://www.vmmedical.com/ Email: info@VMMedical.com Email: order@VMMedical.com http://www.vmmedical.com/vitaminerals_patient_price_list.htm

Laboratory Services

Name Website Address Phone Numbers Online Contact Product List/Cross References
Analytical Research Labs, Inc. http://www.arltma.com/ 2225 W. Alice Avenue, Phoenix, Arizona 85021 USA 602-995-1580 Phone Number 800-528-4067 Toll-Free Phone Number 602-371-8873 Fax Number Information: information@arltma.com Sales/Customer Service: service@arltma.com http://www.arltma.com/HairAnalysis.htm http://www.arltma.com/Supplements/index.html
Direct Labs http://www.directlabs.com/ 4040 Florida St. Suite 101 Mandeville, LA 70448 Local: (985) 624-9186 Toll-Free: (800) 908-0000 Fax: (985) 626-4020 Toll-Free Fax: (800) 728-9048 Email Customer Service: contact@directlabs.net http://www.directlabs.com/OrderTests/tabid/55/language/en-US/Default.aspx
Health Tests Direct http://www.health-tests-direct.com/ 3303 Harbor Blvd., Bldg. G-2 Costa Mesa, CA 92626 U.S.A. Call us: 949.764.9301 x206 800.456.4647 x206 Fax: 949.764.9306 Email: Operations@OHSinc.com http://www.health-tests-direct.com/ordering-page
Lab Tests Online http://labtestsonline.org/ No Physical Address Listed http://labtestsonline.org/contact http://labtestsonline.org/site/

Index

A

B

C

R

Figures

Tables

www.ingramcontent.com/pod-product-compliance
Lightning Source LLC
Chambersburg PA
CBHW071730220326
R18016900001B/R180169PG41598CBX00002B/1

9780963591968